CHALLENGING
HIV AND AIDS

CHALLENGING HIV AND AIDS

A NEW ROLE FOR CARIBBEAN EDUCATION

EDITED BY

MICHAEL MORRISSEY

WITH

MYRNA BERNARD
AND DONALD BUNDY

FOREWORD BY

SIR GEORGE ALLEYNE

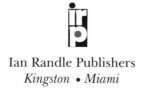

Ian Randle Publishers
Kingston • Miami

Kingston Office

United Nations
Educational, Scientific and
Cultural Organization

Published jointly by
The United Nations Educational, Scientific and Cultural Organization (UNESCO)
7 place de Fontenoy
75007 Paris, France
and
Ian Randle Publishers
11 Cunningham Avenue
Box 686
Kingston 6, Jamaica
www.ianrandlepublishers.com

Response of the education sector in the Commonwealth Caribbean to the HIV/AIDS epidemic © International Labour Organization 2005. Reproduced with permission.

Is learning becoming taboo for Caribbean boys? © Commonwealth Secretariat 2007. Reproduced with permission.

An HIV/AIDS workplace policy for the education sector in the Caribbean © International Labour Organization and UNESCO 2006. Reproduced with permission.

Declaration on education, HIV and AIDS © CARICOM 2007. Reproduced with permission.

HIV and AIDS education through Health and Family Life Education for 10-14-year olds © CARICOM 2007. Reproduced with permission.

Graduate programme in health and human relationships: Masters in education (health promotion) © The University of the West Indies 2007. Used with permission.

ISBN 978-923-104-151-8 UNESCO
ISBN 978-976-637-353-5 (pbk)

The designations employed and the presentation of material throughout this publication do no imply the expression of any opinion on the part of UNESCO concerning the legal status of any country, territory, city or area or of its authorities, or the delimmitation of its frontiers or boundaries.

The authors are responsible for the choice and presentation of the facts contained in the book and for the opinions expressed therein, which are not necessarily those of UNESCO and do no commit the Organization.

National Library of Jamaica Cataloguing in Publication Data

Challenging HIV/AIDS: a new role for education/edited by Michael Morrissey…[et al]
    p. ; cm.
      Includes index
      ISBN 978-976-637-353-5 (pbk)
1. AIDS (Disease) – Caribbean Area   2. HIV infections – Caribbean Area
3. AIDS (Disease) – Prevention – Study and teaching   4.   HIV infections – Prevention – Study and teaching   5. Health education

I. Morrissey, Michael

362.1968792009729

Cover photograph by Chris Hamilton
Book design and cover design by Ian Randle Publishers
Printed and bound in the United States of America

TABLE OF CONTENTS

SECTION 3: TOWARD POLICY AND CONCERTED ACTION

LIST OF TABLES

LIST OF FIGURES

LIST OF BOXES

Foreword

First, I must congratulate the editor, Professor Michael Morrissey and the authors on addressing this topic which by all accounts has to be one of the most complex in health. 'AIDS and Education' generates 124 million entries when searched in Google. This shows the importance of the issue as well as the tremendous global effort that has been put into divining the relationship between HIV/AIDS and education as a sector as well as the extent to which the whole educational process can be involved. I suppose this should not be surprising, given the fact that education broadly conceived has to be involved in all aspects of human endeavor and the control of this recent pandemic has become central to much of human endeavor.

The multiple ways in which HIV and education interact are exemplified by the range of topics covered in the book. But the uniqueness of this publication and I am sure the driving force behind adding yet another publication on HIV/AIDS to the world literature is that it is necessary to be locale specific and the problems of the Caribbean are unique enough to merit special attention from predominantly Caribbean scholars or at least scholars working in the Caribbean. Thus, for example, it is gratifying to see that the aspect of sexuality in schools is dealt with in the specific context of Jamaica and the Caribbean. The impact of AIDS on the human resources in the education sector is related specifically to the Caribbean and does not paint a picture in terms of some apocalyptic or almost eschatological scenario as is done sometimes in relation to Africa. While it is important for the Caribbean to learn from experiences in other places, it is good to see the work centred on the Caribbean experience which actually may be of relevance to other countries with similar characteristics.

I am sure that all persons who have thought about this issue have come to the obvious conclusion that education must be involved and there are perhaps two main approaches that I find most relevant and which also find echo in the book. The education sector can be the 'victim' of the epidemic and there are numerous accounts in the literature of the impact on all aspects of the sector, but predominantly on its human resources. But I find it refreshing that more emphasis is placed here on the instrumental role of education in the control of the epidemic. I like to think of education in its pristine and proper role of leading society out of ignorance and by so doing addressing the root causes of the epidemic or perhaps as is appropriate for a population-health approach, the causes of the causes. I see education as having three major functions as through reducing ignorance and correcting misperceptions it can be effective in preventing the infection, reducing stigma and discrimination and improving the quality of life of persons living with HIV and not only those with AIDS. In addition, simply staying in a formal educational setting is preventive in terms of reducing the prevalence of HIV and other sexually transmitted infections in the young.

The book emphasises the obvious truth that education is a lifelong process and every encounter among people can be a forum and an opportunity for education. Thus we find considerable emphasis on education in the workplace as an ideal entry point for promoting universal access to prevention, treatment and care. However, one of the chapters makes perhaps the most cogent case for the instrumental value of education when it points out that apart from infection transmitted from mother to child, primary infection is rare or extremely low in the very young. Thus this is the correct time at which the educational process can inculcate the information that leads to the knowledge which can produce optimum results in prevention. This is not to decry the possibility of information being useful and relevant throughout the life cycle, but the returns can be higher if the process is begun in the young and reinforced continually during other stages. I would also add that this is of critical importance in relation to the second reason for involvement of the educational sector- the reduction of stigma and discrimination. These are learned behaviours and while they may be 'unlearned', it is clearly better that education inoculate the young against them at an early age. The third function of education-improving the quality of life of persons living with HIV is probably best addressed through education more generally.

We must never ignore the fact that there may be huge externalities to be garnered from appropriate education of the young in that they live not only in the formal domain of the educational institution, but also move in the domain of the family and community. It is in the latter that they can be powerful agents for change of attitude and practice.

Considerable attention is given to the efficacy of the programmes of Health and Family Life Education and one cannot escape the sensation of some disquiet as to whether these programmes as currently structured and applied are effective in addressing the epidemic. In many cases the curriculum may need to be restructured and in others there is simply not enough attention paid to resourcing these programmes adequately and according them the necessary place in the curriculum. While it is important that these programmes be adequately structured and resourced, I have often wondered if they should not be accompanied by a process of incorporating HIV education into other aspects of the curriculum. Why should data from HIV programmes not be part of the exercises in mathematics and statistics for example? Why should the programmes in nutrition not deal with HIV? I also confess to being attracted to the view put forward so well by Professor Rex Nettleford that the old fashioned hygiene which was taught in schools might have a place in our modern curricula in that it dealt with all aspects of being healthy and as such would touch on the various manifestations and ramifications of HIV/AIDS. I am pleased to see that the issue of availability of suitable educational materials is addressed and that the Caribbean publishing fraternity is playing an active role in ensuring this.

The fact that education on HIV to be effective has to start at a very young age always brings into question the sensitivity of matters of sexuality, as there are many who in spite of evidence of early initiation of sexual activity in the Caribbean are uncomfortable with these issues being addressed in schools.

Perhaps the relevant chapters in the book might make clearer the difference between sexuality and the physical aspects of sex. The drive of sexuality is a normal and healthy one which cannot be eliminated, but it need not always result in the sex act. Of course if it does, then the aspect of prevention comes to the fore.

I have found in my discussions on this topic that there is not ready acceptance of what is common knowledge for behavioural scientists; that the exploratory behaviour of the young is a normal phenomenon not restricted to humans. The young explore their bodies, they explore their emotions, they explore their environments and they explore risky behaviours with the insouciance that derives from the feeling of immortality or invulnerability that characterises that age. Educational and other approaches have the responsibility not to try to curb this natural phenomenon, but to point out the risks and ensure that knowledge of the proper preventive measures is inculcated. Of course we have now passed the stage where there is any credence given to the myth that education about sexuality leads to precocious sex or unhealthy sexual practices; indeed, it is just the reverse.

It is gratifying to see the Ministerial Declaration on HIV, AIDS and Education included as it is important for it to be known that there is political commitment. However, this Declaration has to be translated into very specific actions with budgets so that agreements can have the possibility of being translated into programmes. The political commitment is important for another reason. Even if the educational process were optimally effective in changing behaviours, this will not produce the best results unless it is accompanied by the environmental change that can only be effected through governmental action. The government has at its disposal the levers of legislation and regulation and these have to be employed as well. Education about stigma and discrimination cannot be effective when these practices find homes in the laws of the land.

I am very pleased to have been asked to write this foreword and I hope the book is widely circulated and serves to inform policy and practice in the Caribbean.

George A.O. Alleyne
December 19, 2006

Preface

UNESCO is particularly proud to co-publish this important book with Ian Randle Publishers. It is the result of five years of UNESCO support to the Caribbean to strengthen the response of the education sector to the most alarming spread of HIV and AIDS and attendant stigma and discrimination. These five years have seen the blossoming of partnerships between UNESCO and several other cosponsors of UNAIDS, the joint response of the United Nations to the global epidemic.

Our principal UNAIDS partners have been the United Nations Children's Fund (UNICEF), the International Labour Organization (ILO) and the World Bank. Other critical partners have been the CARICOM Secretariat, the Caribbean Network of Seropositives (CRN+), the Caribbean Publishers Network, the Commonwealth Secretariat, the University of the West Indies (UWI) and the InterAmerican Development Bank (IDB). The 25 chapters of this book are the result of the combined effort of these organisations to galvanise the promise and responsibility of the education sector in halting this epidemic.

Ten of the chapters were originally commissioned to inform CARICOM Ministers of Education at their special meeting on HIV and AIDS in June 2006. The Declaration of Port of Spain was an outcome and is reproduced in full on pages 265-267. The World Bank partnered with UNESCO and UWI to support the CARICOM Secretariat in planning and actualising this critical meeting. The Bank arranged for two important studies for this meeting and raised funds from the United Kingdom's Department for International Development which enabled distribution of this book to stakeholders and libraries.

Sir George Alleyne, the UN Secretary General's special envoy to the Caribbean on HIV and AIDS, and also Chancellor of the University of the West Indies, kindly agreed to write a foreword. His reasoned endorsement of this book and its content is sweet music to the ears of UNESCO and its partners: our effort to raise the profile of the entire education sector as partner in the AIDS response is no longer a voice in the wilderness.

With the exception of Sir George, I have referred only to organisations and institutions in my acknowledgements. We know, of course, that it is the dedicated professionals affiliated with these organisations and many others who have cooperated in various ways to whom the real credit must be given. UNESCO would not have been able to publish this work without them. We hope our joint effort will prove invaluable to the education sector of this region and beyond in the years to come.

S. T. Kwame Boafo
Director, UNESCO Office for the
Caribbean Kingston, Jamaica
February 2007

Acronyms and Abbreviations

AIDS	Acquired Immune Deficiency Syndrome
API	AIDS Policy Index
ART	Antiretroviral Therapy
ARV	Antiretroviral
CAREC	Caribbean Epidemiology Centre
CARICOM	Caribbean Community
CCHI	Caribbean Cooperation in Health Initiative
CCNACP	Caribbean Coalition of National AIDS Programme Coordinators
CDC	Centers for Disease Control (USA)
CFPA	Caribbean Family Planning Affiliation
CIDA	Canadian Interantional Development Agency
COHSOD	Council for Human and Social Development
CRN+	Caribbean Regional Network of Seropositives
CSME	Caribbean Single Market and Economy
CXC	Caribbean Examinations Council
EC	European Commission
EDC	Education Development Centre
EI	Education International
EU	European Union
FBO	Faith-based Organisation
GFATM	Global Fund to Fight AIDS, Tubercolosis and Malaria
GNP+	Global Network of People Living with HIV/AIDS
GOJ	Government of Jamaica
HFLE	Health and Family Life Education
HIV	Human Immunodeficiency Virus
HPS	Health Promotion Specialist
HRT	HIV/AIDS Response Team
IATT	Inter Agency Task Team (on Education)
IDB	Inter-American Development Bank
IEC	Information, Communication, Education
ILO	International Labour Organization
IPPF	International Planned Parenthood Federation
JBTE	Joint Board of Teacher Education
JICA	Japanese International Cooperation Agency
JN+	Jamaica Network of Seropositives
JOCV	Japan Overseas Cooperation Volunteer
MoEY	Ministry of Education and Youth
MoEYC	Ministry of Education, Youth and Culture
MoH	Ministry of Health
MTCT	Mother-to-Child Transmission
NACC	National AIDS Coordinating Committee

NFE	Non-formal Education
NFPB	National Family Planning Board
NGO	Non-Governmental Organisation
NHSCPP	National HIV/STI Control and Prevention Programme
OECS	Organisation of Eastern Caribbean States
OPEC	Organization of Petroleum Exporting Countries
PAHO	Pan-American Health Organization
PEP	Post-Exposure-Prophylaxis
PEPFAR	President's Emergency Plan for HIV/AIDS Relief
PIOJ	Planning Institute of Jamaica
PLWHA	People Living with HIV and AIDS
SIRHASC	Strengthening Institutional Response to HIV/AIDS and other Sexually Transmitted Diseases in the Caribbean
STD	Sexually Transmitted Disease
STI	Sexually Transmitted Infection
TB	Tuberculosis
TOT	Trainer of Trainers
UNAIDS	Joint United Nations Programme on HIV and AIDS
UNDCP	United Nations Drug Control Programme
UNESCO	United Nations Educational, Scientific and Cultural Organization
UNGASS	United Nations General Assembly Special Session
UNICEF	United Nations Childrens' Fund
USAID	United States Agency for International Development
UTECH	University of Technology
UWI	University of the West Indies
UWI HARP	UWI HIV/AIDS Response Programme
V(C)CT	Voluntary (and Confidential) Counselling and Testing
VCT	Voluntary Counselling and Testing
WB	World Bank
WHO	World Health Organization

SECTION 1

ASSESSMENT: THE RESPONSE AT MID-DECADE

Response of the education sector in the Commonwealth Caribbean to the HIV/AIDS epidemic: A preliminary overview

Michael Morrissey

University of the West Indies and Senior Consultant, UNESCO Office for the Caribbean, Kingston, Jamaica

This analysis of the response of Education to the HIV and AIDS epidemic was electronically published in March 2005 by the International Labour Organization, which commissioned it in preparation for development of a Caribbean HIV/AIDS workplace policy for the education sector (for the policy, see Chapter 20). In the two years that followed this overview, more detailed analytical work was undertaken, much of which in included in this book, and a number of critical actions have been accomplished that address a response that the author concludes at the time as insufficient and ineffective. Although the analysis may be dated in some respects, it opens this book to paint a broad picture of the situation in mid decade.

BACKGROUND

The states and territories considered part of the Commonwealth in the Caribbean (hereafter Commonwealth Caribbean) comprise 15 small island developing states (ten are independent and five are British Overseas Territories) and two independent countries on the mainland of South and Central America respectively: Guyana and Belize. All but four of the British territories are member of the Caribbean Community (CARICOM), but this community also includes two non-Commonwealth members, Suriname and Haiti. The level of the HIV/AIDS epidemic is at a critical stage, rising unarrested and becoming generalised, losing former social and geographical concentrations.[1]

This overview provides a situation analysis of the general response of the education sector in the Commonwealth Caribbean to the HIV/AIDS epidemic as of early 2005, with particular reference to HIV/AIDS education in the workplace. There has been no systematic country-by-country survey of this subject, although the ILO has undertaken mapping exercises of responses to the epidemic in some countries, which include references to the education sector.[2]

This overview has therefore been based on: (i) fact finding undertaken in 2003[3] by a team engaged by the UNESCO Office for the Caribbean and the Inter-American Development Bank (IDB); (ii) responses of four Commonwealth Caribbean countries in the *Global Readiness Survey* of the Education Sector to the HIV/AIDS epidemic conducted in 2004 by UNESCO's International Institute for Educational Planning (IIEP) for the Inter-Agency Task Team (IATT) on HIV/AIDS & Education (note 3);[4] and (iii), most importantly, since 2001, the author's[5] expert consultancy work in this field.

In broad terms, the education sector in the Commonwealth Caribbean had until recently been unresponsive to the growing and generalised epidemic. This was the conclusion of the author after region-wide discussions in 2002 and was confirmed in the situation analysis conducted in 2003 by the team of UNESCO/IDB consultants engaged to design a technical cooperation project to build education capacity in this field.[6]

Although it is 'early days', it would seem, however, that as a result of advocacy efforts focussed on this sector by UNESCO, UNICEF, the Pan-American Health Organisation (PAHO), and other UN partners, there has been a perceptible change in the 'Education & HIV/AIDS' landscape of some of the CARICOM counties in the last two years - notably in Barbados and Jamaica - although even in these two countries, it must be emphasised, the shift is at the embryonic stage and little has yet changed at the classroom level.

The next sections will review the development of the education sector response, from Health and Family Life Education (HFLE) and Non-governmental organisation (NGO) interventions that began more than a decade ago, through current efforts at engaging the sector systemically and plans for the near future to build sector capacity. Focus will be given to the extent that workplace training has been included in these initiatives, the interest of the ILO as one of the UNAIDS co-sponsors and the underlying focus of this report.[7]

THE HFLE APPROACH

Prior to 2002, the response of the education sector was limited to a curriculum reform that embedded HIV/AIDS prevention as a small element within health promotion. For over two decades from 1983, a small band of enthusiasts, supported particularly by PAHO/WHO and UNICEF worked with the CARICOM Secretariat and selected Caribbean countries in development of a regional curriculum, HFLE, targeted to lower secondary grades (grades 7 to 9). Within this initiative, sexuality education and HIV/AIDS prevention constituted a small element.

Efforts focussed on achieving an outline of curriculum and content, a regional commitment at the political level through endorsement by CARICOM Ministers of Education & Health, and piloting elements of the new curriculum in a smattering of schools, in a few of the countries. The philosophical background and impetus for this movement is outlined by Cheryl Vince Whitman of the Education Development Centre Inc. (EDC), in an article that appeared in a special issue of *Caribbean Quarterly* dedicated to 'HIV/AIDS & Education in the Caribbean' in 2004.[8]

After a decade of HFLE efforts, however, there was little to show for this initiative at the school level, as agreements in principle had not been translated into action at sector management or classroom levels. Teachers' Colleges across the region had not changed their training curriculum to reflect the need for HFLE. Commercial publishers of learning materials – the litmus test of school demand – had not published any instructional materials for HFLE or HIV/AIDS. As HFLE had not become a reality by the early 2000s – and this was the only mechanism on the table for HIV/

AIDS prevention education in the formal curriculum – it was clear that the response of the formal education system in response to the epidemic was negligible. Moreover, even in the few schools where HFLE had been piloted, the average classroom teacher would not have had skill nor desire (bearing in mind the silence and the universal stigma related to HIV/AIDS in the region) to effectively meet any HIV/AIDS objectives.

In 2002, however, there was a renewal of commitment to HFLE on the part of the CARICOM Secretariat and a renewal of UNICEF support in several of its offices in the region (Barbados/Organisation of Eastern Caribbean States [- OECS], Jamaica, Guyana). The new energy resulted in a renewed political commitment in 2003 by the regional CARICOM Council for Human & Social Development (COHSOD) and development of a new curriculum framework and prototype lessons for four HFLE themes, one of which was HIV/AIDS. The Education Development Centre (EDC) was engaged by CARICOM and UNICEF to support this development and to follow up through piloting work between 2005–2008 in four Caribbean countries, Barbados, Grenada, St Lucia and Antigua & Barbuda. The four-theme detailed curriculum was completed in early 2005[9] and classroom activity to evaluate is about to commence. A parallel effort has been led by responsible officers in the Ministries of Education of Jamaica, Trinidad and Tobago and Guyana, but implementation everywhere is stymied by the lack of teacher readiness or preparation, and the absence of HFLE in the core (and examinable) curriculum of schools.

There has been some recent movement forward in teacher preparation for HFLE. For several years, the Reproductive Health Unit of UWI's School of Continuing Studies has been engaged in professional development in HFLE with teachers across the region, but in small numbers in each country – work led by Dr Phyllis McPherson-Russell, a guiding light in the HFLE initiative from its inception. Then from 2003, all teacher trainees in the UWI School of Education on the St Augustine campus (Trinidad) have been required to complete an HFLE module as an element of teacher preparation. UNICEF and EDC supported the UWI Cave Hill Campus (Barbados) to deliver a course in HFLE in the summer of 2004 in which 35 teachers were trained as potential leaders in this subject. In 2005, the UWI Institute of Education on the Mona Campus (Jamaica) began a process of developing an HFLE curriculum and instructional materials for Jamaican teachers' colleges, with the support of the UWI HIV/AIDS Response Programme (HARP), an initiative funded by the European Union (EU).

This recent activity gives hope that HFLE may one day be embedded in the curriculum of Caribbean schools, and that HIV/AIDS prevention will form part of it. However, what is being done relates largely to the three years of lower secondary education, in a region where a significant proportion of the population is sexually active in the upper primary age cohort, and discussion on inclusion of HIV/AIDS prevention at this level has hardly been initiated. The same holds true for upper secondary education (where the curriculum focus is on the 16+ examinations) and in teacher education institutions and universities – direct HIV prevention training is the exception rather than the norm.

In the case of UWI, a regional institution that is accountable to 15 Caribbean governments, an effort has been made to renew the curriculum between 2002–2005 with European Union assistance referred to above under SIRHASC (Strengthening Institutional Response to HIV/AIDS and other Sexually Transmitted Diseases in the Caribbean) and a blueprint of what could be done was outlined in 2002.[10] While much was accomplished,[11] the university has not succeeded in developing a mechanism to ensure AIDS-competence among all of its staff and students (one of the key recommendations of the blueprint referred to above).

In essence, at the beginning of 2005 in a region reportedly second in the world in its level of HIV prevalence and in a region generally with no downturn in prevalence trends, generations of students are passing through its primary, secondary, tertiary and teacher education institutions with no preparation through the formal curriculum of the institutions for the world of sexuality and the prevention of HIV infection. In the classroom, the stigma that has surrounded this epidemic from its inception in the region in 1981 continues to be a barrier to prevention education. The ensuing silence by teachers generally continues to fuel stigma, discrimination and ignorance, as the author's discussions with Ministry of Education and other education sector actors in recent years tends to confirm.

In relation to this paper's main subject, HFLE and other curriculum initiatives, such as UWI's programming adjustments supported through SIRHASC, have increased readiness and sensitivity, but have not resulted in wholesale preparation of teachers and lecturers in the education workplace.

A DECADE OF NGO & FBO INTERVENTION

In the absence of a response through the formal curriculum, donors and UN agencies have supported interventions by NGOs through the formal education sector, as well as through non-formal channels, targeted at young adolescents. The United States Agency for International Development (USAID), for example, channelled considerable resources through contractors, such as Family Health International (FHI), to a Jamaican performing ensemble, *Ashe*, that has delivered HIV/AIDS prevention messages to young people in the school setting, and trained selected teachers and peer counsellors in 'edutainment' methodology. Between 1996 and 2004, Ashe worked with schools in ten Caribbean countries and published methodology manuals. However, such efforts are dependent on evolving donor philosophies and funding allocations, and – in spite of positive evaluations[12] – *Ashe's* contract was not renewed in 2005 when USAID undertook a review of its Caribbean strategy.

As well as secular bodies, faith-based organisations (FBOs) have been active selectively. USAID, UNICEF, and – most recently – the Ministry of Education of Trinidad & Tobago, have channelled funding through faith-based NGOs to deliver HIV prevention education, but messages are often related to the beliefs of the faith in question. FBOs, such as the *Seventh Day Adventists*, have worked within their denominational schools, but again, prevention messages are couched in the belief system of the religion rather than based on public health principles. Generally in the region, teachers are church, mosque or temple-goers, and their HIV/AIDS knowledge may be more related to what is preached than to scientific knowledge.

In addition to the sustainability of such interventions, issues of content and quality of NGO and FBO-delivered training have frequently surfaced. For example, the Ministry of Education, Jamaica, withdrew all *Ashe* materials from its schools in 2000 and required changes to the portrayal of sexuality (particularly homosexuality). The messages of FBO-related organisations, such as the 'Governor's Program on Abstinence Louisiana, USA', that has been communicating fundamentalist messages in Trinidad & Tobago since 2004 in a programme funded by the Government,[13] may be contrary to the policy advocated by a country's national AIDS committee.

In general, ministries of education (MOEs) do not have clarity of policy nor the capacity to monitor NGO and FBO HIV prevention efforts through the formal sector, and by so permitting them under such circumstances, are often in derogation of their responsibilities under national education acts – and therefore liable in the event of public concern or complaint.

In any event, NGO and FBO coverage is not only unmonitored, but also patchy, intermittent and unevaluated in any objective sense. To address these issues, one of the components of a CARICOM/ Inter-American Development Bank (IDB) /UNESCO technical cooperation project that will begin in mid-2005[14] will be to work with one pilot MOE which has significant NGO/FBO involvement in HIV/AIDS in its sector to develop procedures to ensure effective management, quality assurance and efficient utilisation of resources. The project anticipates disseminating the approach developed, if successful, to other Caribbean countries.

Clearly the HFLE effort and NGO/FBO effort have been curriculum and prevention-oriented, and could not, even incidentally, be viewed as contributing to comprehensive workplace education. At best, these efforts may have sensitised school settings where they have been active. It was not until 2002, that effort began to develop an approach to a comprehensive sector response, inclusive of workplace education.

TOWARD A COMPREHENSIVE SECTOR RESPONSE

In 2002, the UNESCO Office for the Caribbean undertook an informal assessment of the role of the education sector *vis-à-vis* the HIV/AIDS epidemic across the region in the context of its own mandate to support Governments to achieve *Education for All* (EFA) commitments and education-related *Millennium Development Goals* (MDGs).

It appeared indisputable that the sector had – in general terms – not responded whatever to the HIV/AIDS epidemic, with the exception of timid advances on the HFLE front, and enabling entry of NGO players as summarised above. In the region of the world with the highest HIV prevalence outside sub-Saharan Africa, UNESCO viewed this situation as untenable as it threatened EFA advances and MDG achievement. In this context, UNESCO sought the mandate of Caribbean Ministers of Education who jointly subscribed to the Havana Commitment of 2002.[15]

UNESCO has also developed a medium-term education strategy for the Caribbean (2002–07) that emphasised support to the education sector's HIV/AIDS response as a priority,[16] and subsequently elaborated a detailed Education & HIV/AIDS strategy for 2004–05.[17] Resolve followed strategy, and the work of UNESCO in the Caribbean on this front was viewed as a model for other UNESCO field offices by a 2004 independent evaluation of UNESCO's response to HIV/AIDS globally.[18]

In developing and implementing its strategy, UNESCO has collaborated with other UNAIDS cosponsors active in the education sector in the region, particularly with UNICEF, WHO/PAHO, UNDP, the World Bank and beginning in 2004, with ILO. A record of the evolving contribution of UNESCO, other UNAIDS cosponsors and non-UN partners has been recorded in the eight quarterly reports electronically distributed to date throughout the region under the banner *Education & HIV/AIDS*.[19]

UNESCO's approach has been: (i) to foster a comprehensive response by the sector, balancing prevention and mitigation roles, and comprehensive in scope (from early childhood to university, formal and non-formal); (ii) to reach the ministries of education of all 20 countries that its Caribbean office serves; and (iii) to find the resources necessary to accomplish this through partnership-building and fund-raising.

What has been accomplished at the country level as a result of this new level of effort since 2002? In the absence of a formal Caribbean evaluation, the following indicators provide evidence of a quantum leap forward in the education sector perspective and response over the three years:

- Political commitment through signature by all Ministers of Education of the *Havana Commitment* in 2002.
- Positive reaction region-wide to, and acceptance of, the justification and framework for a comprehensive sector response first published by UNESCO in 2003 under the title *Education & HIV/AIDS in the Caribbean*,[20] evidenced, *inter alia* by independent book reviews in newspapers in Jamaica and Trinidad and Tobago, congratulatory messages from regional specialists and highly positive comments of the co-directors of the Mobile Task Team of southern Africa.

- Inclusion of HIV/AIDS as an element of the 2003–04 strategy of the Caribbean Publishing Network (CAPNET)[21] and sensitisation of CAPNET membership on the need for a publishing response to HIV/AIDS in the annual conference in 2003.[22]

- Publication of the first (and still the only) Caribbean instructional textbook focussed on HIV/AIDS prevention and mitigation.[23]

- Cabinet approval in Jamaica in 2004 for an education sector *Schools' HIV/AIDS Policy* that guides school boards, school principals, teachers and parents in a rights-based and prevention-oriented national policy.[24] This is the first such sector policy in the Commonwealth Caribbean, and provides a climate for workplace education.

- Publication of a manual in 2004 by the teachers' union in Trinidad & Tobago, but this has not to date received Government endorsement and distribution, and therefore its impact is uncertain.[25]

- Active and frank self evaluation by four Ministries of Education in the Commonwealth Caribbean that participated in a global survey of education sector 'readiness' to respond to the epidemic in 2004,[26] two of which claimed to be advanced in workplace HIV/AIDS programmes and their implementation, and two indicating a lack of action.

- Establishment in 2004 by the Ministry of Education in Jamaica of a prototype dedicated *HIV/AIDS Response Team*, integrated into the ministry's six region administrative structure, to disseminate its HIV/AIDS & Schools policy, provide workplace training and promote the curriculum response. A preliminary evaluation of the team's initial impact was undertaken in early 2005.[27]

- Mobilisation of the teacher training system in Jamaica by the Institute of Education, UWI, in 2004 to commence formulation of a comprehensive institutional response.

- School-level assessment in 2004-05 of the effectiveness of sub-Saharan Africa HIV/AIDS instructional materials in formal and non-formal situations in Guyana and Jamaica, to begin addressing the absence of learning support tools in this sphere.[28]

- Holding of an international conference and training for Caribbean educational publishers on publishing for HIV/AIDS.[29]

There is much more to be done, and UNESCO launched in February 2005 an *Advocacy & Leadership Campaign* that will design a strategy for delivery to all Caribbean ministries of education to: (i) ensure that each one recognises the role it must play in a national multi-sectoral strategy; (ii) create in the sector the demand for capacity building in this new field for key leaders and officials; and (iii) create in the education sector the demand (currently weak to non-existent) for central resources (such as those provided by the World Bank and the Global Fund). This campaign will include advocacy of workplace training in the sector. It is expected that by the end of 2005, six countries will have benefited from this campaign, with remaining countries reached in 2006.[30]

In respect of workplace training in the education sector, action has been limited to the effort of Educational International's Caribbean regional organisation in 2004–05 to sensitise key union members across the region to the need for such training. Quite separately, in Jamaica, with World Bank support, there was some training in the sector in 2004, but this was limited to a handful of headquarters staff; more recently an interest has been expressed on the part of the World Bank to discuss its involvement in future regional activities. Across the Caribbean region, it would not be an exaggeration to say that workplace training is yet to begin.

Of potential importance in this respect is the inclusion of five Caribbean countries (Barbados, Belize, Jamaica, Trinidad & Tobago and Guyana) in an initiative launched in mid-2004 by the ILO with United States Department of Labor (USDOL) support for workplace training in selected sectors, to be determined at the national level. Sectors have not been pre-selected and selection will be on a needs/demand basis. It is anticipated that the UNESCO-funded *Leadership & Advocacy* project will prioritise ILO/USDOL countries in its first wave of targets so that education sector leaders will be sensitised to the urgency of workplace training in their own sector and will, as a result, make a strong case for ILO/USDOL support in education. Through such efforts, it is hoped that education managers will come to recognise the role of workplace training as one element of a broad education sector response.

CAPACITY BUILDING FOR EDUCATION SECTOR MANAGERS

While advocacy will increase the resolve and influence policy, the reality is that capacity in the Caribbean education sector to respond to HIV/AIDS is undeveloped. To address this, there is a plan in 2005 to support professional development in this field during 2005 in a comprehensive, integrated and sustained way, beginning with in-depth training of selected key MOE officials. Based on results of a mission to the region by the co-directors of the South Africa-based *Mobile Task Team* (MTT) on HIV/AIDS & Education in late 2004 and their consultations with Ministries of Education across the region, UWI and UNAIDS co-sponsors,[31] programmes developed for sub-Saharan MOEs would be adapted to Caribbean epidemiological and cultural settings and mobilise experienced university professors to deliver such training. This innovative programme will, among many skills, enable MOEs to plan and implement workplace training suitable to their conditions, giving priority to national epidemiological 'hot spots'. Through both the advocacy and capacity building initiatives, an MOE environment conducive to successful workplace programmes would be sought with UNESCO and ILO support.

In preparation for this undertaking, UNESCO has made plans to provide professional development for selected university professors and other senior resource persons in a range of disciplines to orient them to the need for and requirements in capacity building for education sector personnel. The concept of workplace training will form a part of this professional development exercise and prepare experts to be able to deliver technical assistance to MOEs in this and other areas. The Organisation of American States has agreed to support UWI & UNESCO in the preparation of the necessary team of professional trainers.

To provide sustained leadership to such activities and the need for research, UWI

has established a *UNESCO/Commonwealth Chair in Education & HIV/AIDS* that will report to the Vice Chancellor, and it is expected that the first professor will take up the Chair (the first globally) in mid-2005.[32] The Chair will have a broad mandate for the response of the sector, through leadership in research, professionalising the area and capacity building for MOE officials, including workplace training.

A new UNAIDS thrust of 2005 is the agreement of co-sponsors to launch the UNESCO-led *Global Initiative on HIV/ AIDS & Education.* This initiative aims to accelerate a comprehensive education sector response in all critically affected countries, beginning with a first wave of pilot countries in 2005. The initiative has the support of all ten UNAIDS co-sponsors, including ILO, and includes promotion and execution of workplace training in the education sector with the concept. It is anticipated that one Caribbean country will be included in the first wave of six countries. The initiative will provide resources for rapidly developing a model MOE response in the Caribbean for replication elsewhere in the region. The initiative will formalise the contributions of several UNAIDS cosponsors at the country level as well as attempt to integrate efforts of civil society organisations and donors in a sector response.[33]

The ILO also launched in 2004 an initiative to draft a model education workplace policy based on the *ILO Code of practice on HIV/AIDS and the world of work*, accompanying guidelines on applying such a policy and suitable training materials for use by education authorities, public and private, teachers' unions and other stakeholders in the region.[34]

In the Caribbean, the establishment of national coordination bodies on HIV/AIDS is well-advanced, as is the development of national HIV/AIDS strategies. This is mirrored on the regional level by a CARICOM regional strategy, an association of national HIV/AIDS coordination authorities (CCNAPC) and a regional alliance of national Persons Living with HIV and AIDS (PLHA) networks – the Caribbean Regional Network of Persons Living with HIV and AIDS (CRN+).

However, due to the lack of recognition of the education sector as a key player – both of itself and by other sectors – until very recent years, regional and national plans, and the authorities that implement them, grossly under-reflect education sector professionals. With the efforts underway as noted above, the goal is for this situation to be corrected by 2006, as national education sectors better understand the role to be played and the urgency of playing it. The development of a Caribbean model under the Global Initiative will, it is hoped, create a methodology that can be rapidly replicated across the region.

The same applies to teachers' unions and principals' associations, which have been slow respectively to recognise the implications of the epidemic for union membership and for school leadership and management. While there have been some sensitisation workshops at regional level organised by the Caribbean regional organisation of the largest international federation of teachers' organisations, Education International (EI), an EI/WHO/EDC training programme on HIV prevention begun in Guyana, and some sensitisation of school principals at selected national and regional meetings, these interventions have merely scratched the surface. As of early 2005, there was virtually no sustained pressure from unions for workplace training in Caribbean countries

and no pressure for HIV/AIDS policy & management training from associations of school managers. There is considerable scope therefore, for initiatives such as those highlighted above by UNESCO, ILO, UNAIDS, EI and WHO to increase advocacy and build capacity for workplace and management efforts to deal with the epidemic.

BEACONS OF EVOLVING GOOD PRACTICE

This preliminary report attempts to broadly portray the situation across the Caribbean region in terms of a comprehensive response by Education to the epidemic, with particular reference to the extent to which HIV/AIDS workplace training has been implemented. In respect of this particular focus – development of comprehensive workplace policies and the training of every education official and teacher in an education system to be HIV/AIDS competent and non-discriminatory – the picture is bleak: to the author's knowledge, this has not been accomplished, nor has it been planned for, in any Caribbean country.

Nor has much been accomplished towards this end in the major regional university, the University of the West Indies, in spite of a grant of US$2.5 million to strengthen its institutional capacity in this field. The project will terminate in mid-2005, yet comprehensive workplace training has not been established, nor a workplace-wide approach piloted. This institution of 50,000 staff spread across 15 countries of the region remains largely in denial that the epidemic is within its walls. An external review of UWI's response will be undertaken in early 2005 as part of a UNESCO global study of 12 universities across the world.[35]

Nevertheless, the education sector is wakening to the challenges and in several countries there are instances of evolving practices that will facilitate the development of more comprehensive responses and workplace training policies. Three examples will illustrate.

First, the Jamaica team of health promotion officers integrated into MOE's six-region structure, with two dedicated officers in each region, presents a vehicle for nationwide workplace training and monitoring. The HIV/AIDS response team was initially dedicated to building capacity of the regional office in the Ministry's Schools Policy on HIV/AIDS, disseminating the policy through training, and monitoring its implementation. The team is funded by a mix of Government and donor resources (financing from UNICEF, UNESCO, World Bank, Japan International Cooperation Agency (JICA) and the Global Fund) that promise to sustain it. The preliminary evaluation of the HIV/AIDS Response Team's effectiveness, referred to earlier, is positive in its conclusion. The team presents a readymade framework for national workplace training, alongside the teachers' union, head teachers' associations and other players.

In Barbados, the Chief Education Officer was trained as an HIV/AIDS Leader under a regional UNDP-organised programme in 2003, and this resulted in her involvement in the training-of-trainers and a plan for sensitising all teachers at primary and secondary levels beginning in late 2003. About 63% of primary teachers and 44% of secondary teachers have been sensitised to date. Additional activities planned for the 2004–05 school year include the training of teachers in behaviour modification strategies. The Ministry of Education also plans to work in partnership with the Ministry of Labour and Social Security during 2004–05 to conduct training for staff in managing HIV/AIDS in the workplace, which will include the distribution of first aid kits, and the inclusion of such issues as the female condom and sexual rights in the workplace. In addition, the Barbados Community College, an institution that feeds a large portion of its students directly into the labour force has plans for staff orientation sessions to sensitise the staff on a volunteer basis on the impact of HIV/AIDS in the community, including a discussion of workers rights.[36] The efforts in Barbados, as a result, are likely to present a welcoming environment for the more intensive workplace effort that has to follow the initial sensitisation.

The Commonwealth of the Bahamas was subject to a higher level of prevalence than other Caribbean countries a decade ago, and its Ministry of Education acted more decisively from the mid-1990s to utilise NGO services in all secondary schools in a prevention campaign. Statistics suggest a declining prevalence in this country over the past few years, but there is no evidence to suggest a link between the two. In the Bahamas, as in most other Caribbean countries, the levels of stigma, denial and discrimination are severe, and a concerted effort will be needed to change the situation, a change essential if the epidemic is to be contained. It is likely the Bahamian Government will welcome accelerated workplace training in view of its national readiness.

CONCLUDING REMARKS

In education, and particularly in values education, it is widely held that teachers cannot communicate skills, foster attitudes nor nourish values unless they have and hold these themselves.[37] This premise is critical to the role of schools in prevention and in the inclusion of those infected and affected in education (both as receivers and deliverers).

HIV/AIDS workplace training universally delivered is therefore critical, if teachers are to be agents to promote safe practice, rights and tolerance. It is also urgent, if the level of the epidemic is to be contained below sub-Saharan African levels. Across the region, direct training would be impossible to effect and culturally-sensitive cascade approaches will need to be developed, beginning in countries such as those referred to in this paper where the levels of readiness and need are higher than in others.

NOTES

1. See Caribbean Epidemiological Centre: 'The Caribbean HIV/AIDS Epidemic epidemiological status - success stories: a summary' by Bilali Camara et al., CAREC Report Volume 23 Supplement 1, October 2003. Available on CAREC website www.carec.org and reproduced in part in 'Our Challenge HIV/AIDS: The Caribbean Presence in Bangkok - Handbook for Caribbean participants at the XVth International AIDS Conference', published by UNESCO Office for the Caribbean, July 2004.

2. 'HIV/AIDS in the World of Work: Mapping Exercise and Situational Analysis Barbados', prepared for ILO-Barbados by Sarah Adomakoh, September 30, 2004; 'Status Report and Situational Analysis: HIV/AIDS in the Workplace (Legislation, Policies, Programmes) Mapping Exercise', prepared for ILO-Belize by Michael Rosberg; 'HIV/AIDS and the World of Work: Guyana' (author not indicated)

3. CARICOM Secretariat, UNESCO, and the Inter-American Development Bank (IDB), 2003. Cooperation in the Preparation of a Caribbean Education Sector HIV/AIDS Response Capacity Building Programme: Joint Programme Identification Study, April-May 2003, prepared by Roger England

(Team Leader), Jennifer Sancho and Inon Schenker.

4. UNAIDS Inter Agency Task Team, 2005. Report on the Education Sector Global HIV/AIDS Readiness Survey 2004, commissioned of the Mobile Task Team on the Impact of HIV/AIDS on Education (MTT). Commonwealth Caribbean country responses were from Barbados, Guyana, Jamaica and Trinidad and Tobago.

5. In a 2002 Concept Paper that contributed to strengthening the institutional response of the Jamaica Ministry of Education to the HIV/AIDS epidemic, the author provoked discussion on the following proposition: 'Recognition by the Ministry that a central responsibility in an era of global epidemic is to protect its workforce and contribute to health promotion (wellness, virus containment), national population goals (life expectancy maintenance, HRD investment protection), human rights, etc'. Paper included in Michael Morrissey, 2003. Final Consultancy Report to UNICEF Kingston on services provided to the Ministry of Education, Youth & Culture, Jamaica. During the period 2001–2004, the author made specific contributions to the efforts of UNICEF, CAPNET and ILO in this field. The author acknowledges the editorial assistance of Bill Ratteree, Senior Education Specialist, ILO, Geneva, in producing this note.

6. CARICOM Secretariat, UNESCO, and the Inter-American Development Bank (IDB), 2003. *op. cit.*

7. UNAIDS has regional representation in the Commonwealth Caribbean with an office in Trinidad and Tobago, and national representation in Guyana and Jamaica. There are UN Theme Groups on HIV/AIDS that include all UNAIDS cosponsors, in Jamaica, Barbados and OECS, Trinidad and Guyana.

8. Cheryl Vince Whitman, 2004. 'Uniting Three Initiatives on Behalf of Caribbean Youth and Educators: Health & Family Life Education and the Health Promoting School in the Context of PANCAP's Strategic Framework for HIV/AIDS', *Caribbean Quarterly*, Volume 50, No.1, March 2004.

9. CARICOM Secretariat, UNICEF Caribbean Area Office and Education Development Centre Inc., 2005. HFLE Regional Curriculum Framework for Ages 9–14.

10. Brendan Bain and Michael Morrissey, 2002. The Caribbean HIV/AIDS Epidemic: 14-point proposal for priority curriculum and programming responses by UWI, The University of the West Indies HIV/AIDS Response Programme. Commissioned by UWI under the EU-funded SIRHASC project.

11. European Union, 2004. Report on External Mid-term Evaluation of the project 'Strengthening the Institutional Response to HIV/AIDS/STI in the Caribbean' (SIRHASC).

12. Ashe Performing Ensemble, 2004. A decade of Excellence. Includes section on Ashe Edutainment Transformational Model of Teaching.

13. 'Abstinence: the other "Safe Sex"', The *Daily Express*, Trinidad, March 15, 2005, Section 2 page 1.

14. Inter-American Development Bank, 2003. Plan of Operations for the Caribbean Regional Education Sector Capacity Building in Response to HIV/AIDS Technical Cooperation project. IDB Kingston's Social Sectors Division, for the CARICOM Secretariat.

15. The Havana Commitment on Education & HIV/AIDS, 2002. Reproduced in Michael Kelly & Brendan Bain. 2003. *HIV/AIDS and Education in the Caribbean*. First published for the UNESCO Office for the Caribbean by IIEP, and republished for UNESCO in 2004 by Ian Randle Publishers, Kingston, Jamaica.

16. UNESCO Office for the Caribbean, 2002. Medium-term Strategy for the Caribbean 2002–2007 & Caribbean Programme Priorities, 2002–2003, including HIV/AIDS Strategy. Formulated by Michael Morrissey, Senior Consultant.

17. UNESCO Office for the Caribbean, 2004. Programme to build education's response to HIV/AIDS in the Caribbean, 2004–2005. Formulated by Michael Morrissey, Senior Consultant.

18. Kim Forss & Stein-Erik Kruse, 2004. An evaluation of UNESCO's Response to HIV/AIDS. Centre for Health and Social Development, Oslo.

19. UNESCO Office for the Caribbean, 2003–2004. Education & HIV/AIDS: Quarterly Report to UNTG and other partners in the Caribbean. Issues 1-8.

20. Michael Kelly & Brendan Bain. 2003. Op. cit.

21. Caribbean Publishers' Network, 2002. CAPNET Strategic Plan 2002–2003, including HIV/AIDS Strategy. Developed by Michael Morrissey on behalf of the CAPNET President and Executive Council.

22. Graham van der Vyver. 2004. 'Commercial Publishing's response to the HIV/AIDS Epidemic: A report on a UNESCO/CAPNET workshop', *Caribbean Quarterly*, Volume 50, No.1, March 2004.

23. Angela Ramsay, 2003. *Literacy & Life Skills Workbook 1: Understanding HIV/AIDS and Drug Abuse*, Morton Publishing, Trinidad & Tobago, under contract with the UNESCO Office for the Caribbean.

24. Ministry of Education, Youth & Culture, Jamaica. 2004. *Schools HIV/AIDS Policy*.

25. Trinidad & Tobago Unified Teachers' Union (TTUTA), 2004. *Guidelines for Teachers on HIV/AIDS*.

26. According to individual country responses, Barbados & Jamaica are well advanced in terms of Workplace HIV/AIDS programmes (awareness programmes for employees, guidelines on universal precautions, non-discrimination & confidentiality policies) whereas Guyana and Trinidad and Tobago indicated that these were not in place, op cit, 4.

27. Claudia Chambers, 2005. Preliminary Evaluation of Jamaica's HIV/AIDS Response Team. Commissioned by the UNESCO Office for the Caribbean and Ministry of Education, Youth & Culture, Jamaica.

28. Evaluation of African HIV/AIDS Instructional Materials for primary & lower secondary students and out-of-school literacy students is being undertaken by the Ministry of Education in Guyana and Jamaica under UNESCO-funded projects to build sector capacity in HIV/AIDS, 2004–05.

29. The first-ever conference devoted to the educational publisher's role in response to HIV/AIDS, organised by CAPNET, was announced for Jamaica, May 28–June 2, 2005. See CAPNET website www.capnetonline.com

30. Education Development Centre Inc., 2005. Inception Report to the UNESCO Office for the Caribbean on the Advocacy & Leadership Campaign to Advance the Education Sector Response in the Caribbean, prepared by Cheryl Vince Whitman and Connie Constantine.

31. Mobile Task Team, 2004. Caribbean Consultancy on HIV/AIDS Impact on Education and Regional Capacity Building Options: Report on Caribbean Mission of December 2004, prepared by Peter Badcock-Walters & Jonathon Godden.

32. The University of the West Indies, 2004. Proposal for the Establishment of a UNESCO Chair in the field of Education & HIV/AIDS.

33. UNESCO/IIEP, 2005. Information Note: Global Initiative on HIV/AIDS and Education, prepared for a meeting of Global Coordinators, Geneva, 8–9 February 2005.

34. Sectoral Activities Department, ILO, Geneva, 2004. 'Improving responses to HIV/AIDS in education sector workplaces: Sectoral approach to HIV/AIDS in the workplace', concept note.

35. UNESCO, 2004. UNESCO Review of Universities' Responses to HIV/AIDS: Study Protocol.

36. 'HIV/AIDS in the World of Work: Mapping Exercise and Situational Analysis Barbados', op. cit.

37. King, R., P. Morris, M. Morrissey, and P. Robinson. 1983. *Social Studies Through Discovery*, Longman: Harlow, UK

ACKNOWLEDGEMENT

William Ratteree, Education sector specialist, International Labour Organization, Geneva

2

HIV in Caribbean schools: The role of HIV education in the second most severely affected region in the world

David Plummer

Commonwealth/UNESCO Regional Chair in Education (HIV/AIDS), University of the West Indies

This chapter analyses the need for HIV-prevention programmes in the Caribbean during the school years. It also explores what programme characteristics would be the best suited to be vehicles for such education. The analysis considers the following questions:

- *Is HIV education relevant for school-aged children?*
- *Is achieving sustained, widespread protective behaviours realistic, given that sexual behaviours are so deep seated?*
- *Is it appropriate to have programmes that aim to produce widespread protective behaviours during the school years?*
- *Is there evidence that these programmes will have positive effects on children and the epidemic?*
- *What would such programmes look like?*
- *How well positioned is the Caribbean education sector to contribute?*

The evidence in support of HIV programmes that target school-aged children is compelling.

INTRODUCTION

After a quarter of a century of a world with AIDS, many societies are only now coming to confront the potential importance of the education sector in our response to HIV. In this chapter a series of questions will be analysed that form the stepping stones for educational policy development and HIV. Are widespread protective behaviours realistic, given that sexuality is so deep seated? Why target young children, given that AIDS is largely a disease of sexually active adults? Is there evidence that sex education works, or will it simply worsen the situation? What are the implications for the Caribbean education sector?

The analysis concludes that the evidence in support of HIV programmes that target school-aged children is compelling. Nowhere is this more so than in the Caribbean – the second most severely HIV-affected region in the world.

WHAT HAVE SCHOOL CHILDREN GOT TO DO WITH IT?

Children of primary school age have among the lowest HIV rates of any age group. For example, the low HIV prevalence during the early school years in the Bahamas is illustrated in Figure 2.1. The other Caribbean nations have broadly similar patterns. These low HIV levels raise the important possibility that if children can be kept uninfected into adulthood, then HIV can be largely removed from a population within as little as a generation. Because of the potential population health benefits – even in the presence of a severe generalised epidemic – this period of low HIV prevalence during childhood is referred to by the World Bank as the 'window of hope' (World Bank, 2002).

Second, after a period of low prevalence during early childhood, the epidemiology shows that the risk of infection increases dramatically in adolescence and early adulthood. Indeed, it is fair to say that during adolescence young people abruptly enter a period of 'hyper-risk' – a period in which their risks are unlikely to be exceeded at any other time in their lives. Thus, it is also the case that HIV education during the school

ages has an important role of preparing young people to enter this high-risk period and to remain uninfected. Without such preparation, some of them will face certain death.

Third, while the epidemiology varies in different parts of the Caribbean, the average age of sexual debut is invariably early and women, in particular, face considerably higher odds of becoming infected at a young age than do young men. For example, in 2004 the Caribbean Technical Expert Group (quoted in UNAIDS/WHO 2005) reported a survey in which one quarter of 15–29-year-old women in Barbados said they had been sexually active by the time they turned 15. Furthermore, the country reports of the 2006 United Nations General Assembly Special Session on HIV/AIDS (UNGASS) reveal that in a recent Guyanese survey just over 30 per cent of young men and around 12 per cent of young women had their sexual debut before the age of 15; in St Vincent and the Grenadines the figure was 63 per cent of young men and 37 per cent of young women;

FIGURE 2.1
CUMULATIVE HIV INFECTIONS IN THE BAHAMAS BY AGE AND SEX TO END 2005

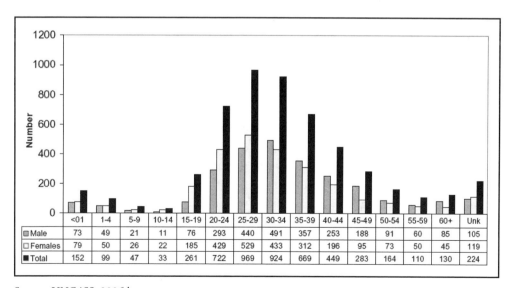

	<01	1-4	5-9	10-14	15-19	20-24	25-29	30-34	35-39	40-44	45-49	50-54	55-59	60+	Unk
Male	73	49	21	11	76	293	440	491	357	253	188	91	60	85	105
Females	79	50	26	22	185	429	529	433	312	196	95	73	50	45	119
Total	152	99	47	33	261	722	969	924	669	449	283	164	110	130	224

Source: *UNGASS, 2006d*

and in Haiti the figures were 28 per cent of young men and 12 per cent of young women (UNGASS, 2006a; 2006b; 2006c).

The early age of infection of young women should be of particular concern for educators: the so-called 'feminisation' of the epidemic. In Trinidad and Tobago, HIV infection levels are six times higher among 15–19-year-old females than among males of the same age (Inciardi, Syvertsen and Surratt, quoted in UNAIDS/WHO 2005). Studies in the Dominican Republic showed that women younger than 24 years were almost twice as likely; and teenage girls in Jamaica were two-and-a-half times more likely to be HIV-infected, compared to their male counterparts (MAP 2003, quoted in UNAIDS/WHO 2005).

This early age of sexual debut unequivocally places the spotlight for effective prevention squarely on the school years. Indeed, as the prominent Jamaican Health and Family Life advocate, and former Minister for Education, Dr Phyllis MacPherson-Russell emphasises, programmes at this stage should focus on the *formation* of safe behaviours from the outset rather than attempting to *change* entrenched risky behaviours later (personal communication). For all of these reasons, early interventions during the school years are essential and every effort needs to be made to ensure that these programmes are effective.

CAN RISKY BEHAVIOURS BE CHANGED?

The next question to be answered is can sexual behaviour be changed on a widespread, sustainable basis? Of course, in everyday life, people change their behaviours constantly and the intuitive answer to this question is 'yes', otherwise even our systems of education would have no foundation.

However, on closer examination, behaviour change for HIV appears to be a special case. First, HIV has spread inexorably around the world for more than quarter of a century despite substantial national and international investments in prevention. Second, despite near-universal levels of AIDS awareness, HIV policymakers and grassroots workers repeatedly complain that risk behaviours are widespread and that there continues to be a substantial gap between awareness and behaviour. Third, it has been known for some time that knowledge does not have a perfect correlation with behaviour change. Fourth, we are seeking to change deeply rooted human behaviours, most notably human sexuality, which is reputedly the result of extremely powerful drives. Therefore it is important to ask whether there is any realistic hope of promoting widespread sustained protective behaviour change that will have significant impacts on HIV at the population level.

To answer this question we need to seek cases where there is definitive evidence of sustained widespread behaviour change that can be confirmed epidemiologically. Indeed, even being able to identify a single case will be sufficient to conclude that sustained widespread change is possible.

Fortunately, there is such a case, and it is one that I am personally very familiar with – I was there when it happened. The case I refer to is the dramatic shift in HIV incidence that occurred in my home country of Australia during the mid-1980s. Figure 2 documents the incidence of HIV in Australia from 1980 to 1993. The graph is based on robust data produced by the National Centre for HIV Epidemiology and Clinical Research. The figure demonstrates that after a steep rise in the four years from 1980 to 1984, the number of new HIV infections dropped steeply for the next four years followed by a steadier decline from 1988 to 1993 and it has been flat until very recently.

There are several possible explanations for this HIV incidence pattern. The first is that antiviral drugs changed the epidemiology of HIV. However, as Figure 2.2 shows, the first anti-viral drug was not introduced until late in the decline of new HIV infections. The second explanation is that the 'natural history' of the HIV epidemic spontaneously exhausted itself soon after arriving in the country. This explanation is unlikely as such a pattern has not occurred elsewhere and Australia continues to have sizeable active gay, sex worker and injecting drug using populations. The third possibility is that the epidemiological pattern is due to wholesale protective behaviour change. This latter explanation does indeed appear to be the case. Australia had an early, pragmatic response to HIV based on 'harm minimization' principles. Moreover, the almost completely flat graph from 1993

onwards confirms that these changes have been sustained for many years (for more detail, see Plummer and Irwin, 2006). The message for educators is that widespread sustained behavioural change is possible, even for powerful sexual behaviours and Australia is one of a number of cases where this can be clearly demonstrated.

DOES SEX EDUCATION WORK?

Of course, although sex education in schools makes perfect public health sense, there is always the possibility that such programmes are either not effective or worse still, that they can have adverse outcomes. To explore this possibility, Kirby, Laris and Rolleri (2005) undertook a comprehensive review of sex and HIV education programmes from around the world. The authors examined 83 programmes conducted in school, clinic or community settings including 18 from developing countries, namely Belize, Brazil, Chile, Kenya, Jamaica, Mexico, Namibia, Nigeria, South Africa, Tanzania,

FIGURE 2.2
THE NUMBER OF NEW CASES OF HIV PER YEAR IN AUSTRALIA (1980–1993)

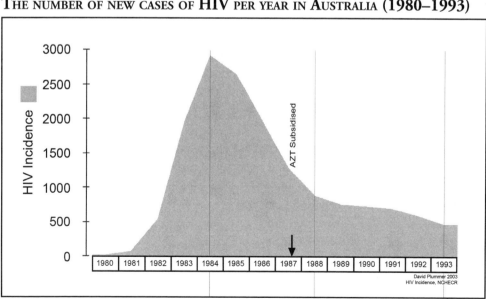

Source: *Plummer and Irwin, 2006*

Thailand and Zambia. The review specifically examined the impact of sex education on pregnancy, HIV and sexually transmissible infections (STI). The authors asked:

1) What are the effects, if any, of curriculum-based sex and HIV education programmes on sexual risk behaviours, STI and pregnancy rates, and mediating factors such as knowledge and attitudes that affect those behaviours?

2) What are the common characteristics of the curricula-based programmes that were effective in changing sexual risk behaviours? (Kirby, Laris and Rolleri 2005)

The outcomes of these studies fell into eight key categories: impact on the age of initiation of sex, the frequency of sex, the number of sexual partners, condom use, contraceptive use, sexual risk taking, pregnancy rates and STI rates. A summary cross-tabulation of the effects of the various programmes can be found in Table 2.1.

The results of the meta-analysis are reason for optimism. Although unwanted outcomes were identified, these occurred in only a minority of cases, and the health benefits of sex education clearly outweighed the risks. The authors conclude:

> Overall, these studies strongly indicate that these programs were far more likely to have a positive impact on behaviour than a negative impact. Across all 83 studies, two-thirds (65 percent) found a significant positive impact on one or more of these sexual behaviours or outcomes, while only 7 percent found a significant negative impact on one or more of these behaviours or outcomes. (Kirby, Laris and Rolleri 2005)

In addition, on the question of whether there were gender or locational differences, the authors reported broadly similar findings in both developed and developing countries; in urban and rural areas; in both low- and middle-income youth; for both sexes; at all age levels; and in school, clinic and community settings.

Importantly, the authors also found that the programmes they evaluated did not lead to increased sexual behaviour as some critics had feared:

> To the contrary, nearly half (45 percent) of the studies that measured impact on sexual initiation, frequency of sex, or number of sexual partners found positive results: the programs either delayed sex or reduced the frequency of sex or the number of sexual partners. Almost all of the rest had no effect. Only one of 52 programs measuring the impact on the initiation of sex reported earlier sexual initiation. (Kirby, Laris and Rolleri, 2005)

HIV AND THE CARIBBEAN EDUCATION SECTOR

So far we have established that targeted HIV education for children makes public health sense; that sustained widespread protective behaviours are achievable; and that the benefits of HIV and sex education for young people outweigh the risks in a wide variety of settings. It remains for us to consider the implications of these findings for the Caribbean education sector.

At first glance, the logical vehicle for HIV education in the Caribbean is the regional Health and Family Life Education (HFLE) strategy. However, because the stakes for HIV in the Caribbean are high, it is important to test this proposition.

TABLE 2.1
NUMBER OF STUDIES REPORTING EFFECTS ON DIFFERENT SEXUAL BEHAVIOURS AND OUTCOMES BY STUDY SETTING

Outcome	Number of studies	Developing country studies (n=18)		All studies (n=83)	
		Negative outcome	Positive outcome	Negative outcome	Positive outcome
Delayed sexual debut	52	0	6	1	22
Reduced frequency of sex	31	0	2	3	9
Reduced partner numbers	34	0	3	1	12
Reduced sexual risk taking	28	0	0	0	14
Increased condom use	54	0	7	0	26
Increased contraceptive use	15	0	0	1	6
Reduced pregnancy (self report)	9	0	0	1	2
Reduced pregnancy (lab report)	4	0	1	0	1
Reduced STI (self report)	5	0	0	1	0
Reduced STI (lab report)	5	1	0	1	2

Source: *Kirby, Laris and Rolleri, 2005*

Is HFLE really the best vehicle for HIV education? Is the HFLE strategy designed in such a way that significant HIV effects can be anticipated? Is HFLE rollout sufficiently advanced, and do the various HFLE curricula have the capacity to make a difference to HIV? Are modifications to HFLE required in order to maximise its impact on HIV? Are there interventions above and beyond HFLE that are necessary to bring about more effective HIV education?

CAN HFLE ACCOMMODATE HIV?

HFLE did not have its origins as a response to HIV. While this fact might be self-evident, it does serve to focus our attention on whether HFLE is suitably designed to have an impact on HIV and whether there is sufficient space in the HFLE curriculum to accommodate the demands of this relative newcomer.

According to Joycelyn Rampersad from the University of the West Indies, the origins of HFLE can be traced back to the 1970s in programmes for health education and family life (Rampersad 2007). By 1981, these earlier programmes were combined and formalised as HFLE (Vince Whitman 2004). Since 1981, the strategy has undergone various iterations. As recently as 2004, the HFLE strategy was reviewed in order to strengthen the HIV content, presumably because the previous HIV content was not considered to have been sufficient.

The HFLE strategy divides HFLE into four theme areas.

1. Self and interpersonal relationships
2. Sexuality and sexual health
3. Eating and fitness
4. Managing the environment

Of these, theme two (sexuality and sexual health) is directly relevant to HIV, and, based on the evaluation of programmes elsewhere by Kirby, Laris and Rolleri (2005), we can reasonably expect positive outcomes for HIV, providing there is a well designed curriculum, full implementation and skilled delivery.

In addition, theme one (self and interpersonal relationships) has contextual and indirect relevance for HIV. The question here is whether contextual material and material of indirect relevance will have an impact on HIV outcomes. While exploring this area with Caribbean HFLE experts, it was argued that there is significant 'indirect' content in HFLE which, while not HIV-specific, will benefit HIV education nevertheless. Unfortunately at this stage there is no data to verify these claims. Indeed, it should be noted that the programmes studied by Kirby, Laris and Rolleri (2005) that were shown to have positive impacts were specific and targeted in nature, and even in that case, the benefits, while consistent, were not necessarily of great magnitude. Indeed, the authors raise a note of caution that finding robustly favourable outcomes should not be confused with magnitude or duration of impact. This leaves us with two opposing possibilities that can only be answered

through further research and evaluation: first, that certain contextual curriculum material and material of indirect relevance will serve to strengthen outcomes in relation to issues like HIV; and/or that at least some of this material will be too remote to be relevant. Clearly, the impact of contextual and non-HIV specific materials should be made a priority for the HFLE and HIV education research and evaluation agenda.

The question as to whether the content of HIV-relevant materials is sufficient to have an impact goes well beyond the regional HFLE strategy itself. Until now, the vehicle for implementing the regional HFLE strategy has been through the various national curricula of the CARICOM member states. While this is a pragmatic arrangement, it is not without its drawbacks, some of which have implications for HIV control. A review of national HFLE strategies reveals that HFLE curricula are extremely broad and they aim to cover a large range of issues. Moreover, there is a wide variation in references to HIV, ranging from little or no mention in some countries through to numerous references, as is the case, for example, in Jamaica. Given that directly relevant material has been linked to positive outcomes, all national curricula should be reviewed to ensure comprehensive coverage of HIV, as should the new regional curriculum currently being developed.

IMPLEMENTING HFLE

Considerable effort over many years has been put into developing HFLE strategies and curricula by Caribbean governments, CARICOM, UNICEF and their other development partners.

However, while HFLE has been in development since the late 1970s, my inquiries confirm that the vast majority of countries in the Caribbean are yet to implement HFLE programmes in all government schools across the majority school years (see Table 2.2). In short, full HFLE rollout has been slow and it continues to be at the stage of piloting in specific schools in key countries. These findings are similar to those reported by Boler and Jellema (2005) in their monograph titled *Deadly inertia: A cross-country study of educational responses to HIV/AIDS*. In the meantime, a rapidly moving epidemic of a viral sexually transmissible disease – HIV – has emerged from obscurity to take its place among the world's most deadly epidemics.

At the grassroots too, there are important barriers to fulsome HFLE implementation. Feedback from country HFLE/HIV coordinators confirms that there are significant barriers to HFLE implementation at the school level. These barriers relate to insufficient teacher training in HFLE; reluctance and lack of confidence when delivering HFLE; perceived community resistance; available time and resources; and the sensitive and taboo nature of some subject material. Work in the UWI School of Education, St Augustine, by Rampersad and Reece-Peeters and my own inquiries reveal that there is some hesitancy by teachers to teach on issues that are technically complex and taboo. The risk therefore, is that the less sensitive 'easier' components of HFLE curricula are taught more fully and those dealing with sexual health will be handled less well. These findings are supported by research elsewhere such as the work by Pelzer and Promtussananon in South Africa (2003) who found that while teachers had the knowledge and ability to teach about HIV and were moderately comfortable with the subject matter, they nevertheless felt that they lacked the material and community support to do so.

TABLE 2.2
CURRICULUM DEVELOPMENT AND IMPLEMENTATION IN TEN CARIBBEAN COUNTRIES AT JUNE 2006

	Curriculum developed	Implementation primary	Implementation secondary
St Kitts	K - 11	50%	40%
Bahamas	1 - 12	70%	75%
St Lucia	K - 11	100%	100%
Guyana	1 - 9	1%	1%
Antigua	K - 9	80%	20%
Belize	1 -6	5%	NA
Trinidad	1-5	-	-
Surinam	7-10	pilot	pilot
SVG	K-9	100%	100%
Barbados	K-11	100%	100%

Source: *Data collected directly from the respective ministries*

STATUS OF HFLE

An area where HFLE appears to be disadvantaged relates to the professional status of the field. In addition to having to compete in a crowded curriculum, HFLE does not appear to enjoy the same regard as most traditional subjects. In part this is due to the taboo nature of the subject matter, but it also reflects the non-compulsory, non-examinable status of HFLE. In a competitive school environment, especially in the latter years, non-examinable non-compulsory subjects will understandably command a lower priority – even though they have profound importance for personal health and the social and economic well-being of the nation.

For teachers too, HFLE does not enjoy the same status as the co-called 'hard' traditional subjects. Instead, HFLE has an image of being 'soft' and it deals with awkward subject matter. This reputation is aggravated because, unlike conventional subjects, there is no tradition of advanced training and research in HFLE and career paths for staff are ill-defined and largely ad hoc. During my consultations with workers in the field I came across several reports of staff who were allocated HFLE as part of their workload despite a lack of training, experience or indeed any interest in the field. It is likely that, far from being an advantage, some staff continue to view HFLE as a career liability. The area is badly in need of professionalisation.

THE FUTURE ROLE OF HFLE AND BEYOND

The response of the education sector to HIV need not be confined to HFLE. Indeed, the evidence presented above suggests that relying solely on HFLE to address HIV has certain risks. The analysis suggests at least two additional approaches: to further strengthen HFLE, including in relation to HIV; and second, to identify what else is required to ensure a comprehensive HIV response by the education sector, beyond HFLE.

The incomplete rollout of HFLE to date raises important questions about the capacity of HFLE to make significant inroads into the HIV epidemic. Clearly, patchy regional and national coverage by HFLE militates against a comprehensive response to HIV. Moreover, the status afforded to HFLE needs elevating so that it can assume an equal place alongside more traditional subject areas. The threat posed by HIV is such that HFLE should be seen as a cornerstone of a healthy, vital society – something that many other subjects cannot make claim to. HIV education must no longer be thought of as an optional add-on to school education: it is core business.

An inescapable conclusion of the present analysis is the need to strengthen HFLE. A Caribbean-wide curriculum should be expedited. A timetable and a fixed deadline for universal coverage of Caribbean schools should be agreed upon. It is also appropriate that HFLE strategies and curricula be reviewed to ensure that HIV-related content is sufficiently foregrounded. Moreover, the curricula of traditional subject areas should be revisited and their HIV content be strengthened where possible. It is worth putting on record that HIV makes an excellent model for teaching in many areas – from biology to the arts. It is also worth noting that teaching about HIV should consist of much more than merely recounting a death toll and forecasting doom. To capture the imagination of young people, HIV education needs to be innovative, creative and have a vision for a better future.

Box 2.1
CARIBBEAN EDUCATION SECTOR RESPONSES TO HIV: DIFFICULTIES THAT NEED TO BE ADDRESSED

- Regional and national HIV strategies remain relatively silent about the role of the education sector.
- HFLE was not intended primarily to address HIV; HFLE did not originate with HIV in mind; there is considerable variation in how well HIV has been accommodated in HFLE programmes.
- HFLE rollout has been slow, incomplete and implementation is uneven.
- Specific reference to HIV is a small part of HFLE documentation. One out of the four HFLE thematic areas is directly relevant to HIV; one is contextually relevant; some country curricula deal with HIV more directly than others.
- The school curriculum is very crowded with important priorities against which HFLE has to compete for time.
- HFLE suffers from lack of status; HFLE is not compulsory; HFLE is not examinable.
- HFLE is not professionalised in the way that other disciplines are; HFLE does not have a tradition of advanced qualifications, training and research; HFLE career paths are ad hoc and not well defined.
- HFLE deals with taboos and sensitive social issues with political implications; this generates 'self censoring' dynamics.
- There is a lack of evidence concerning impact and outcomes of HFLE.

Finally, apart from generalities, regional and national HIV strategies have been found to be lacking in their analysis and plans for the role of the education sector in HIV. The role and responsibilities of the education sector need to be written into these documents in meaningful and concrete ways.

Beyond HFLE, there are additional areas that need to be addressed. Education should be understood as a lifelong process that is not and never was confined to the classroom. Many of the powerful dynamics that can promote HIV (and others that can sustainably protect against HIV) arise in peer groups in the school grounds and beyond the school walls. Done well, peer interventions are a vital part of the educational response to AIDS. Informal education, educational outreach to marginalised populations and

education in the workplace are also essential elements of a complete educational picture.

Finally, there is a clear risk that staff working in HFLE will become isolated and their capacity to deliver results will be undermined. Staff will need much greater peer and professional support and HFLE needs a greatly enhanced professional status. Strengthening this status will require a number of steps, including:

- Making HFLE a core subject, and therefore compulsory;
- Revisiting the issue of making HFLE examinable. Of course, examining 'values' is fraught with difficulties, but there is clearly a role for addressing factual deficiencies in HIV knowledge

Box 2.2
HIV EDUCATION IN THE SECOND MOST SEVERELY AFFECTED REGION OF THE WORLD: POINTS FOR ACTION

- Sex education during the school years makes public health sense and is in the national interests.
- A timetable is needed to achieve universal coverage of sex education in Caribbean schools.
- Curricula should be revisited and adjusted to ensure adequate HIV focus.
- Additional HIV content should be added to school curricula outside of HFLE
- Attention should be directed to extra-mural, informal and peer-based education settings.
- Impacts of one-off sex education may be short-lived; ongoing reinforcement in a supportive environment will be necessary.
- Regional and national HIV strategies should be revisited and the role of the education sector should be written in concrete and meaningful ways.
- Sex education programmes conducted elsewhere should be systematically reviewed to identify best practice and possible reasons for negative outcomes.
- Social dimensions that serve to entrench HIV risk (e.g. peer group dynamics, gender roles, stigma and discrimination) should be studied and addressed.
- Programmes should be evaluated and adjusted accordingly.
- Research into producing sustained outcomes is needed.
- HFLE needs professionalising; career path development; a sound academic basis; advanced recognised professional qualifications; and dedicated research and evaluation capacity.

and examinations do not need to be conventional;
- Material, professional and emotional support for HFLE staff;
- A legitimate career path for HFLE staff;
- Advanced training and qualifications for HFLE; and
- Academic support through research and evaluation of HFLE.

CONCLUSIONS

In summary, sex education during the school years makes public health sense and is clearly in national and regional interests. It is also clear that achieving sustained widespread protective behaviours are possible, even in the case of deeply entrenched sexual practices. Sex education programmes have been shown to be effective, but careful attention to curriculum development and delivery is required. Single sessions and limited exposure to programmes do not appear to be sufficient for sustained outcomes. Regional and national HIV strategies should be reviewed to ensure that the education sector is 'written in' in meaningful and concrete ways. Likewise, regional and national HFLE strategies should be reviewed to ensure that HIV is 'written in'. Specific strategies should be developed for HIV content beyond HFLE and for education outside of the classroom. There is a pressing need to professionalise HFLE; to formalise HFLE career paths; to elevate its status as a school subject; to develop strong academic foundations; to institute advanced training and formal qualifications; and to sharpen research and evaluation. There is also a pressing need for a timetable and deadlines to expedite universal Caribbean coverage of HFLE and HIV education.

REFERENCES

Boler, T. and Jellema, A. 2005. Deadly inertia: A cross-country study of educational responses to HIV/AIDS. Brussels: Global Campaign for Education.

Kirby, D., Laris, B.A. and Rolleri, L. 2005. Impact of sex and HIV education programs on sexual behaviors of youth in developing and developed countries. North Carolina: Family Health International.

Pelzer, K. and Promtussananon, S. 2003. HIV/AIDS education in South Africa: Teacher knowledge about HIV/AIDS: Teacher attitude about and control of HIV/AIDS education. Social Behaviour and Personality 31(4):349–56.

Plummer, D. and Irwin, L. 2006. The relationship between grassroots activities, national initiatives and HIV prevention: What explains Australia's dramatic early success in controlling the HIV epidemic? *International Journal of STI & AIDS*, 17: 787–93.

Rampersad, J. 2010 Health and Family Life Education in the Formal Education Sector in the Caribbean. *Challenging HIV and AIDS: A New Role for Caribbean Education.* Paris: United Nation Educational, Scientific and Cultural Organization (UNESCO); and Kingston: Ian Randle Publishers, 26–57.

UNAIDS/WHO. 2005. AIDS epidemic update: December 2005. Geneva, Switzerland: UNAIDS.

UNGASS. 2006a. Follow-Up to the Declaration of Commitment on HIV/AIDS (UNGASS): Haiti Country Report. Port of Prince: Government of Haiti.

UNGASS. 2006b. Follow-Up to the Declaration of Commitment on HIV/AIDS (UNGASS): St Vincent and the Grenadines Country Report. Kingstown: Government of St Vincent and the Grenadines.

UNGASS. 2006c. Follow-Up to the Declaration of Commitment on HIV/AIDS (UNGASS): Guyana Country Report. Georgetown: Government of Guyana.

UNGASS. 2006d. Follow-Up to the Declaration of Commitment on HIV/AIDS (UNGASS): Bahamas Country Report. Nassau: Government of the Bahamas.

UNICEF. 2006. HFLE in Caribbean schools: new approaches, prospects and challenges. Barbados: The United Nations Children's Fund.

Vince Whitman, C. 2004. HIV/AIDS Education in the Commonwealth Caribbean. *Caribbean Quarterly* 50(1):2–30.

World Bank. 2002. Education and HIV/AIDS: A window of hope. Washington DC: The World Bank.

ACKNOWLEDGEMENTS

The School of Education, University of the West Indies, St Augustine, Trinidad

Network of Caribbean Ministries of Education HIV Coordinators

The Commonwealth Secretariat

Geoffrey Ijumba, UNICEF, Guyana

Elaine King, UNICEF, Barbados

Michael Morrissey, UNESCO Office for the Caribbean

3

Health and Family Life Education in the Formal Education Sector in the Caribbean: a Historical Perspective

Joycelyn Rampersad

Lecturer, Faculty of Humanities and Education, The University of the West Indies, St Augustine Campus

The development of health and family life education (HFLE) programmes for schools in the Commonwealth Caribbean is traced from the era of independence in the 1960s and 1970s through to the present day. Lobbies and situations that promoted such programmes are analysed as are factors that put a brake on realisation. The chapter is organised under the following headings:

- *Expansion and restructuring of the education and health sectors in the 1960s and 1970s;*
- *Impact of foreign-debt crises, structural adjustment policies, unequal income distribution, and attempts to build human capital and meet basic needs during the 1980s;*
- *Impact of economic recovery and socio-economic development challenges during the 1990s; and*
- *Impact of changing global realities, 2000 to 2006.*

The chapter concludes with the author's view of challenges ahead for HFLE.

Two important contributors to the human capital and by extension, the economic growth and development of the Caribbean region are education and health. While there has been considerable investment in education and health over the past decades, with significant returns in terms of accessibility and quality of education and health services, the changing health profile of the region has come under considerable scrutiny in recent times. A recent report of the Caribbean Commission on Health and Development (CCHD) reveals that while non-communicable diseases (heart disease, cancers, stroke, and diabetes) are the leading causes of death, the prevalence rate for HIV/AIDS, a major communicable disease gives cause for concern. A mortality analysis for the year 2000 showed AIDS in 5th position as a leading cause of death. The data also reveal that in CAREC member countries, AIDS had become the second leading cause of death among men aged 25-34 years, and the fifth and fourth leading causes of death among women aged 15-24, and 25-34 years respectively. Additionally, violence and injury together were the major causes of death in the 15-24 age-groups for the year 2000 (CCHD, 2005).

Susceptibility to most of these diseases is increased by health-compromising behaviours established during youth (Kolbe, 1993, cited in Mohammed & Jing-Zhen, 2000). These diseases also contribute to an as yet to be fully acknowledged significant economic cost for governments through increased expenditure on health care. For example, the projected minimum additional expenditure to reverse trends for HIV/AIDS alone in Trinidad and Tobago has been estimated to be 4% of present national output, which works out to be TT$1.8 billion. The estimated overall cost of an annual response to HIV/AIDS in Caribbean countries has been estimated at between US$ 60 to US$ 573 million dollars (Theodore, 2001). These figures do not include emotional and other social costs to young people, their families, and communities.

Schools have always been one of the key settings of efforts to improve the health and wellbeing of children and youth. Traditionally, they served as institutions for the delivery of school health services and other basic needs, and as referral points for dental, diagnostic, and counselling services. In recent times, the school has begun to play a more important role in facilitating the acquisition of knowledge, attitudes and skills by children and young persons, to better position them to make choices conducive to their healthy growth and development, and to the prevention and reduction of specific health problems. In order to strengthen Caribbean schools and other educational institutions to discharge this role, governments of the Caribbean Community and Common Market (CARICOM), with the support of the international donor agencies and regional institutions, have implemented the CARICOM/UN Multi-Agency Health and Family Life Education (HFLE) Project. The rationale was to provide the supportive environments and programmes that would reduce risk factors,

and facilitate the development of behaviours that would improve health status, and maximise learning potential.

This chapter attempts to trace the development of Health and Family Life Education (HFLE) in the CARICOM Caribbean, from its initial conceptualization to the present. (The CARICOM Caribbean comprises 13 Caribbean countries and 3 mainland countries of Central and South America.) The organizing framework used is an historical trace from 1961 to 2006. Within this framework, significant global events impacted the political process in the region and influenced the course of economic growth and development. These events provide the contexts for an examination of the central issues that impacted on health and human well being, and the types of responses by the various sectors and interest groups at both country and regional levels to bring about change in the health status of citizens of the region. Important milestones in HFLE development are juxtaposed with key global events that were taking place simultaneously, and which were impacting on education and health in the region.

The chapter is organized under the following headings:
- The expansion and restructuring of the education and health sectors in the 1960s and 1970s
- The impact of foreign-debt crises, structural adjustment policies, unequal income distribution, and attempts to build human capital and meet basic needs during the 1980s
- The impact of economic recovery and socio-economic development challenges during the 1990s
- The impact of changing global realities – 2000 to 2006.

THE EXPANSION AND RESTRUCTURING OF THE EDUCATION AND HEALTH SECTORS IN THE 1960S AND 1970S

Prior to the 1960s, the pre-independence era for many of the countries in the Caribbean, gastro-intestinal, helminthic, and other communicable diseases, contributed to high rates of infant mortality, and low levels of health in children and young people. These were problems traditionally associated with developing countries, and were directly related to conditions of living that existed at the time such as poor hygienic and sanitary practices, unhealthy environmental conditions, inadequate nutrition, and unsafe water (see Waldron, 1997); and to colonial health policies.

MacPherson (1982), in his thesis on *Social Policy in the Third World,* posits that the imperative of economic expansion and exploitation during the colonial period determined both the nature and extent of social provision in "third world" countries. MacPherson refers to three major components of medical care during the colonial era – the urban hospital, the rural dispensary, and the hygiene or public health element. Colonial administration hospitals were built initially to meet the needs of Europeans and their families, and were in the major centres of European settlement and economic activity. In terms of public policy the essential objective of the colonial policy was to provide a 'safer' environment for the Europeans both in residential areas and areas of economic activity such as estates and plantations. The legacy of colonialism was not only inadequate services that were poorly distributed and irrelevant to the needs of the majority, but an approach to health that was inimical to the development of an appropriate health system.

The role of the school in health education was acknowledged during this pre-independence period in the region. Personal hygiene, physiology of the body, causes of infectious diseases, basic sanitation measures, or some other aspect of health education, were compulsory components of the school curriculum, particularly at the primary level in most countries (PAHO/WHO, 1985). For example, the *Syllabus of Work for Primary Schools* in Trinidad and Tobago in the pre-independence era contained 14 subject areas including hygiene (Harvey, 1988). At primary schools, teacher inspection for cleanliness of hands, ears, hair, clothing, and so forth, was routine. Health education was also a compulsory component of general education in the apprenticeship training schemes for teachers as obtained, for example, in Guyana, Trinidad, Grenada, and a number of the other English-speaking countries. While the focus was on acquisition of knowledge, these programmes were in direct response to prevailing conditions and the need to improve health and human living, and by extension productivity.

As countries moved towards independence and associated statehood in the 1960s and 1970s, there was an imperative for the educational sector to expand, and to increase equity to access. This expansion thrust brought with it a reorganization of priorities, of ways of doing things, and a retargeting of values. Governments and leading educators were of the view that Caribbean education systems should move beyond their historic roles as vehicles for personal growth and advancement to address development priorities and contribute to social and economic changes (PAHO/WHO, 1985). This argument is supported by Miller (1998a, p.4), who posits that "imperatives of the political sovereignty in the case of the independent countries, or full internal self-government in the case of the still dependent territories, had fuelled their own waves of educational reform in the 1960s and 1970s." These reform initiatives were backed by international lending agencies who could now, as part of the whole human capital orientation to education, justify their investments. For example, following its independence in 1962, Trinidad and Tobago, with technical assistance from UNESCO, was able to access loans from the World Bank and the Inter-American Development Bank to finance its 15-year (1968-83) *Draft Plan for Educational Development* (Alleyne, 1996).

Social demand, political will, and favourable economic circumstances up to the mid 1970s, facilitated the expansion and restructuring of the education system in all countries in the region. This included the refashioning of the design and content of the curriculum to make it more broad-based and culturally relevant to national and Caribbean needs, the reorienting and strengthening of teacher training programmes, the development of Caribbean examination systems, and the production of teaching/learning materials that reflected local realities (PAHO/WHO, 1985). The expansion and restructuring of the education system had one positive health outcome, that is, improved sanitation conditions. However, the value of health in terms of its importance to the education system was not part of the political discourse at the time.

Political independence and associated statehood made little difference to health policies of countries in the region. Newly independent states attempted expansion of their health systems, but essentially in the form developed under colonialism. This "neo-colonialism" was responsible for perpetuating the injustices of health care systems in the Caribbean. According to Gish

(1979), cited in MacPherson (1982), the rhetoric of post-independence health plans emphasised preventive and rural priorities at the same time that expenditures were overly curative and urban. Antrobus (n.d.) concedes that there were "gaps" between the newly formulated national development and health plans and the existing "old structure" to implement the plans, but argues that the gaps may be attributed to a lack of human, technical, and financial resources, as well as the application of a management mechanism. Health care during this era, therefore, focussed on building/refurbishing large hospitals, and the expansion of health services. Emerging from this was a bio-medical model of health with emphasis on responses to physical manifestations of ill health. Preventive health education was not an aspect of practice, and countries' expenditures during this period revealed that they were not budgeting for any serious health prevention education.

Two significant events in the 1970s signaled changes for education and health. The first was the oil shock in 1974 when the Organization of Petroleum Exporting Countries (OPEC) exercised its control on the price of crude oil, following the Arab Oil Embargo. The immediate increase in the price of oil generated a lot of money for those countries that were oil-producing, but impacted negatively on the economies of those that were oil-importing. This had implications for the countries of the region, especially the smaller countries, and aggravated the existing problem of generating internal capital for development (PAHO/WHO, 1985) which in turn limited the resources that could be allocated to education and health.

International concerns about health in developing countries, however, and a view of development that focused on the needs of the most impoverished, especially their nutritional and basic health needs (WHO, 1973) pointed to a need for a shift in emphasis to basic health care services. This re-focusing led to the enunciation of the principles of primary health care by the Director General of the World Health Organization in 1975 (WHO, 1975) and resulted in *The Declaration of Alma-Ata* in 1978, the second significant event of this period. This Declaration established primary health care as the model of health development for the majority of developing countries, and the strategy to reach the goal of *Health for All* (HFA) in 2000 (WHO, 1978). In 1978, therefore, following on the Declaration of Alma-Ata, the Caribbean Ministers with responsibility for Health issued the *Declaration on Health for the Caribbean Community*. These two Declarations had a beneficial impact on the evolution of national health systems, as well as infrastructural development for the delivery of health care at the community level in the region (Moss, 1997).

In spite of the renewed interest in the health of the Caribbean Community during the 1970s, there was reduced emphasis on health education in schools during this period. One reason was the refocusing of development priorities as a result of educational expansion. Another, was the perceived improvement in the health status of children as a result of initiatives such as immunisation programmes, provision of maternal and child care services, improvement in basic environmental services, and provision of safe water supplies. In spite of reduction rates in infant mortality and the elimination of some communicable diseases, however, there continued to be a number of health-related issues that needed to be addressed (Antrobus, 1978). In young children, the continuing

presence of gastro-intestinal diseases, and the visible evidence of malnutrition was cause for concern. Antrobus (n.d.) in a discourse on the health needs of Caribbean youth during the 1970s identified teenage pregnancy, and the unknown incidence of abortion and its attendant morbidity. In the absence of empirical data based on research studies, the evidence provided was based on increasing bed occupancy in the gynaecology wards of hospitals, medical school records, and school drop out. He also referred to the limited knowledge of the role of early pregnancy/ abortion as cause or effect in relation to behavioural disorders. Antrobus suggested that the absence of, or inadequate school health education and family life education services had a strong, predisposing influence on the nature and magnitude of the health problems that were characteristic of youth during the 1970s.

There were a few countries in the region that were implementing programmes addressing health and family life issues in the formal education sector during this period. There is, however, no available data on the effectiveness or "adequacy" of such programmes for addressing the prevailing health problems. A survey carried out by PAHO/WHO in 5 Caribbean countries in the 1970s revealed that Guyana, St. Vincent, and St. Kitts had such a programme as a separate subject in their schools and teachers' colleges. The findings, however, revealed that the approach was generally "ad hoc" and irregular due to difficulties related to identification of content areas and availability of trained staff (PAHO/WHO, n.d.). There is no evidence from the data collected of any approach to treat with the risk factors that precipitated these problems, or to provide the kinds of information in formal or informal educational settings, that might have informed positive health practices.

Attempts were made by the health sector, however, to treat with health problems as they were identified. This reactive approach to addressing health problems was the stimulus for a teacher development initiative in Guyana in the early 1970s. This initiative by the health sector, expanded on the existing health education component of the teacher preparation curriculum, and included links to health services, teacher inspection, the creation of supportive environments, and a resource manual for teachers. While this initiative was knowledge-based in approach and limited in scope and reach, it was an initial attempt at an integrated approach to programming that went beyond instruction. Although the initiative came from the health sector, it was important in that it established a model for teacher development in the area of health-related education, as well as a network between nurses and teachers, and was a hallmark in intersectoral collaboration.

The health sector continued to drive the thrust for health education, and recognised the importance of collaboration among the sectors. The need for the inclusion of health education in the school curriculum was expressed as early as 1973 at the Conference of Caribbean Ministers with Responsibility for Health. Resolution No. 20 challenged Ministers to "take the initiative to ensure the development of a joint school health policy between the Ministers of Health and Education" (cited in PAHO/WHO, 1978, p.1). At the Conferences of Ministers of Health in 1974, 1975, and 1976, resolutions were again adopted for the inclusion of health education in the school curriculum, and a request was included in Resolution No. 18 of 1976, that "each health administrator ... take action on resolutions on this subject adopted in 1973, 1974, and 1975" (PAHO/WHO, 1978, p.2; PAHO/WHO, 1985).

At the same time that the health sector was bringing some pressure to bear on the education sector with respect to development of a joint school health policy, new problems were surfacing. Changing demographics during the 1970s revealed an increase in the youth population (Antrobus, n.d.; PAHO/ WHO, 1985). This increase coincided with a rise in social problems, which were at the core of mental, emotional and physical health manifestations in this cohort. The increase in social problems precipitated another call from the health sector for programmes to address these problems. At their 1977 Conference, Health Ministers expressed concern about the implications for health and social development of the increasing proportions of youth in the total Caribbean population. They noted that the health problems of youth were multi-dimensional, and that their solutions required the involvement of many disciplines and sectors (PAHO/WHO, 1985).

A recommendation was made to the CARICOM Conference of Heads of Government that higher priority be assigned to programmes in family life education, social and community development services, sex education in schools, and special programmes for pregnant schoolgirls (PAHO/WHO, 1978, pp.2-3; PAHO/ WHO, 1985). Requests were specifically made to a) health administrators to cooperate with other ministries (including the Ministry of Education) to carry out programmes concerned with school health, family life and nutrition, and to include financial provision for a health education component in the preparation of budgets; and b) to the Pan American Health Organization (PAHO) to assist in the implementation of short-term courses in health education for tutors, and to assist countries in the development of their health education programmes (PAHO/ WHO, n.d.).

The thrust for family life education also came from private organisations. Among the private organisations taking the lead in the English-speaking countries of the Caribbean in the mid 1970s was the family planning services. According to Saint-Victor (1991), family planning workers recognised that their services needed an educational and motivational component to increase contraceptive usage, and that the approach to reducing the high incidence of teenage pregnancy was through education. Family life education was seen as the vehicle to do this.

In the latter part of the 1970s, therefore, private sector family planning organisations as well as those within various Ministries of Health began to implement out-of-school family life education programmes and projects. These out-of-school programmes and projects became associated with a model of instruction that focussed on knowledge acquisition in areas related to human reproduction and sex education, social problems, problems associated with adolescence, child care, and interpersonal family relationships. The United Nations Fund for Population Activities (UNFPA), with Pan American Health Organization/World Health Organization (PAHO/WHO) as the executing agency, was the major force among the external agencies, in the promotion of family life education in the region, facilitating projects in 9 countries during this period. These initiatives were later strengthened by contributions from international and Caribbean agencies, such as the United States Agency for International Development (USAID), the CARNEGIE Corporation, the International Planned Parenthood Federation (IPPF), and the Caribbean Family Planning Affiliation Limited (CFPA), along with its local affiliates (Saint-Victor, 1991).

The initiative for a regional approach to curriculum development in the areas of health education and family life education was driven by PAHO/WHO. This was informed by concerns about the increase in health-related problems in children and young people, the models of health care that were emerging, the low priority given to preventive health education in country budgets, and the resolutions of the Ministers of Health (PAHO/WHO, 1978). The need for health and family life education in all schools began to emerge as an important issue of health development with Caribbean countries.

In the work plan of its Family Health Division for 1977, PAHO/WHO proposed that a sub-regional workshop in Family Life Education (FLE) be held in the Caribbean area. In 1978, PAHO/WHO as the executing agency for UNFPA, and in collaboration with the Government of Guyana sponsored the "Caribbean Workshop on Health Education and Family Life Education" in Guyana. Among the participants at the two-week workshop, were thirty-nine (39) representatives from a cross section of sectors from fifteen (15) Caribbean countries, and twelve (12), from regional and international agencies (PAHO/WHO, 1978).

This "benchmark" workshop has been regarded as the beginning of an organized campaign to introduce health and family life education in schools throughout the region. The purpose was to formulate a framework for the establishment of effective family life education and school health education programmes in order to promote through schools, the development and maintenance of desirable health practices in children, youth and families in the Caribbean. Some of the objectives were: "to arrive at common terminology and description of family life education and school health education and identify their inter-relationship; to determine general concepts to be incorporated into the school curricula...; and to prepare broad curricula outlines...." (PAHO/WHO, 1978, p. 4.) It was at this workshop that the term *Health and Family Life* was formally adopted as appropriate terminology for a single programme that would attempt to address key interrelated health issues.

The 1978 Guyana workshop created the opportunity for a multi-sectoral approach to a critical examination of the issues that were impacting children and youth in the region and attempted to prioritize them. A curriculum framework (*Family Life Education and Health Education*) was developed around eleven broad areas. Each area was further developed to specifically address each of three levels in the education sector - primary, secondary, and tertiary. In addition, a statement of policy, and regional and in-country strategies were identified for moving the project forward. The regional strategies considered the following: coordination within and between relevant ministries; further development of curriculum and of teacher units; teacher training; and materials and media development (PAHO/WHO, 1978). This was a milestone in regional curriculum development, and took into account the scope of HFLE, as well as strategies for coordination, policy development, teacher training and materials development. However, it did not lead to immediate development of policies, and implementation of the plans and strategies for strengthening HFLE by the education sector for at least two reasons.

The first reason relates to events that occurred at the workshop. As one of the funding agencies for the workshop, UNFPA tabled the issue of *family planning*, and this inadvertently impacted workshop outcomes. The emerging issue of teenage pregnancy in the Caribbean, while part of the prevailing

culture at the time, was not accepted as a normative strand by the UNFPA in its global thrust to promote family planning. The family planning issue generated much debate and many participants were unable to see health education or family life education beyond the issue of sex education. Thus the broader purpose of the workshop was obscured. The overall result was a major setback in the thrust to have an integrated programme that addressed inter-related health issues, and the fallout has remained up to the present, so that "FLE became a euphemism for family planning" (Saint-Victor (1991). Saint-Victor further suggests that the FLE/family planning promotion/sex education controversy soon found its way into religious and political discourse, and garnered much negative public response. As a result, there was considerable resistance by some Ministries of Education in the Caribbean to the introduction of FLE (or any programme that included sex education) in schools for almost a decade.

The second reason that impacted the progress of the HFLE movement was the apparent lack of follow-through by the co-ordinating agency on decisions made during the 1978 workshop. Donor agencies continued to prioritise, plan, and fund health-related projects as mandated within their particular operational frameworks, often duplicating projects within and across agencies. Both reasons are in a sense related and must be examined within the broader context of donor frameworks. In the first instance, donor agencies operate within the mandates of international frameworks which determine priority areas for intervention, and these may not necessarily be aligned to the socio-cultural realities of a Caribbean society. In the second instance, follow-through would have called for some level of co-ordination among agencies and across sectors, requiring adjustments in work plans, and development of a management strategy.

In spite of the attempt at a conceptual shift to a *Health and Family Life* focus at the 1978 Guyana workshop, FLE continued to be the preferred terminology used with reference to health-related programmes in the region. Even within agencies or organizations that facilitated curriculum development or workshops for in-service training of teachers, reference was sometimes made to FLE programmes, at other times to HFLE programmes, and the terms were often used interchangeably. Thus the first attempt to conceptualise the scope and focus of a regional HFLE programme was not very successful, and the scope and focus became blurred during subsequent developments.

In summary, global and regional developments in the 1960s and 1970s resulted in a number of responses that impacted on the development of HFLE. Health-related curricula were given low priority in the education reform thrust; some of the gatekeepers in the education sector took a hands-off approach to the issue of health and family life education in schools; and donor agencies and other organisations outside the education sector took the lead in the development and funding of projects to address perceived needs related to health and psycho-social issues of young people.

The slow response by the education sector to the various resolutions passed at the Conferences of Caribbean Ministers of Health between 1973 -1977 might be explained from two perspectives. One was a lack of vision with respect to the potential for rates of return in terms of capital accumulation that could result from investment in both the education and the health of citizens (Todaro & Smith, 2006). The education sector at the time did not seem

to have the same conceptualisation of the intersecting roles of health and education in the development and attainment of potential of young people, and by extension overall economic development. The second could be attributed to a dearth of strong leadership capacity within the education sector to mobilise the resources necessary for policy and programme development in health-related education, as well as the associated training needs and implementation issues. While there were financial constraints that might have set limits to budgetary allocations for development of policies and programmes, this could have been offset through a partnership approach between the donor agencies and the governments of the day. Such an approach would have given national governments and their agents more control over the scope and focus of HFLE, and would have positioned them to assume ownership of HFLE.

At the close of the 1970s, therefore, attempts to organize and implement a comprehensive school health and family life programme were largely unsuccessful. However, the fallout as a result of events occurring during the next decade put considerable pressure on the education sector, and led to a reconsideration of its position.

THE IMPACT OF FOREIGN-DEBT CRISES, STRUCTURAL ADJUSTMENT POLICIES, UNEQUAL INCOME DISTRIBUTION, AND ATTEMPTS TO BUILD HUMAN CAPITAL AND MEET BASIC NEEDS DURING THE 1980S

The 1980s saw a reversal of some of the strides made in the region during the 1960s and 1970s in education and health as a result of two significant events. The first was the second oil shock at the beginning of the decade (1983) with the decrease in oil prices. This resulted in low economic growth, macroeconomic crises with inappropriate fiscal policy responses and ensuing debt accumulation, deficiencies in the labour market, and deterioration in the quality of social services (Baker, 1997; Downes, A. S. 1992). The responses to macroeconomic instability incurred some social and economic costs, such as increases in levels of poverty, increases in crime and violence, retrenchment of workers, skewed income distribution, and changes in family structures (Baker, 1997). By the late 1980s, countries like Barbados, Guyana, Jamaica, and Trinidad and Tobago, had International Monetary Fund-backed, market-oriented economic stabilisation and structural adjustment programmes in place. This debt crisis had implication for budgetary allocations, resulting in severe contraction in resource availability for investment in education, health, and other social infrastructure (Tsang, Fryer, & Arevalo, 2002).

This decline in economic growth occurred at a critical period when regional governments were developing action plans to promote health. For example, by the beginning of the 1980s, Caribbean governments had already joined the international community in adopting the goal of *Health for All* (HFA) by the year 2000. In commitment to this goal they endorsed the *"Primary Health Care Strategy"* as the key to its achievement, and developed the *"Caribbean Plan of Action"* for its implementation at the St. Lucia Conference on Primary Health Care in 1981 (PAHO/WHO, 1985). The *Primary Health Care Strategy* identified intersectoral action, and the education and active involvement of individuals, families, and communities in

health development activities as indispensable measures for the achievement of HFA by the year 2000.

Following the adoption of the Ottawa Charter for Health Promotion in 1986, the Caribbean Ministers with responsibility for Health launched the Caribbean Cooperation in Health Initiative (CCHI) as a joint framework for health action in 1986. Although the implementation of the *Caribbean Plan of Action* was severely constrained by the prevailing economic circumstances following the second oil shock, the *Primary Health Care Strategy* had underscored the importance of the education sector in achieving HFA. This provided additional impetus for the institutionalisation of HFLE in the formal education sector in the region. Resolutions were again passed by the Conference of Ministers responsible for Health in 1980 and 1982 for the inclusion of FLE in schools (CARICOM, 1986).

The second significant event of the 1980s was the fall of the Berlin Wall in 1989. The fall of the Berlin Wall and the end of the Cold War, brought with it a high expectation of a new world order, and the prediction of a "peace dividend." It was felt that reduced expenditure on defense would be redeployed to the cause of poverty eradication and economic development. According to Billie Miller, the expected peace dividend never materialized for Caribbean countries. Rather, the effect of the vacuum caused by the disintegration of the east-west balance led to a period of instability in international affairs, and economies of the Caribbean were further marginalized (Miller, 2001). Errol Miller also refers to a set of international paradoxes that manifested themselves in the post-cold war period. For example, the prospect of global peace was accompanied by an unprecedented increase in crime, and the triumph of capitalism over communism was accompanied by increasing poverty (Miller, 1998b).

All of these converging events had a direct impact on the poor in the region in terms of access to health care and living conditions conducive to good health. While mortality due to communicable diseases decreased, the prevailing health problems impacting young people during this period included vector-borne diseases, teen-age pregnancies, sexually transmitted diseases, and the recurring issue of malnutrition in children (Brandon, 1987). In the adult population, the emerging problems of serious concern included HIV/ AIDS, and chronic non-communicable diseases such as cardiovascular diseases and cancer. As a result, the health status of individuals, families, and communities continued to be a growing concern (Holder & Lewis, 1997).

Simultaneously with global and regional initiatives to attain the goal of *Health for All*, moves were also afoot to strengthen the role of education in the development process. For example, by the beginning of the 1980s, the world's multilateral agencies had adopted the "basic needs approach" and the significance of education to the development process was seen as threefold. Education was identified as:

- a basic human need (a condition for the ability of the individual to identify with the prevailing culture)
- a means of meeting other human needs (influencing, and in turn being influenced by, access to other basic needs such as adequate nutrition, safe drinking water, health services etc.), and
- an activity that sustains and accelerates overall development (World Bank, 1980).

The education reform thrust in the region, however, had more than one paradoxical effect. For example, while the fundamental values and goals underpinning the reform efforts had implications for opportunities for institutionalising and strengthening HFLE, in actual fact, the rapid changes had resulted in some unintended outcomes. Four of these outcomes were highlighted in a 1985 PAHO/ WHO project proposal to the CARNEGIE Corporation (PAHO/WHO, 1993). These were:

- The emphasis given in practice to cognitive mastery and acquisition of knowledge (with a focus by schools on examinations) - academic achievement had become synonymous with educational attainment
- The allocation of financial resources - expenditure in the main was devoted to ensuring and maintaining the requisite pool of teachers, and a small cadre of managers was available to oversee the reform efforts (including the promotion and support of HFLE)
- The institutionalisation of mass schooling – the shared roles between home and school for the education and socialisation of children had become sharply demarcated, with pre-eminence given to schools. In the context of rapid social change, fragmentation of communities, and the construction of new and larger schools, organisational reform had created, both literally and figuratively, physical and social distance between schools, homes and communities.
- The expansion of the school curriculum by continual addition of new subjects over the years – the issue of curriculum overload had become a point of contention for some educators and even some parents.

The combination of all of these unintended outcomes, therefore, had tended to deflect or undermine any consistent attention to those components of the curriculum concerned with the affective and developmental aspects of children and young persons, such as HFLE.

By the mid 1980s, as a result of continuing pressure from the health sector, there was gradual acceptance by Ministries of Education for school health and family life education programmes in schools. The degree of acceptance, however, varied from country to country. An informal survey of country representatives at a sub-regional workshop in 1981 to assess the extent to which school health and family life education had been further developed in the school system (PAHO/WHO, 1985) revealed that 7 of the 17 countries present had *active* programmes (my emphasis). Of these, Dominica, Anguilla, St. Vincent, St. Kitts and Nevis, Montserrat, and the British Virgin Islands had initiated curriculum development using the 1978 Guyana prototype as a guide. It is note-worthy that while participants may have perceived their programmes to be active, there were no empirical data presented as to classroom impact or positive health outcomes. The remaining 10 countries present at the workshop were at varying stages of readiness for implementation of HFLE curricula on a systematic basis.

With the introduction of HFLE-related curricula, a few countries were also pro-active with respect to policy development. For example, as early as 1982, St. Kitts and Nevis had clearly enunciated policies that placed the health of the nation as a top priority in the government's overall socio-economic development plan, and ensured that appropriate family life education programmes were implemented at all levels of the education system, including the teacher's college. Policy implementation was facilitated by the coordination of health and education matters under a single Ministry of Education and Health (CARICOM, 1987).

As the school-based thrust made some inroads in the various countries, it became necessary to obtain feedback on what was happening at both the school level and the teachers' college level. A survey of teachers' colleges in the Eastern Caribbean was undertaken in 1983 by PAHO/WHO in collaboration with the School of Education, UWI, Cave Hill, Barbados (PAHO/WHO, 1983). The purpose of the survey was to document what existed, and to determine strategies for establishing and maintaining HFLE within the teachers' colleges. Two years later, in 1985, PAHO/WHO commissioned a short-term consultant to make an assessment of the state of FLE in the region over the previous ten years (CARICOM, 1986). The recommended approach for delivery of HFLE from the 1983 survey was that of integration within other subject areas. This was based on the argument that a) integration of "health education and related aspects" had been successfully implemented in "other third world" countries, b) integration into well established subject areas should improve the status of HFLE, and c) analysis of HFLE curricula, and the curricula of existing subjects, had shown that it was feasible (PAHO/WHO, 1983).

Similarities in findings between the two surveys included the lack of rationalisation with respect to what constitutes HFLE and how it should be promoted; the different configurations of arrangements that existed for its implementation at both schools and colleges; and the low status given to the programme. The latter impacted negatively on resource allocation for development of policy measures to move HFLE forward. These recurrent findings in the 1985 survey highlight the slow response by national governments/education sectors to take action on the recommendations made previously at the various sub-regional fora. The issue of terminology for the curriculum was still to be resolved. Both surveys were executed by the same agency, yet one report spoke to HFLE and the other to FLE. The main recommendations coming out of the 1985 survey were:

- Improvement in teacher education with accredited certification
- Standardisation of FLE curricula, particularly at primary and secondary levels
- Establishment of a regional institution that could fulfil the functions of a data bank and a clearing-house for FLE information, materials and resources
- A Regional Conference to consider and endorse the proposals and carry forward the planning for implementation (CARICOM, 1986).

There was up to this time no specific qualification/accreditation that HFLE teachers/teacher educators in the region could access, or even consensus about the competencies that were desirable for such persons. While this was an opportunity for dialogue among the regional universities, the teachers' colleges, and representatives from the key sectors with a view to addressing this anomaly, no immediate action was taken. In addition, procedures for taking recommendations (coming out of the various surveys) forward were either non-existent or poorly structured in light of the suggestion for a Regional Conference to carry forward the planning for implementation.

The findings from the 1983 survey, together with the field experiences of PAHO/WHO personnel and other educators in the region, prompted PAHO to identify a number of constraints impacting the institutionalisation of HFLE in the school system. These included differences in orientation of health and education sectors to health and education issues, limited finances, different approaches to training, and inadequately trained teachers. It was concluded that there was a need for a comprehensive and systematic approach to strengthening the role of the school in HFLE (PAHO/WHO, 1985). It is noteworthy that many of these constraints had been identified at various fora beginning in the 1970s, and were still being reiterated almost 10 years later.

The subject of HFLE/FLE in schools was again referred to the CARICOM Standing Committee of Ministers responsible for Education (SCME) in 1986 in an effort to formulate and implement a regional strategy for teaching the subject in schools and teachers' colleges (CARICOM, 1986). The Committee was requested to:

- endorse the establishment of FLE as a teaching area within the education system
- note the recommendations of the PAHO/WHO consultant
- approve activities proposed in the action plan for the promotion of FLE in schools, and
- support the proposal to seek external assistance for the establishment of a regional training programme in FLE education.

The last was a direct appeal to the international donor community for both technical expertise, and funding.

In the meantime a number of initiatives aimed at strengthening and supporting HFLE curriculum reform and implementation were taking place. Some of these were duplicating efforts, and some had competing goals. For example in 1986 PAHO with funding from CARNEGIE implemented a 3-year project to promote HFLE in schools and colleges in selected Eastern Caribbean countries (PAHO/WHO, 1993), while the PAHO 1985 survey was still in progress. The initial objectives of the 1986 PAHO project were to promote the formal development of policy; revision and reform of school health and family life curricula of primary schools; and the development, production and distribution of reference materials to support and reinforce continued implementation of the revised curriculum. While this project was still being implemented, a sub-regional workshop, organized by other agencies, was taking place.

This 1987 sub-regional workshop, jointly sponsored by UNFPA and CARICOM, was in keeping with the mandate of the SCME. The main aim of the workshop was to explore ways in which FLE could be infused into the curriculum and learning experiences of Caribbean schools. While the focus of both the PAHO/CARNEGIE project and the UNFPA/CARICOM workshop was on curriculum review/revision, there seemed to be no coordination between the various agencies, since the aims were diametrically opposed. On the one hand the PAHO/CARNEGIE project was attempting to strengthen and support HFLE as a separate curriculum subject, while on the other hand the sub-regional workshop was exploring the issue of integration of HFLE into the general curriculum.

While the issue of integration of HFLE had been one of the recommendations in the 1983 survey of teachers' colleges report (PAHO/WHO, 1983), the challenges presented by such an approach had already been identified in the 1985 survey report (CARICOM, 1986). It is reasonable to assume that some kind of antecedent change had occurred in the outlook of those proposing the new approach. It was now

felt that the strategy of infusion as a form of integration would be economical in terms of addressing time and human resource constraints.

A significant event at the 1987 workshop was the case made by Brandon (1987) for expanding the scope and focus of FLE by placing it within the broader context of health and related social issues in the Caribbean, and examining the implications for curriculum development. The rationale for education for [improving] health was based on the research evidence that showed health as both a condition for, and a consequence of, personal and societal development. While Brandon's position presented some advantages (examination of causes and responses to health and social issues to facilitate change) as well as disadvantages (possibility of overlooking or de-emphasising key issues), there is no evidence that any of the arguments put forward were considered in the processes leading up to workshop outcomes. This is an example of how differences in the conceptualisation of health and related issues by the two main sectors, and of how these should be treated, impacted the curriculum development process.

One outcome of the 1987 workshop was the *"Curriculum Guidelines for Family Life Education in the Caribbean: Education for Living"* document which was endorsed by the SCME in 1988 (Steward, n.d.). This was the second regional document on HFLE curriculum guidelines produced within the space of a decade, and events leading up to its production demonstrate the circuitous process of HFLE development, and the challenges involved in its implementation up to this period. Table 1 below gives a comparison of the content areas in the 1978 Guyana curriculum outline, and the 1987 Education for Living curriculum guidelines.

As can be seen in the table, the 1988 document was much wider in scope than the 1978 document. Details were provided in the new document on the processes involved in integration through infusion, and suggestions were given for its organization across subject areas, and on the logistics of timetabling (Steward, n.d.). Emphasis was given to emerging health issues such as STDs and chronic non-communicable diseases, and an entire sub-section under "Sexual Well-Being" was devoted to "HIV Infection and AIDS". However, there was no reference to the importance of behaviour change methodologies either in the teaching or evaluation strategies suggested.

In order to address the shortage of trained educators, the Advanced Training & Research in Fertility Management Unit (ATRFMU) of The University of the West Indies, Mona, Jamaica, with considerable funding from Germany, developed a training design in 1989. The purpose was to prepare resource personnel in three sectors – Health, Education, and Community Services – to deliver HFLE at different levels in their respective sectors (ATRFMU, 1996). This was the first regional initiative to train a large cadre of professionals to strengthen HFLE programmes across sectors and within countries.

A curriculum was developed by ATRFMU in 1989 (and later revised in 1990) for use in the preparation of these HFLE *trainers*. This was yet another attempt at curriculum development to meet perceived needs. While

TABLE 3.1
COMPARISON OF THE 1978 AND 1988 CURRICULUM OUTLINES

Health Education and Family Life Education Curriculum Outline (PAHO/WHO, 1978)	Education for Living – Curriculum Guidelines for Family Life Education in the Caribbean (Steward, n.d.)

▯ Human Growth and Development
▯ Food and Nutrition
▯ Environmental Health
▯ Human Relationships
▯ Mental Health and Drug Abuse
▯ Consumer Education
▯ Health and Social Services
▯ Population Education
▯ Safety and First Aid
▯ Dental Health
▯ Health Problems
    o Recognition
    o Prevention
    o Management
	▯ Health and Well-Being
	    o Intrapersonal Health
	    o Interpersonal Health
	    o Growth and Development
	    o Environmental Safety
	    o Environmental Health
	    o Disease Control and Prevention
	    o Sexual Well-Being
	    o Consumer Health
	▯ Family
	    o Functions
	    o Roles and Relationships
	    o Problems
	    o Legal Issues
	    o Management
	▯ Population Education
	    o Variables and Characteristics
	    o Dynamics
	    o Techniques
	    o Management and Related Issues
	▯ Work and Leisure
	    o Career Choices
	    o Occupational Clusters
	    o Self Assessment
	    o Preparation for Employment

the intersectoral approach to training was in keeping with the recommendations of the SCME in 1986, the training model developed did not take into account the model/s already existing at the teachers' colleges and other educational institutions, or the recommendations put forward in the 1988 Curriculum guidelines. This was yet another example of duplication of effort as well as resources. In retrospect, a critical issue is whether ATRFMU was the appropriate lead agency for the task of training HFLE educators, with respect to a) its human and technical resources capability for execution of the task, b) its lack of accreditation for conferral of certification, a need that had been voiced previously, and c) its involvement in the area of fertility management. With respect to the latter, the progress of HFLE development and implementation in the region had already been negatively impacted by its association with family planning promotion and sex education.

In summary, the responses to the development challenges in the 1980s included: a) commitment by governments to the goals of HFA by 2000, and the recognition of the need for inter-sectoral collaboration in order to realise these goals; b) commitment by the education sector to policy changes that allowed HFLE programmes to become part of the formal education system in most countries; and c) increased donor interest and funding of HFLE projects, including the development of HFLE curricula guidelines that explored options for HFLE curriculum delivery (integration versus specialisation), and the preparation of HFLE "trainers" to address the shortage of trained personnel across sectors.

While the economic downturn in the 1980s impacted on the availability of resources that could be allocated to sectors for

HFLE development, there was little progress with respect to maximizing the human resource potential for moving HFLE forward in the region. A crucial question is whether there was a fundamental flaw in the process utilised that undermined the implementation of HFLE from the beginning. The process seemed to be locked into a continuous cycle of situation analysis followed by strategy document development, and so on.

Of the three HFLE curriculum guidelines developed up to this period, only the 1988 curriculum was produced as a separate document for wide circulation within the formal education sector (Steward, n.d.). In all three cases, however, the approach to curriculum development was what is described in the literature as the "top-down" approach (see Schubert, 1986), in which a curriculum is expected to be implemented by persons who were not involved in its formulation. In the absence of a) clearly articulated policies for HFLE curriculum implementation in all countries, b) in-country pilot studies to monitor and evaluate implementation, c) on-going development programmes to develop teacher capacity, and d) a strong support system for HFLE teachers/educators, it is plausible that the implementation process was slowed because adopters of the curriculum were unwilling or unable to see the potential of HFLE for empowering young persons to manage their health, and enhance the quality of their lives. It is also plausible that the absence of feedback on the progress of HFLE at the ground level, lack of communication across sectors and agencies, and shifting priorities of the donor agencies drove the curriculum development process into a cycle that prevented forward progress.

A major issue that also impacted the forward progress of HFLE was the absence of a central authority to coordinate, mobilise, organize, and manage the different aspects of HFLE at a regional level. The logistics of managing an initiative in a complex system such as CARICOM, involving several countries, require the kind of organisational leadership that could forge synergy and coherence. The absence of such leadership results in overload and fragmentation (Fullan, 1999). This was evidenced by the failure of local systems to effectively mobilise for HFLE implementation, the duplication of efforts, and the wastage of resources, in a period when the health and psychosocial needs of the region were escalating.

Thus, while the importance of HFLE as an intervention in the formal education sector was acknowledged, there was up to this period no agreement by key players as to its scope and focus, or how it should move forward. In order to bring some resolution to these issues, a number of response strategies were developed and executed during the next decades.

THE IMPACT OF ECONOMIC RECOVERY AND DEVELOPMENT CHALLENGES DURING THE 1990S AND BEYOND

The 1990s were characterised by a number of development challenges that demanded creative policy responses to stimulate and sustain economic growth in the region. Some of these challenges included global economic changes in trade and capital markets, the erosion of preferential market access, vulnerability of the tourist industry, and decline in capital flows from bilateral sources. In spite of these challenges, there were varying levels of economic recovery from the severe economic crises of the 1980s, with actual growth occurring in some countries. For example, between 1990 and 1994, there

were increases in per capita income, with countries such as Antigua and Barbuda, Belize, Guyana, St. Lucia, St. Kitts and Nevis, and St. Vincent and the Grenadines, high on the spectrum in terms of real gross domestic product (GDP) growth rates, while others like The Bahamas, Barbados, Suriname, and Trinidad and Tobago, were low on the spectrum. While economic growth is linked to poverty reduction, poverty continued to be pervasive in the region. Countries such as Belize, Dominica, Guyana, Haiti, Jamaica and Suriname, that registered medium or low economic growth during this period, experienced high levels of poverty. Trinidad and Tobago, in spite of increases in economic growth, continued to experience medium levels of poverty. The social and economic costs associated with poverty such as increasing levels of crime and violence, impacted on the social health of communities in the region, and diverted scarce financial resources that could have been invested in health and education (Baker, 1997).

Problems such as poverty, and escalating crime and violence, constrain efforts by countries to meet basic learning needs. This situation was not unique to the Caribbean during this period of development. In recognition of the place of education in human development, *The World Declaration on Education for All: Meeting Basic Learning Needs* was adopted by the World Conference on Education for All in Jomtien, Thailand in 1990. This was an expanded vision of education, and recognition that essential learning tools and basic learning content were prerequisite for humans to survive, to develop their full capacities, to participate in development, and to improve the quality of their lives. Some of the premises on which this Declaration was based were that education was a fundamental right for all; that education could help ensure a safer, healthier, more prosperous and environmentally sound world; and that sound basic education was fundamental to the strengthening of higher levels of education (UNESCO, 1994). Following on the Jomtien Declaration, there was a refocusing on education in the region, particularly in the area of access at all levels of the system.

In spite of the varying levels of economic recovery during the early 1990s, it was still difficult for governments to expand health facilities and services in response to increasing health demands, and competing demands from other sectors. The epidemiological profile of the countries during this period revealed that chronic non-communicable diseases were becoming the major causes of ill health and mortality, and were placing additional demands on an already over-burdened health sector. In addition, the resurgence of communicable diseases including food borne illnesses, tuberculosis, and malaria (in some countries), and the emergence of new communicable diseases such as HIV/AIDS, Hepatitis C, and human papillomavirus (HPV), were largely affected by high-risk behaviours (Theodore & Greene, 1997).

These development challenges had a negative impact on children and youth. There was increasing vulnerability to violence (self and interpersonal), substance use (alcohol and illicit drugs), HIV/AIDS and STDs (early sexual initiation, sexual abuse, commercial sex), under-nutrition (related to pockets of poverty), and homelessness (the appearance of street children). School failure increased with associated dropouts, and the safety and quality of the school environment were severely compromised by increasing school violence and teacher frustration. In addition, there was limited family support

and supervision related directly to changes in family structures as a result of fragmentation of families and communities (Brandon, 1999).

In spite of the widespread acknowledgement of the importance of HFLE as a school based intervention to meet some of these challenges, there were still a few Caribbean countries that had not introduced it into school curricula at the beginning of the 1990s. This period, therefore, was characterised by a number of response strategies for addressing all the health and social issues that were being presented, in a more focussed way. These strategies are discussed below.

Re-thinking the Scope and Focus of HFLE in Schools

Re-thinking the scope and focus of HFLE was imperative because of the conflicting perspectives and understandings that were coming from the two main sectors (education and health), as well as from interest groups that were involved in training initiatives and curriculum planning. Two reports coming out of the region during this period reflect this re-thinking.

The first report was on a 1990 PAHO/WHO survey of HFLE/FLE in the Caribbean over a 15-year period. It sought to document the changes in the conceptualisation of FLE from its narrow view as a mechanism for family planning information, to its newer focus as a vehicle for the acquisition of knowledge, skills, and attitudes to equip young people to adopt constructive behaviours (Saint-Victor, 1991). The second, the summary report of the PAHO/CARNEGIE project (PAHO/WHO, 1993), spoke directly to the need for rethinking the concepts of *education* and *health* by the two sectors.

The latter report acknowledged that while there had been shifts in the paradigms of the two main sectors, it was apparent that the roots of the concepts of *education as cognition* and *health as disease* still ran deep and had given rise to organisational structures and pressures within the educational system which had created forces that ran counter to the principles and approaches that were requisite for health and family life education (PAHO/WHO, 1993). The report also called for a paradigmatic shift in the thinking of administrators, national coordinators, principals and teachers. This shift required new approaches and strategies, since HFLE as delivered was making no significant inroads with respect to positive behavioural outcomes in the school population. In re-thinking the scope of HFLE in schools, it was important to broaden the narrow concepts of health that still underpinned existing curricula and recognise that health status was mediated by behaviours and conditions of living. It was therefore necessary to shift focus from knowledge to skill and action, in order to bring about behaviour change, and to place emphasis on the creation of safe social and physical settings to facilitate the change (Brandon, 1999).

RE-CONCEPTUALISING A HEALTH AND FAMILY LIFE CURRICULUM FRAMEWORK

An adjunct to the PAHO/CARNEGIE project was the establishment of an inter-agency committee to advocate for the development of materials. Among the documents produced was the *Core Curriculum Guidelines for Strengthening the Teaching of Health and Family Life Education in Teachers' Colleges in the Eastern Caribbean* (PAHO/WHO, 1992). This curriculum guide was an off-shoot of an initiative to re-conceptualise a realistic HFLE curriculum framework for the teachers' colleges. At the time there were around eighteen health-related curricula in use at teachers' colleges addressing specific health issues such as "violence", "STDs", "AIDS", "drug use", and "obesity". The new approach to curriculum development took into account a broader vision of health that linked health, education and development benefits. It focussed on the common underlying risk behaviours that contributed to current and emergent health and health-related issues, curriculum overload and duplication, acquisition of skills and the creation of settings and policies to reinforce the skills, the personal and professional preparation of teachers, and the management capabilities of the training colleges. The related health issues were collapsed under *"five behavioural themes."*

The justification for the thematic areas was based on the following conceptual framework:

- *Promoting Health, Wellness, and Human Living* - Health is "behaviour" which is shaped by how people think about health, and how they act about health
- *Developing Emotional and Social Skills* - Health problems have a basis in human behaviour. Crime and violence, mental health, and suicide, are all related to individual capacity to form emotional and social relationships
- *Protecting Sexual Health* - Risks for STDs, including HIV/AIDS, are related to sexual choices
- *Promoting Appropriate Eating and Fitness* - Problems with obesity that increase the risk of chronic non-communicable diseases, are related to food choices and levels of physical activity
- *Managing the Environment* - Problems with the environment (degradation or hazards) have to do with how the environment is managed.

This approach saw a shift in focus from knowledge acquisition to one of pro-action, awareness of factors shaping choices, and accentuated wellness. Participatory, active learning strategies and broader assessment measures were also promoted.

A substantial portion of the section of the guide on human sexuality was devoted to HIV/AIDS, and explored issues ranging from transmission and treatment, options for reducing risks, to emotional aspects including discrimination and stigmatisation. The "Core Curriculum Guide" was formally adopted by the Eastern Caribbean at the Eastern Caribbean Standing Conference on Teacher Education in April 1995 to aid instruction in HFLE (ATRFMU, 1997) and became the reference document for HFLE in the teachers' colleges of the Eastern Caribbean by September of 1995.

Strengthening Coordination and Partnerships

The most important initiative in this area was the establishment of the CARICOM/ Multi-Agency HFLE Project. A resolution was passed at the 1994 meeting of the SCME giving support for the development of a comprehensive approach by CARICOM and the UWI to HFLE. This new approach was supported by the United Nations agencies working in the region and included other regional organizations working in the area of health (see CARICOM/UNICEF, 1996). With the establishment of the Project, the CARICOM Secretariat assumed overall responsibility, while UNICEF assumed responsibility for its coordination (UNICEF, 1999). Principles for coordination among agencies were later developed and accepted in September, 1995 (CARICOM, 1995), and at a meeting of Heads of Agencies in November 1996, recommendations were made for maintaining inter-agency collaboration. These included the development of a communication strategy. UNICEF and

UNDP were given the responsibility to ensure that the recommendations were pursued.

At the request of the SCME at its 1994 meeting, UNICEF assisted CARICOM and the UWI in the development of a strategy document for strengthening HFLE in the region (UNICEF, 1995). The document, endorsed by the SCME and the Ministers responsible for Health at their respective meetings in 1996, set out the process for implementation of the multi-agency Project. The objectives of the strategy document were to:

- develop policy, including advocacy and funding for the overall strengthening of HFLE in and out of school
- strengthen the capacity of teachers to deliver HFLE programmes
- develop comprehensive life-skills based teaching materials, and
- improve co-ordination among the agencies operating at the regional and national levels in the area of HFLE.

The Ministers reaffirmed their commitment to HFLE as a priority for achieving national development goals. Some of the proposals agreed to were policy formulation to include HFLE as a core curriculum area, establishment of mechanisms for national co-ordination as well as co-ordination across sectors, allocation of resources to establish/strengthen programmes, and according priority to the development of materials and curricula in the area of HFLE. With respect to the latter proposal, it was underscored that attention be paid to AIDS and drug use (CARICOM, 1996).

Mechanisms were established by CARICOM to ensure and support collaborative efforts at all levels. These included the establishment of a Regional Working Group to oversee the implementation of the Project, establishment of national inter-sectoral groups to coordinate national efforts, and periodic meetings with Chief Technical Officers (CTOs), CMOs, and CEOs of the various countries to apprise them of developments, and enlist their support at the national level for strengthening the Project. In keeping with the mandate, therefore, the joint meeting of CEOs and CMOs in 1997 (CARICOM 1997b) made a number of key recommendations in the areas of policy development, teacher training, procuring and development of materials, and health promotion in schools, for "taking HFLE beyond endorsement to full implementation."

There seemed to be a number of barriers, however, that impeded the transformation of these recommendations into implementation at the country levels. One barrier was the wide variation in programming arrangements at teachers' colleges. For example, there was still no clear policy with respect to HFLE as a foundational element of training programmes; many college tutors lacked training; and there was a dearth of resources. To overcome this barrier, there was the expressed need for the development of a fully structured HFLE programme for all teachers colleges, in-service training, and recognition of this training for the purposes of remuneration, promotion, and accreditation (university programmes). It was also suggested that governments ensure that HFLE be included in school improvement plans and the general reform process in education.

Another barrier identified was the management capability of college administrators. In order to support the emotional, mental, and professional health of teachers, there was need for good leadership (administrative and instructional). Principals,

therefore, needed to have management training to interact effectively with a range of partners, and to facilitate the development of the physical and psycho-social environments that support change.

The extent to which the 1997 recommendations of CEOs and CMOs could be operationalised, however, was directly related to their commitment to the Project, and their abilities to mobilise the necessary mechanisms and resources at the national levels. The issue of training and building teacher capacity, programming issues at the colleges, and the dearth of resources to support the delivery of HFLE were old issues that had been raised earlier. That the issue of teacher training was still being raised, even after the ATRFMU training project which began in 1989, speaks to the design and organisation of the training programme.

IMPROVING THE DATA BASE TO INFORM PLANNING AND EVALUATION

Attempts had been made to gather information on the implementation of HFLE through country reviews during sub-regional workshops held in 1981 and 1987, surveys (PAHO/WHO 1985; St. Victor, 1991), or direct interventions (PAHO/WHO, 1993). While the move to begin documenting the happenings in HFLE was indeed commendable, either because of funding constraints or lack of technical expertise in the area of evaluation, the methodologies used to determine outcomes were not always transparent. For example, the St. Victor 15-year survey, did not mention the methodologies used to collect data, or limitations if any, of the data gathering process. The report on the PAHO/ CARNEGIE intervention admitted to the absence of formal evaluation instruments.

The latter project, according to the report, was assessed on the extent to which strategies were implemented and sustained, and concepts and principles internalised (PAHO/WHO, 1993).

A cross-country needs assessment study was commissioned by the CARICOM Multi-Agency Project in 1996. The study, funded jointly by PAHO/WHO and UNICEF, was implemented by UWI, Cave Hill Campus. The purpose of the study was to determine the needs of the English-speaking Caribbean with respect to HFLE, and thus increase awareness among policy makers and technicians of the gaps in programme design and implementation. Seven countries (Belize, Jamaica, Antigua, Barbados, Guyana, St. Lucia, and Trinidad and Tobago) participated in the actual study. Comprehensive summaries of the findings and recommendations were published (UWI, 1998).

Another major data-gathering strategy was the PAHO funded survey of adolescents in the Caribbean undertaken in 1999. The purpose was to generate data on youth health and its associated risk and protective factors. Nine countries took part in this survey (Antigua, Bahamas, Barbados, The British Virgin Islands, Dominica, Grenada, Guyana, Jamaica, and St. Lucia). The entire report was published through funding from the Kellogg Foundation (WHO Collaborating Centre on Adolescent Health, 2000). These two studies together, provided a significant data-base to inform the CARICOM/Multi-Agency HFLE Project. While there is evidence that the data-base contributed to the development of the rationales for HFLE as an intervention in national policy documents, there is little evidence to show how or if the data were used to inform other HFLE initiatives, including curriculum development in the various countries.

Evaluation of HFLE programmes presented a greater challenge. This was in part due to the frequent changes or modifications to HFLE curricula, and to the continued focus on knowledge outcomes, rather than on skills competence and behaviour change. The lack of a clear vision or definition of the desired attributes to be fostered, as well as appropriate indicators and strategies to measure change, were limiting factors in the collection of any meaningful data to demonstrate HFLE programme effectiveness, and/or its contribution to overall development.

FACILITATING THE TRAINING OF TEACHERS AND COMMUNITY EDUCATORS

Training of trainers continued to be carried out as part of the second phase of the initial ATRFMU training project. In 1996, with funding from UNICEF, ATRFMU embarked on a training course for the Northern and Southern Caribbean countries (Barbados, Belize, Jamaica, Guyana, Suriname, and Trinidad & Tobago) which had been omitted in the earlier training programme (UNICEF, 1997).

One of the objectives of this training programme was to review/revise the curriculum for HFLE *trainers* (ATRFMU, 1996). The rationale for reviewing the existing curriculum was to align it with the PAHO HFLE curriculum framework. Suggestions were also made for making the "Core Curriculum Guide" operational not only at the college level, but also at the school level. This was commendable, as it implied recognition of the PAHO HFLE framework as the model for training, and for provision of in-school learning experiences.

An examination of the ATRFMU revised curriculum for HFLE *trainers,* however, revealed that while there was an attempt to incorporate the five thematic areas of the PAHO HFLE framework, its underpinning philosophy was not fully understood. New areas such as *family, family law, crisis issues, counselling, population dynamics, philosophy and goals of family planning,* and *contraceptive technology,* were added. In addition, the objectives still focused on knowledge acquisition. It seemed, therefore, that the facilitators and participants either had not made the paradigm shift with respect to the rationale and philosophy that had informed the PAHO HFLE curriculum framework, or that they were ensuring that areas related to their particular mandates/interests remained in order to justify their continuing involvement in the Project.

The continuing focus of training programmes on outcomes that did not extend beyond knowledge acquisition to include action competence, was a point of concern at the regional level. The importance of life skills training and learner-centred methodologies in HFLE programmes was highlighted at the CARICOM/UNICEF Consultation in 1996 and it was proposed that a series of regional training programmes be conducted by ATRFMU once more to build teacher capacity in these areas (CARICOM/UNICEF, 1996).

UNDCP, as a result of a resolution passed in May 1996 to endorse the development of drug eradication as part of HFLE, provided funding for the training. The intention was that this new group of facilitators would provide the critical mass of resource persons/ trainers at the national and regional levels, to accelerate the achievement of the aims of the CARICOM/Multi-Agency Project in the formal and non-formal educational sectors over the period 1998 – 2000 (ATRFMU, 1997). While the phases of the training did

not all proceed as planned (31 participants from 10 countries participated instead of the projected 182), for the first time, training focused on life skills acquisition, and the methodologies required for making the shift from acquisition of information to behavioural outcomes. The thematic areas from the original PAHO HFLE framework were utilised (ATRFMU, 2000).

The UNDCP evaluation report of the overall 3-year training programme revealed mixed reviews on the quality of the training. Some participants felt that the training had not been targeted to their needs. The response by ATRFMU was that selection of country participants did not meet the criteria given and so participants were at different levels of development/knowledge; some were not in a position to make decisions, thus thwarting attempts to operationalise action plans or develop programmes in-country; and pressure from countries with respect to the release of participants had also resulted in a reduction of training time, thus impacting on the quality of training received. In addition, changes in governments in some countries during the 3 year period had resulted in changes in top personnel, so that lists of participants changed frequently (UNDCP, 2004). The changes in key personnel attending workshops had been, and continue to be a perennial problem in the region, frustrating attempts to build on what had been done previously.

The logistics of conducting training at a regional level to meet the needs of three sectors simultaneously, also presented challenges. Facilitators in the formal education sector needed more intense training to properly internalise the various theories and methodologies to which they were exposed in order to be able to train others and/or competently plan appropriate classroom experiences. For example, participants at the workshops conducted in 2000 did not feel that they had gained the requisite competencies to move forward since they requested follow-up training in the use of the life skills methodologies, and access to experts in curriculum development. Two limitations of the ATRFMU regional training initiative were later identified as a) the flaw in the training design that impacted on development of life skills competencies, and b) the lack of follow-through in-country. There were several reasons for this, including the competence of the technical resource persons, conflict between sectors in-country, lack of confidence/skills by members of country teams, or general lack of direction (UNDCP, 2004).

Simultaneously with the UNDCP training project, ATRFMU, in collaboration with the Institute of Education, UWI, Mona, Jamaica, undertook an initiative in 1998 to promote HFLE in teacher education institutions of the Northern Caribbean (Belize, The Bahamas, and Jamaica). There were at this time 14 teacher institutions altogether in the Northern Caribbean with different configurations of training models which included pre-service and in-service training, as well as different arrangements for providing HFLE-related learning experiences. Up to this point, HFLE was not offered as a full course for teacher trainees in any of the teacher training institutions in Jamaica (UNICEF, 1997).

The objectives of this ATRFMU initiative, were to a) develop a strategy to move towards a core HFLE programme for all teacher-trainees in teacher education institutions; b) determine how pre-service and in-service HFLE programmes could be articulated, and c) develop action plans for strengthening HFLE programmes (ATRFMU, 1998). Of

interest, is that while attempts were being made to streamline HFLE programmes in the colleges of the Northern Caribbean, colleges in the Eastern Caribbean, under the governance of the School of Education, UWI, Cave Hill, Barbados, had either established, or were planning to establish HFLE-related programmes. However, there had been no collaboration between the Institute of Education at Mona and the School of Education at Cave Hill to ensure articulation between their programmes. The colleges in the Southern Caribbean, as well as the School of Education, UWI, St. Augustine, Trinidad and Tobago, had also independently developed and implemented their own programmes.

Teachers from the various colleges and institutions in the region, therefore, were exiting the system with different understandings of HFLE and different competencies with respect to knowledge, skills, and attitudes required for its in-school implementation. This was an indictment against the models of teacher development that were being used in the training institutes in the region, and also against the UWI, a partner in the Project, for not giving more direction and leadership in this important area. In addition, the expected educational and health outcomes were not being realised.

ADVOCATING AND SUPPORTING POLICY DEVELOPMENT

Policy development had already received a fillip in the 3 countries (one country opted out of the project), Dominica, St. Kitts and Nevis, and the British Virgin Islands, that participated in the PAHO/CARNEGIE project (PAHO/WHO, 1993). The call for national policy development, however, was made at the Regional Consultation in Barbados in 1996 (CARICOM/UNICEF,

1996). Policy development was identified as one of the strategies to move the Project forward and give legitimacy to HFLE programmes. It was also necessary to bring some order to the seemingly ad hoc implementation of decisions taken at various fora. UNICEF, through a short term consultant, offered technical assistance to various countries for policy development (CARICOM, 1997a). In spite of progress towards national policy development, there was a tardy response by the various governments with respect to the ratification of policies.

In the absence of policy development at national levels, or ratification of policies which had been developed, national coordinating committees were disempowered. They were therefore unable to fulfil their roles with respect to making recommendations to governments for budgetary requirements for funding programmes, for strengthening the human resource base through in-country training, for development of materials to support teaching and other initiatives, or for development of communication strategies to strengthen HFLE, and mobilize support from the wider population. Funding for HFLE initiatives, therefore, continued to be provided primarily by the donor agencies. This was a reflection on the political will (or lack thereof) and level of commitment to the Project by the various governments, which in turn impacted on the ability of the CARICOM Secretariat to effectively execute its responsibility to the Project.

SUPPORTING CURRICULUM REFORM AND IMPLEMENTATION

A proposal had also been made at the CARICOM/UNICEF Consultation in April 1996, for the "Core Curriculum Guide" to be revised, and for the development of additional guides for the different levels of the school system (CARICOM/UNICEF, 1996). No action was taken in the 1990s on revision of the "Core Curriculum Guide." However, the process for common curriculum and materials development to support the teaching of HFLE at pre-primary, primary, and secondary levels began at the Regional Curriculum Planners Workshop in 1998 with support from UNICEF. The intentions were to place emphasis on skills development, and culminate in the development of a regional curriculum framework for different stages in the system. Countries would then use the framework to develop their national curricula.

In support of this initiative, an alternative framework for more efficient learning experiences in HFLE was offered at the workshop (Brandon, 1998). The three-phase framework was based on principles of partnership and participation, was outcomes driven, and emphasised both processes as well as outcomes. The rationale that informed the PAHO HFLE framework was the suggested approach to curriculum planning at the school level. It was recommended that UNICEF in collaboration with the partner agencies develop a communication strategy to promote this framework. This was necessary to facilitate ready understanding and acceptance by principals, teachers and other stakeholders, and gain its acceptance by the other funding agencies as the recommended model for HFLE programming.

Curriculum reform at the school level was a natural progression. Most countries began developing or revising their own curricula, initially with technical guidance and funding from external agencies such as UNICEF and USAID, in addition to the financial input from their respective governments. By1998/9 countries such as Grenada, St. Lucia, and Jamaica had begun to develop and/or implement revised HFLE primary school curricula. In spite of the experiences and guidelines provided at the curriculum planners' workshop, however, the new curricula did not reflect the shift to skills acquisition and behaviour modification.

In summary, the responses to the development challenges, survey reports, and recommendations of stakeholders resulted in the implementation of a number of key strategies to move the HFLE process forward. However, by the end of the 1990s, the continuing lack of coordination among the key players in the region had resulted in unresolved curriculum issues, vicarious approaches to training, and lack of commitment by some governments with respect to policy development and implementation. These all had implications for the institutionalisation and sustainability of HFLE. In addition, there was very little attempt to look beyond the individual components of the Project to the bigger goal of investment in human development. The challenges of the new millennium saw some attempts to streamline the HFLE curriculum, and build teacher capacity at various levels of the system, but it also brought with it new health crises that threatened to derail the HFLE movement in the region.

THE IMPACT OF CHANGING GLOBAL REALITIES – 2000 TO 2006

The end of the 1990s into the beginning of the new millennium saw the region in a state of transition. The increases in competition stemming from global economic changes in trade and capital markets; the erosion of preferential market access (implementation of the North American Free Trade Agreement (NAFTA), and policies of the European Economic Community); the vulnerability of the tourist industry to fluctuations in the global economy, competition from other destinations, and the effects of natural disasters; as well as the decline in official capital flows from bilateral sources, all presented difficult challenges for the Caribbean (Baker, 1997). While the development of the Caribbean Single Market and Economy (CSME) is likely to bring new opportunities and policies to deal advantageously with the global economy (CCHD, 2005), countries in the mean time have had to diversify and develop new areas, for example service industries. This has meant adjustment or loss of job opportunities, and substantial investment in the retraining and retooling of persons.

The region, at the same time, has been undergoing a major health transition. While non-communicable diseases are still major causes of mortality, the enhanced interaction and inter-connectedness of globalisation has facilitated the movement of people that have contributed to the spread of HIV/AIDS. AIDS, which had already reached epidemic proportions in some Caribbean countries since 1982 (e.g. Haiti), is now a leading cause of death in other Caribbean countries. The incidence rate among young people is increasing along with the growing number of children infected/orphaned as a result of HIV/AIDS. Models of the economic impact of HIV/AIDS show the region losing much of its work force in key sectors such as agriculture and manufacturing (CCHD, 2005). This has implications for the quality of life and health status of persons and families infected/affected by HIV/AIDS, and by extension, the quantity and quality of human capital.

Globalisation, through the opening up of markets, has also widened the gap between rich and poor at both country and individual levels. This has accentuated the plight of the poor, and migration, either within or across countries, has contributed to further instability in social structures. The accelerated pace of social change has resulted in increased pressure on young people, taking a toll on their mental and emotional health. Managing emotions and social relationships is now a major challenge for young people. Increasing violence (self and interpersonal) is a manifestation of their inability to cope (Brandon, 1999).

This period, to date, has been characterised by attempts at both regional and national levels to address these two important health threats to young people, that is, the HIV/AIDS epidemic and the increasing levels of violence and injury. There has also been a renewed emphasis on building teacher capacity, development of regional HFLE curriculum frameworks, and further support for curriculum development. To this end sub-committees (with responsibilities in these areas) were established at the 2004 Regional Working Group Meeting (CARICOM, 2004). There has also been a renewed commitment to drive the Project at the level of CARICOM. The key events occurring to date and their implications are discussed below.

DONOR FUNDING AND **HIV/AIDS**

Aggressive approaches to stemming the spread of HIV/AIDS have been taken at both regional and national levels. This has been largely due to the amount of donor funding available to countries in the Caribbean. Regional organizations receiving funding include the UWI HIV/AIDS Response

Programme (UWI/HARP), an accelerated institutional response to the HIV/AIDS epidemic funded by the European Union Commission; and the Pan Caribbean Partnership Against HIV/AIDS (PANCAP), a coordinated network of regional and international governments, organisations, and donor agencies established in partnership to reduce the impact of HIV/AIDS in the Caribbean. Funding in the region for HIV/AIDS has quadrupled since 2001, with the establishment of PANCAP, standing at $US 35 million in 2005.

The availability of project funding for HIV/AIDS has resulted once more in a number of in-school programmes/projects in individual countries, competing with, and threatening to derail HFLE. While HIV/AIDS in the Caribbean is a priority issue and should be treated as such, it is a manifestation of a number of inter-connected issues including socio-cultural characteristics, sexual norms, and media messages that influence sexual behaviours and choices. There is no doubt that the school is well positioned in its role as socialisation agent to address some of these issues. Through its enacted curricula, as well as the "hidden" curriculum – modelling behaviours of staff, the nature of the interactions among staff and students, the messages that are conveyed about gender roles and sexual attitudes and so on – the school, beginning at the pre-school level and continuing, can begin to change those socio-cultural characteristics and "norms" that have been identified as barriers to safer sexual choices. However, piece meal, uncoordinated, or competitive approaches to address intertwined psycho-social and health needs of children and young people can only be counter-productive.

The position that HIV/AIDS should be taught within the framework of HFLE was taken by the sub-committee of the Regional Working Group with responsibility for HIV/AIDS Education and Resource Mobilisation at its 2004 meeting. The recommendation was that where possible, resources from other organizations that funded/supported HIV/AIDS programmes should be meaningfully directed into HFLE programmes (CARICOM, 2004). Even then, it was recognized that the priority areas and peculiar interests of funding agencies would likely affect the redirecting of funds.

The whole approach to addressing HIV/AIDS in the Caribbean therefore, has been another example of a crisis response to an emerging health issue. It has also highlighted the importance of fulfilling the mandate of international donor frameworks, and more importantly the conflict that may arise with respect to meeting individual mandates and fulfilling partnership agreements.

CURRICULUM HARMONISATION

The move towards achieving curriculum harmonisation was another priority. A Working Group Initiative resulted in the development of the Regional HFLE Curriculum Framework for Schools, initially for the age-groups 9-14 years in 2002/3. This was coordinated by the Education Development Centre (EDC) with funding from UNICEF. The rationale for starting with this age group was that it represented a critical period of transition and priority issues such as sexual choices, STDs, HIV/AIDS, and self and interpersonal relationships needed to be addressed at this level.

A sub-regional meeting was held to introduce the framework to countries in 2004, and guidelines were given for countries to review and revise their curriculum documents to align them with the framework. This was an important exercise, but for many

countries it represented a duplication of effort and a drain on human and financial resources, as many of them had only recently developed new curricula to incorporate the life skills approach and interactive methodologies. While some countries still depended on donor funding to help with this exercise, others were able to access national resources. For example, through their relevant ministries, Jamaica contracted three consultants to develop curricula along with relevant instructional materials, while Suriname obtained the services of an independent HFLE consultant.

The process for revision of the "Core Curriculum Guide" for teachers' colleges was also started in 2005 as a PAHO/CARICOM initiative. Technical Working Groups were established, and the outline for the revised curriculum framework was developed using the same format as the framework for schools. This framework has been incorporated into the new draft curriculum guide, which was completed at the end of September 2006 for review and further revision.

ACCELERATING TRAINING IN RESPONSE TO COUNTRY DEMAND

The demand for training for HFLE teacher educators and teachers continues to be high. UNICEF, from its Caribbean Area Office in Barbados, has been one of the lead agencies responding to country requests. In 2001, UNICEF contracted the services of the EDC to coordinate sub-regional training workshops for training college tutors in interactive strategies and alternative assessment. Country coordinators continue to make requests to UNICEF and the CARICOM secretariat for training for teachers at the school level. Since 2003, in-country training of teachers in life skills methodologies and assessment strategies has been facilitated in selected countries by the EDC with funding from UNICEF, and by the National HFLE Coordinator/ Curriculum specialist from St. Lucia, with funding sourced by the CARICOM Secretariat.

A special workshop to improve the technical capacity of the college tutors for organizing and facilitating learning experiences in HFLE using the draft curriculum framework for teachers' colleges (which was still being revised) was held in 2005. This workshop, funded by PAHO/CARICOM/PANCAP, and executed by PAHO, was held at the request of college tutors who felt that they lacked certain competencies to effectively facilitate the achievement of the outcomes in the framework. To date, however, there has been no training model for the region in the area of HFLE teacher development. The design, focus, and quality of training depend on the particular orientation of the technical resource persons as well their levels of competence.

ONGOING INITIATIVES

On completion of the Regional HFLE Curriculum Framework for the 9-14 age-groups, UNICEF funded a 3-year EDC project to implement, monitor and evaluate a common HFLE curriculum in four countries. This project began in 2005 and is expected to be completed in 2008. Two themes from the framework were selected, "Self and Interpersonal Relationships" and "Sexuality and Sexual Health." The revised "Core Curriculum Guide" is almost completed and should be ready for review and piloting by the end of 2006. The completion of the Regional HFLE Curriculum Framework to include the under 9 age-group, and the 15+ age-group is still pending.

Training colleges in the region have restructured or are in the process of restructuring their programme offerings to upgrade certification to associate degrees or in the case of Trinidad and Tobago to a full Bachelor of Education degree. In the process, HFLE has become an optional area for some colleges in the Eastern Caribbean. This move has implications for competencies in the area of HFLE of the graduates leaving these institutions, and puts an additional burden on those agencies that have been funding training programmes for in-school teachers.

CARICOM in its regional work plan for 2004-2006, articulated the goal of successful development and implementation of the HFLE programme, both in and out of schools in all CARICOM member states by December 2006. CARICOM has also committed to strengthening the HIV/AIDS component of the HFLE programme in the region (CARICOM, 2004). In order for CARICOM to achieve these goals any where in the near future, there are some challenges that have to be overcome.

CHALLENGES AHEAD

The first challenge is the need to strengthen commitment by CARICOM governments to HFLE so that the commitment can be turned into actual investment and effective implementation. Lack of commitment by governments has been in part responsible for the circuitous path HFLE has taken in the last thirty years. This lack of commitment has led to under investment in HFLE, which in turn has resulted in weak impact, which has served to reinforce the lack of commitment. Commitment is also a requisite for ownership of HFLE. National policies need to be fully operationalised, with the requisite budgetary allocations and other resources in place to drive a coordinated approach to the institutionalisation of HFLE in the formal educational sector. While a regional strategy is suggested, governments should drive the process.

Strengthening commitment is not an easy task. Heaver (2005) posits that commitment goes beyond influencing politicians to sign agreements. It requires three kinds of skills: a) *skills in strategic communication*. These skills are essential to put across the message that investing in HFLE benefits everyone, and that it is a key intervention to address the issues such as HIV/AIDS and violence that are threatening to derail human development in the region; b) *skills in partnership building*. Key stakeholders, including the UWI, need to come together and develop a memorandum of understanding, since action together is more effective and sustainable than competing actions or action alone; c) *skills in designing, and managing implementing organisations*. These are necessary so that staff at all levels share the same understandings, and are motivated to perform. At issue here is the implementation of HFLE as a core area at all levels of the education system, from pre-school right up to the teachers' colleges.

Another challenge is teacher education. There is a need for the development and implementation of a teacher development model that looks at reform in education and health in a meaningful way. Such a model is critical for building capacity of teachers of HFLE in the area of those pedagogies that support the development, monitoring and evaluation of skills competence and behaviour modification.

The final challenge is to source the funding and technical resources necessary for completion of the Regional HFLE Curriculum Framework for schools. This is a pre-requisite for addressing issues such as HIV/AIDS and violence at all levels; for monitoring and evaluation of programmes; and for the development of a research base to support the institutionalisation and sustainability of HFLE in the region.

REFERENCE LIST

Alleyne, M. H. McD. (1996). *Nationhood from the schoolbag: A historical analysis of the development of secondary education in Trinidad and Tobago.* Available online from http://www.iacd.oas.org/Interamer/Alleyne.htm

Antrobus, K. (n.d.). *The health needs of the youth in the Caribbean.* Unpublished background paper presented at the PAHO/WHO Caribbean Workshop on Family Life Education and Health Education. January 17-28, 1978, Georgetown, Guyana.

Antrobus, K. (1978). *Health education as an approach to school health problems in the Caribbean.* Unpublished paper presented at the PAHO/WHO Caribbean Workshop on Family Life Education and Health Education. January 17-28, 1978, Georgetown, Guyana.

ATRFMU. (1996). *Report of the trainer of trainers course, August 5 – 30, 1996.* Unpublished report prepared for the CARICOM Multi-Agency HFLE Project. Mona, Jamaica.

ATRFMU. (1997). *CARICOM Multi-Agency HFLE Project teacher education strategy: Preparing facilitators to implement new approaches to teaching and learning.* Unpublished paper. Mona, Jamaica.

ATRFMU. (1998). *Teacher education strategy: Strengthening the HFLE programme in teacher education institutions.* Unpublished Report of the three-day workshop. Mona, Jamaica. January 28 -30, 1998.

ATRFMU. (2000). *Facilitators programme – Phase 3 trainer of trainers workshop.* Unpublished report prepared for CARICOM Multi-Agency HFLE Project. Mona, Jamaica. October 2000.

Baker, J. L. (1997). *Poverty reduction and human development in the Caribbean: A cross-country study.* Discussion Paper 366. Washington, DC: World Bank.

Brandon, P. (1987). *Elements of health.* Unpublished paper presented at the UNFPA/CARICOM Sub-Regional Workshop on Family Life Education. ,Bridgetown, Barbados.

November 23-27, 1987.

Brandon, P. (1998). *A conceptual framework for organizing health learning experiences in HFLE in schools.* Unpublished paper presented at the Regional Curriculum Planners Workshop. Barbados, July 8 – 10, 1998.

Brandon, P. (1999). *Health and Family Life Education in the Caribbean: Promoting health and life skills in young people.* Unpublished paper.

CCHD (Caribbean Commission on Health and Development). (2005). *Report of the Caribbean Commission on Health and Development.* Barbados: Author.

CARICOM. (1986). *Sixth Meeting of the Standing Committee of Ministers Responsible for Education.* Unpublished report. Castries, St. Lucia. 12-16 May, 1986.

CARICOM. (1987). *Reports and experiences in integrating family life education into the school system of St. Kitts and Nevis.* Unpublished report prepared for at the UNFPA/CARICOM Sub-Regional Workshop on Family Life Education Workshop. Bridgetown, Barbados. November 23-27, 1987.

CARICOM. (1995). *Principles for coordination among agencies on Health and Family Life Education (HFLE).* Unpublished paper.

CARICOM. (1996). *Recommendations of the CARICOM Standing Committee of Ministers of Education concerning the CARICOM Health and Family Life Education Project.* Unpublished paper.

CARICOM. (1997a). *CARICOM Multi-Agency Health and family Life Education Project: First meeting for 1997 of the Regional Working Group on HFLE.* Unpublished Report. Barbados. March 24 – 25, 1997.

CARICOM. (1997b). *Report on the second meeting of Chief Education Officers and Chief Medical Officers on the CARICOM Health and Family Life Education Project.* Unpublished Report. Barbados. October 27 – 29, 1997.

CARICOM. (2004). *Report of the Health and Family Life Education (HFLE) Regional Working Group.* Unpublished Report. Kingston, Jamaica. February 16 -18, 2004.

CARICOM/UNICEF. (1996). *National implications of the CARICOM Health and Family Life Education Project.* Unpublished paper prepared for the CARICOM/UNICEF

Consultation. Barbados. April 19 -21, 1996.

Downes, A. S. (1992). *Impact of structural adjustment policies on the educational system in the Caribbean.* Paper presented for round table meeting on the Impact of World Bank policies and Intervention on Education in the Caribbean. Available online from http://www.iacd.oas.org/La%20Educa%20116/downes.htm

Fullan, M. (1999). *Change forces: The sequel.* London: Falmer Press.

Heaver, R. (2005). *Strengthening country commitment to human development: Lessons from nutrition.* Washington, D.C.: The World Bank.

Harvey, C. (1988). Educational change and its impact on national development in Trinidad and Tobago 1962-1987. In S. Ryan's (Ed.) *Trinidad and Tobago: The independence experience 1962-1987,* pp. 345-379. St. Augustine, Trinidad and Tobago: ISER.

Holder, Y., & Lewis, M. J. (1997). Epidemiological overview of morbidity and mortality. In *Health conditions in the Caribbean,* Scientific Publication No. 561, pp. 22-61. Washington, DC: PAHO.

MacPherson, S. (1982). *Social policy in the third world: The social dilemmas of underdevelopment.* Brighton, Sussex: John Spiers.

Miller, B. A. (2001). *Managing foreign policy in an interdependent world.* Honors Excellence Occasional Papers Series, Volume 1 – Number 1. Miami, Florida: Florida International University.

Miller, E. (Ed.). (1998a). *Educational reform in the Commonwealth Caribbean.* Washington, DC: Interamer.

Miller, E. (1998b). Commonwealth Caribbean Education: An assessment in E. Miller, Ed. *Educational Reform in the Commonwealth Caribbean,* pp.291-315. Washington, DC: Interamer.

Mohammed, R.T., & Jing-Zhen, Y. (2000). *Comprehensive school health model: An integrated school health education and physical education programme.* Paper presented to the International Commission on Physics Education (ICPE) Proceedings, Barcelona. August 26-27, 2000.

Moss, S. G. (1997). Health legislation and policy. In *Health conditions in the Caribbean,* Scientific Publication No. 561, pp. 91 – 116. Washington, DC: PAHO.

PAHO/WHO. (n.d.). *The status of the teaching of health and family life in the schools and teacher training colleges in five Caribbean countries – The Bahamas, Jamaica, Guyana, St. Kitts and St. Vincent.* Unpublished background paper presented at the Caribbean Workshop on Family Life Education and Health Education. Georgetown, Guyana. January 17-28, 1978.

PAHO/WHO. (1978). *Health and family life: A perspective for schools in the Caribbean.* Unpublished Report on the Caribbean Workshop on Family Life Education and Health Education. January 17-28, 1978, Georgetown, Guyana.

PAHO/WHO. (1985). *Strengthening the role of the school in health development and school health and family life programs in four countries of the Eastern Caribbean – Antigua, British Virgin Islands, Dominica, and St. Christopher-Nevis.* Unpublished project proposal prepared for the CARNEGIE Foundation. Barbados: PAHO.

PAHO/WHO. (1992). *Core curriculum guide for strengthening health & family life education in teacher training colleges in the Eastern Caribbean.* Barbados: Author.

PAHO/WHO. (1993). *Summary report of the school health & family life education project in three Eastern Caribbean Countries.* Unpublished Report prepared for the CARNEGIE Corporation and PAHO.

Saint-Victor, R. (1991). *Family life education in the English speaking Caribbean: 1975-1990.* Unpublished Report prepared for PAHO/WHO.

Schubert, W. (1986). *Curriculum: Perspective, paradigm, and possibility.* NY: Macmillan Publishing.

Steward, L. (Ed.). (n.d.) *Curriculum guidelines for family life education in the Caribbean.* Georgetown, Guyana: CARICOM.

Theodore, K. (2001). *HIV/AIDS in the Caribbean: Economic issues - impact and investment response.* Department of Economics, UWI. Commission on Macroeconomics, Health Working Group 1, March 2001.

Theodore, K. & Greene, E. (1997). Socioeconomic and political context. In *Health conditions in the Caribbean,* Scientific Publication No. 561, pp. 3 - 21. Washington, DC: PAHO.

The University of the West Indies. (1998). *Regional report of needs assessment study.* Unpublished

report prepared for the CARICOM Multi-Agency HFLE Project. Cave Hill, Barbados: Author.

Todaro, M. P., & Smith, S. C. (2006). *Economic development (9th. Ed.).* Boston: Pearson/Addison Wesley.

Tsang, M. C., Fryer, M., & Arevalo, G. (2002). *Access, equity and performance: Education in Barbados, Guyana, Jamaica and Trinidad and Tobago.* Washington, DC: Inter-American Development Bank.

UNDCP. (2004). *Assessment of the Health and Family Life Education training.* Retrieved December 2005, from http://www.unicef.org/evaldatabase/files/CAB_2001_004.pdf

UNESCO. (1994). *World declaration on education for all, and framework for action to meet basic learning needs.* Paris: Author.

UNICEF. (1997). *First meeting for 1997 of the Regional Working Group on HFLE.* Unpublished Report of the Regional Working Group Meeting held on March 24 -25, 1997. Barbados: Author.

UNICEF. (1999). *Health and Family Life Education: Empowering young people with skills for healthy living.* Barbados: Author.

Waldron, E. R. (1997). Health research: Perspective from the Commonwealth Caribbean Medical Research Council. In *Health conditions in the Caribbean,* Scientific Publication No. 561, pp. 158 – 167. Washington, DC: PAHO.

WHO Collaborating Center on Adolescent Health. (2000). A *portrait of adolescent health in the Caribbean.* Minnesota, MN: Author.

World Bank. (1980). *Education sector policy paper.* (3rd ed.) Washington DC: World Bank.

World Bank. (1991). *World development report.* New York: Oxford University Press.

World Health Organization. (1973). *Interrelationships between health programmes and socio-economic development.* Public Health Papers, 49. Geneva: WHO.

World Health Organization. (1975). *Promotion of national health services.* Geneva: WHO.

World Health Organization. (1978). *The Alma-Ata conference on primary health care.* WHO Chronicle, 32 (11), 409 – 30.

4

Preliminary Assessment of Education Ministries' Capacity to Address HIV and AIDS

Cheryl Vince Whitman and Mora Oommen

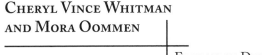

Education Development Center, Inc., Health and Human Development Programs

An assessment of the capacity of Ministries of Education in the Caribbean to respond to HIV and AIDS was undertaken in 2006 by the Education Development Centre under contract to the Caribbean Community Secretariat. The survey also gathered data about the interests and needs for knowledge and skill development among key officials. It was found that Ministries of Education across the Caribbean have taken steps and report progress in building their capacity to respond to HIV and AIDS. However, given the urgency and increase in the prevalence of the disease among the younger age groups, the report concludes that Ministries' response must be more aggressive. An executive version of the findings is presented, followed by the detailed report.

EXECUTIVE REPORT

The purpose of the *Special Meeting of the Council for Human and Social Development (COHSOD) on Education and HIV/AIDS* is 'to provide a forum for Ministers of Education and other stakeholders to: examine the role of the education sector in preventing the spread of HIV and AIDS; mitigate effects of the disease in the Region; and identify modalities for the strengthening of the education sector to provide an appropriate response. The major objectives are to:

1. promote education sectoral leadership;
2. create a supportive policy and financial environment for the education sector response to HIV and AIDS at the national and regional levels; and

3. focus on national priorities for capacity development.[1]

To address these objectives, in March–April 2006 Education Development Center, Inc. (EDC) conducted a preliminary assessment of the capacity of Ministries of Education (MoEs) in the Caribbean to respond to HIV and AIDS. EDC also gathered data about the interests and needs for knowledge and skill development of the members of the new Caribbean Network of Education Sector HIV Coordinators. Fourteen Caribbean Community (CARICOM) member countries and the British and Dutch Overseas Caribbean Territories (OCTs) participated in this assessment. All nine Organisation of Eastern Caribbean States (OECS) member countries are represented in this study. Table 4.7, 'Countries, affiliations and study involvement' (Appendix) describes the data each country provided. Since 2001, eight countries in this sample have received the Multi-Country HIV/AIDS Prevention (MAP) and Control Adaptable Program Lending for the Caribbean Region.

EDC conducted the assessment under the recently awarded CARICOM Caribbean Education Sector HIV and AIDS Capacity-Building Programme.[2] This programme was funded by Inter-American Development Bank (IDB), acting in its capacity as administrator of Japan Special Funds and UNESCO funds. Under contract with CARICOM, EDC, in partnership with The University of the West Indies (UWI), is

developing this programme. The goal is to strengthen the education sector's capacity in leadership and advocacy, policy development, coordination and quality control of services provided by non-governmental organisations (NGOs), selection and implementation of evidence-based interventions and evaluation. Beyond initial intensive work with four countries, EDC/UWI will disseminate the programme's products and lessons learnt throughout the Caribbean Region and provide a range of professional development activities to enhance the capacity of MoEs. The Caribbean Network of Education Sector HIV Coordinators will work closely with the CARICOM Programme as one of the programme's major vehicles for dissemination and capacity-building.

FINDINGS

FIGURE 4.1
A COMPREHENSIVE EDUCATION SECTOR APPROACH TO HIV AND AIDS[4]

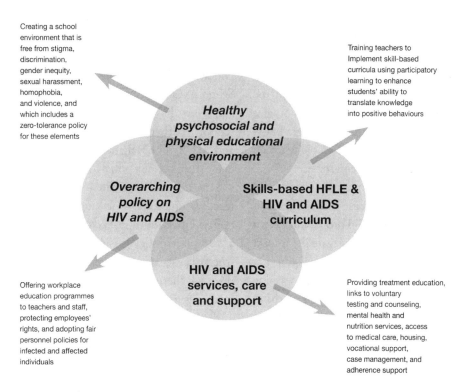

Creating a school environment that is free from stigma, discrimination, gender inequity, sexual harassment, homophobia, and violence, and which includes a zero-tolerance policy for these elements

Training teachers to Implement skill-based curricula using participatory learning to enhance students' ability to translate knowledge into positive behaviours

Healthy psychosocial and physical educational environment

Overarching policy on HIV and AIDS

Skills-based HFLE & HIV and AIDS curriculum

HIV and AIDS services, care and support

Offering workplace education programmes to teachers and staff, protecting employees' rights, and adopting fair personnel policies for infected and affected individuals

Providing treatment education, links to voluntary testing and counseling, mental health and nutrition services, access to medical care, housing, vocational support, case management, and adherence support

Source: *EDC and UNESCO, 2005.*

Improving capacity to respond to HIV and AIDS is a challenge and a remarkable opportunity. Education and health are interdependent. The physical, social and emotional health of teachers and staff affect the quality of the overall system, classroom teaching and learning and academic performance. In turn, academic success and school completion affect the health status of students. While the imminent challenge is to strengthen the education sector's capacity to respond to HIV and AIDS, the opportunity is far-reaching. By strengthening education sector capacity to improve the health of the education work force and students, there will be a much stronger foundation for all efforts in education reform and improvement.[3]

Since 2002, with the establishment of the UNAIDS Inter Agency Task Team (IATT) on Education, convened by UNESCO, there is a growing effort to support accelerated and improved education sector responses to HIV and AIDS.[5] IATT has developed tools to enhance a comprehensive education sector response to addressing the HIV and AIDS epidemic.[6] The comprehensive response takes a systemic management as well as a public health approach to HIV and AIDS in the educational setting. Quality education itself is at the core – creating a system that graduates educated and literate young people who can assume a productive place in society.

In a comprehensive approach to HIV and AIDS, the education sector uses all means at its disposal to promote and protect the health of students and staff and mitigate the impact on the system itself, as illustrated in Figure 4.1. The education sector can do so by developing the following elements: an overarching education policy that reaches out to inform, protect and support students *and* teachers; a skills-based curriculum; a healthy psycho-social and physical educational environment;

and information about and links to services, care and support.

EDC assessed the current status of study participants' efforts in these four areas, as well as coordinators' views of the knowledge, skills, and capacities they require to implement a comprehensive approach. Highlights of the findings follow. Table 4.1 presents a summary of the elements of a comprehensive approach, which MoEs report they have established or are putting in place.

AN OVERARCHING MINISTRY OF EDUCATION POLICY (INCLUDING WORKPLACE POLICY) ON HIV AND AIDS

An overarching policy recognises that schools are both educational environments and workplaces that employ thousands of people in the Caribbean. Across the Caribbean, MoEs are at different stages of developing overarching policies to guide their responses to HIV. Of 15 respondents, only Jamaica and Haiti report the development, ratification and implementation of its policy for the management of HIV and AIDS in schools. Jamaica has developed the National Policy for HIV and AIDS Management in Schools. Haiti's Ministry of Education, Youth and Sports has developed and implements a school health policy, which includes HIV and AIDS. The Bahamas have a draft HIV and AIDS school policy. In two countries – Barbados and Trinidad and Tobago – the teachers' unions have developed a workplace policy. Three additional countries report that a workplace policy exists or is in draft form (the Bahamas, Grenada and Haiti). Moving forward, there is a need for MoEs in many countries to undertake policy development, endorsement and implementation in a strategic and coordinated way. Leadership and support at the highest levels are crucial.

TABLE 4.1
FINDINGS: ELEMENTS OF A COMPREHENSIVE APPROACH

Question	Total (15 responses)			
	Yes	In process	No	Mixed*
Policy Is there an HIV and AIDS policy?	2	4	9	0
Has the policy been implemented?	1	2	12	0
Is there a workplace policy?	3	2	9	1
Curriculum Is there an HFLE policy?	13	1	1	0
Is the ministry using the HFLE Regional Framework Curriculum?	12	1	2	0
Has the ministry invested in training teachers on HFLE?	13	1	0	1
Has the ministry trained teachers to teach about HIV and AIDS?	8	4	3	0
Environment Is there a policy to develop a safe and healthy psycho-social and physical educational environment (free from physical, sexual violence such as bullying, homophobia, sexual harassment and gender bias)?	4	3	8	0
Have there been efforts to sensitize staff in the ministry on issues related to stigma and discrimination towards people infected and/or affected by HIV and AIDS?	10	4	1	0
Have there been efforts to actively gain participation from persons' living with HIV/AIDS in programmes addressing HIV and AIDS?	9	1	4	1
Services Does the ministry provide access to counselling and voluntary testing services?	6	1	8	0
Are there youth-based strategies (such as peer education, youth drop-in centres) that address HIV and AIDS?	11	1	2	1
Are there programmes to address the needs of orphaned and vulnerable children?	8	1	6	0

* Mixed indicates that British and Dutch Overseas Caribbean Territories are at different stages of their responses.

SKILLS-BASED HFLE AND HIV AND AIDS PREVENTION CURRICULUM

A skills-based curriculum is based on effective strategies of behaviour change, skill development and participatory learning. In the Caribbean, there is a long tradition of offering such curricula in the context of health promotion for responsible lifestyles as addressed by Health and Family Life Education (HFLE) and the development of the ideal Caribbean person. Research has shown that teacher training is necessary for effective implementation and to achieve student outcomes.[7] Across the region, HFLE is currently the primary area of the school curriculum that delivers information and develops skills to address HIV and AIDS. Twelve countries in the sample report that they are presently implementing the recently developed, Caribbean Regional Curriculum Framework for Health and Family Life Education for ages 9–14. All ministries, except two, report that they currently have an HFLE policy. All ministries report that they are in the process of training teachers on HFLE: eight have trained teachers, specifically on teaching about HIV and AIDS. Several challenges remain related to the extent to which the curriculum is timetabled and measured, the dosage of activities devoted to HIV and AIDS, and the extent to which an adequate number of teachers are provided professional development and ongoing coaching and support.

A HEALTHY PSYCHO-SOCIAL AND PHYSICAL EDUCATIONAL ENVIRONMENT

A healthy environment is one that is free of fear, stigma and homophobia, one that promotes gender equity and is free of sexual harassment and sexual assault, and one with codes of teacher and student conduct. Facilities and policies to ensure girls' attendance are key factors. Eight ministries report that they do not have a policy to develop a safe and healthy school environment; four ministries do have a policy; and three are in the process of developing one. All respondents describe discrimination against people living with HIV and AIDS as a severe issue across the region. All MoEs, except one, report that there have been efforts to sensitise staff in the ministry on issues related to stigma and discrimination. However, much more needs to be done. Greater involvement of persons living with HIV and AIDS is one effective strategy to be used more.

During the April meeting of coordinators in Jamaica, several reported that the current system of confidentiality of information is not well instituted so people are not willing to come forth and get tested. In addition, multiple countries, including Jamaica, state that students infected or affected by AIDS – or perceived to be so – experience discrimination. A number of previous studies report the high incidence of sexual assault and homophobia in the Caribbean region.

HIV AND AIDS SERVICES, CARE AND SUPPORT

Services to educate staff and students about the benefits of voluntary counselling and testing and life-saving treatment are vital in the response to HIV and AIDS. Ministries and schools can provide information about what is involved and where to find and take advantage of such services. EDC collected information about services, youth-based strategies, and programmes for orphans and vulnerable children. Eight of the 15 respondents report that they do not currently provide information about or access to voluntary counselling and testing services.

These services are provided by the Ministries of Health; in some case MoEs partner with Ministries of Health to refer people. Jamaica, St Lucia and Trinidad and Tobago report that they have trained guidance counsellors and school social workers in counselling people affected or infected by HIV and AIDS. Although some ministries are training their school counsellors in HIV and AIDS, many more need this education and training but resources are scarce. Eleven ministries report that they have youth-based strategies, such as peer education or youth drop-in centres in place. Concerning orphans and vulnerable children, eight countries report that they have a programme in place. However, this assessment could not go into details on the extent and quality of the programmes or determine whether they are targeted towards in-school or out-of-school children.

In the interviews and focus groups for this assessment, HIV coordinators report on the competencies – the knowledge, skills, structures and support – they need to carry out their duties. Coordinators also report on the professional development they need to assist them with their work. The eight managers interviewed state that they urgently need to develop skills in the following three areas: programme planning and policy development; data collection and monitoring and evaluation; and deeper understanding of HIV and AIDS (such as voluntary counselling and testing, treatment and care). They would also like more information on intervention ideas and procedures, and they want to develop additional experience in counselling. As one coordinator commented, 'People are comfortable speaking to me and I need to understand the right thing to say.'

CONCLUSION AND RECOMMENDATIONS

Seminal publications, such as the IATT *Global Readiness Survey 2004* and *Education and HIV and AIDS in the Caribbean* by Professors Kelly and Bain, provide critical information on the rationale and need for building education sector capacities to address HIV and AIDS. As described above, MoEs across the Caribbean have taken steps and report progress in building their capacity to respond to HIV and AIDS. Given the urgency and increase in the prevalence of the diseases among the younger age groups, the response must be more aggressive.

AIDS is the leading cause of death in the 15–44 age group.[8] By 2009, experts estimate that there will be 243,000 new HIV infections and 334,600 new cases of AIDS in the Caribbean. Among these, three per cent (9,400) will be children.[9] Significant work must be undertaken in policy development, advocacy and targeted interventions to reach youth with the knowledge and skills they need and to protect staff throughout the education system. Further, HIV coordinators are seeking professional development, resources, leadership from their ministers, and management support structures to succeed in their vital efforts. Developing these capacities and other key areas such as the meaningful involvement of persons living with HIV and AIDS, programme sustainability and implementing and evaluating evidence-based approaches are all essential components of a comprehensive response to HIV and AIDS. From this study, we recommend that:

- EDC/UWI identify ways to extend the CARICOM Capacity-Building Programme on policy development to more countries immediately through the Caribbean Network of Education Sector HIV Coordinators.

- Ministers of Education and other senior education policy makers lend their vision, visibility and vocal support to building education sector capacity.

- MoEs enhance curricula and environments by: strengthening and integrating HIV and AIDS into HFLE; building no-tolerance policies regarding bullying, sexual harassment, and discrimination into school systems and HFLE; and providing HIV/AIDS training and ongoing coaching to teachers.

- MoEs draw on the principle of Greater Involvement of People Living with HIV/AIDS (GIPA), foster collaborations between Ministries of Education and the Caribbean Regional Network of Persons Living with HIV and AIDS (or country affiliates), using strategies to involve and prepare PLWHA for participation at all stages.

- MoEs allocate resources to hire and train guidance counsellors and social workers to provide a range of mental health, support and HIV/AIDS services.

- MoEs, working with Caribbean Network and Capacity-Building Programme create clearly-defined position descriptions for the newly appointed HIV and AIDS education coordinators, collegial teams to support them and supervisory structures reporting to the most senior level education officials.

- CARICOM, EDC/UWI deepen the synergistic relationship between the newly formed Caribbean Network of Education Sector HIV Coordinators and the CARICOM Education Sector HIV and AIDS Capacity-Building Programme, providing a virtual community and professional development agenda.

THE FULL REPORT

PURPOSE OF THE ASSESSMENT

On April 25–28, 2006, in Kingston, Jamaica, CARICOM Caribbean Education Sector HIV and AIDS Capacity-Building Programme, operated by Education Development Center, Inc. (EDC) and The University of the West Indies (UWI), hosted the First Meeting of the HIV and AIDS Coordinators of Caribbean Ministries of Education in collaboration with UNESCO's Office for the Caribbean. These coordinators have now joined together to form the Caribbean Network of Education Sector HIV Coordinators. The Network will be a significant partner with which the CARICOM Capacity-Building Programme will disseminate information and materials and strengthen the education sector's capacity through professional development activities. In particular, the CARICOM Capacity-Building Programme seeks to strengthen the following capacities of the education sector: policy development; leadership and advocacy; coordination and quality control of ministry work with non-governmental organisations (NGOs); selection and implementation of evidence-based interventions; and using data for planning, tracking and monitoring.

In preparation for this meeting, during March–April 2006, EDC gathered data on the current capacity of the Caribbean Ministries of Education (MoEs) to address HIV and AIDS. This review will inform the design of the dissemination and capacity-building activities of the CARICOM Capacity-Building Programme in support of the coordinators and other audiences.

DATA COLLECTION METHODS

For this assessment, using a common template, EDC requested brief reports from fourteen CARICOM countries (and one combined report from the British and Dutch Overseas Territories). A summary of results from the country reports is provided in Table 4.8 (Appendix). EDC then conducted telephone interviews with eight HIV and AIDS education sector coordinators and convened a focus group discussion with coordinators at the meeting described above. Table 4.7 (Appendix) provides details on the types of data collected.

The 14 Caribbean countries and the British and Dutch Overseas Caribbean Territories (OCTs) were invited to participate in the HIV Coordinators' meeting in Jamaica. All countries sent a representative to the meeting. The OCTs sent a single representative for all the territories. This representative was also responsible for providing country information for the assessment. The following countries participated in the meeting: Antigua and Barbuda, the Bahamas, Barbados, Belize, Dominica, Grenada, Guyana, Haiti, Jamaica, St Kitts and Nevis, St Lucia, St Vincent and the Grenadines, Suriname, and Trinidad and Tobago. All these countries are member states of CARICOM. Antigua and Barbuda, Dominica, Grenada, St Kitts and Nevis, St Lucia, St Vincent and the Grenadines are also members of the Organisation of Eastern Caribbean States (OECS). The British OCTs include the countries of Anguilla (CARICOM associate member; OECS member), British Virgin Islands (CARICOM associate member; OECS member), Montserrat (CARICOM and OECS member), Turks and Caicos (CARICOM associate member) and Cayman Islands (CARICOM associate member). The Dutch OCTs include Aruba and the Netherlands Antilles (which include Curacao, Bonaire, Saba, St Eustatius and St Maarten).

In most cases, the primary source of data is the HIV and AIDS coordinator or the person designated with responsibility for HIV and AIDS in the MoE (referred to as HIV coordinator in this report). Despite the depth of knowledge of the coordinators, it is possible that countries might have activities or mechanisms of which they are unaware.

This preliminary assessment focused on two dimensions: (1) the elements of a comprehensive approach to HIV and AIDS underway in each country; and (2) ministry capacities and coordinators' knowledge and skills to carry out such an approach. A comprehensive approach is one that uses all available means to promote and protect the health of students and staff, while mitigating the impact on the system itself. This approach includes an overarching MoE HIV and AIDS policy; a skills-based curriculum; a healthy psycho-social and physical educational environment; and information about and access to HIV and AIDS services, care and support. The approach involves teachers, students and parent participation in programme design and delivery.

FINDINGS: ELEMENTS OF A COMPREHENSIVE APPROACH

Participants in the assessment provide information about the activities their ministry is currently undertaking to provide a comprehensive approach to HIV and AIDS, as illustrated in Figure 4.1.

OVERARCHING MINISTRY OF EDUCATION HIV AND AIDS POLICY

Overarching policies outline the roles and responsibilities of the MoEs, including workplace policies to protect thousands of employees. Such policies also define the education sector's role, programmes and services along the continuum from prevention to information and education about and links to intervention and care.

An overarching HIV and AIDS policy is essential because it provides guidelines for school administrators, teachers and support staff to protect themselves, the students, and their families from HIV transmission. It can minimise the impact of illness and death. It can also inform employees, parents and students about their responsibilities, rights and expected behaviour while in the school setting.

In April 2006, UNESCO and the International Labour Organization (ILO) released a workplace policy on HIV and AIDS for education institutions in the Caribbean.[10] Representatives from five Caribbean countries (Barbados, Belize, Guyana, Jamaica, and Trinidad and Tobago), including representatives of MoEs, collaborated on the development of this document. Ms Supersad, HIV/AIDS Focal Point at the ILO Subregional Office of the Caribbean presented this new product at the HIV Coordinators' meeting in Jamaica. She urged countries to review and adopt the policy.[11] It provides a framework for addressing HIV and AIDS as a workplace issue in the education sector. The policy covers prevention of HIV; elimination of stigma and discrimination; counselling, care, treatment and support; management and mitigation of the impact in educational institutions; and promotion of safe, healthy and non-violent work and study environments. The document can be used as a basis for a national policy for the education sector and for individual education and training institutions at all levels.

EDC, together with Education International (EI, the global teachers' union) and the World Health Organisation (WHO), funded by the Dutch Ministry of Foreign Affairs, are currently operating programmes in partnership with the teachers' unions across Africa and in Haiti and Guyana. Under the programme, unions receive a grant for policy development, advocacy, research, training and publicity for HIV and AIDS and Education for All. Specifically for HIV and AIDS, the programme emphasises building teacher and learner protective behaviours and fostering advocacy for HIV and AIDS education in the schools.[12]

Haiti and Guyana are the only countries officially participating in this union programme. However, EI has involved teachers' unions from Belize, Bermuda, Grenada, Jamaica, St Kitts and Nevis, St Lucia, St Vincent and the Grenadines, Suriname and Trinidad and Tobago in some of its training activities and planning sessions.

Of the 15 representatives who participated in this assessment, only Jamaica[13] has a National Policy for HIV and AIDS Management in Schools, which has final approval by the Cabinet of Jamaica. Since 2004, the Ministry of Education, Youth and Sports in Haiti has developed a holistic school health policy, including HIV and AIDS. Its HIV and AIDS guidelines address non-discrimination and delivery of prevention education programmes. Other MoEs are at various stages of policy development. Table 4.2 presents the findings for the policy questions.

For example, four countries have begun the process of policy development: The Bahamas, Dominica, Guyana and Trinidad

TABLE 4.2
FINDINGS: POLICY

Question	Total (15 responses)			
	Yes	In process	No	Mixed*
Is there an HIV and AIDS policy?	2	4	9	0
Has the policy been implemented?	1	2	12	0
Is there a workplace policy?	3	2	9	1

* Mixed indicates that British and Dutch Overseas Caribbean Territories are at different stages of their responses.

and Tobago. In two countries, Barbados and Trinidad and Tobago, the teachers' unions have begun to develop workplace policies. Although other MoEs do not have formal policies, they do have guidelines or a strategic plan in place (St Vincent and the Grenadines and the Bahamas).

According to Mr Williams, the representative from Trinidad and Tobago, 'The Ministry of Education has developed a work plan for 2005–2006 and has implemented sensitisation and awareness activities for staff and students. However, the absence of a full-time coordinator has hindered the coordination, monitoring and evaluation of these activities. We very much look forward to our new hire for this role, who should be on board by summer 2006.' Similarly, St Vincent and the Grenadines has a plan that presents a set of policy directions, strategies and targets. The representative commented, 'The primary purpose of these guidelines is to provide strategies for the delivery of education that raises the level of achievement for all learners, enabling them to benefit as individuals and contribute to national and regional development.'

Furthermore, almost all countries have established committees to address HIV and AIDS in the education sector. Such committees are an important first step to begin the process of policy development, which is elaborated below. There is progress on the policy front. However, the increase in HIV prevalence, especially among younger age groups, demands a more urgent and rigorous response.[14]

Jamaica's policy development and dissemination provides a valuable case study. In 2004, the Jamaica Ministry of Education, Youth and Culture (MoEYC) was the first in the region to develop and endorse a national policy specifically for HIV and AIDS management in schools. The policy covers a broad range of issues, including non-discrimination and equality, student admission and staff appointment, disclosure and confidentiality, education on HIV and AIDS, and ways to create a safe institutional environment. Since the policy was endorsed, Jamaica has created the HIV and AIDS Response Team, with funding from the Government of Japan and technical support from the Japan International Cooperation Agency (JICA). Comprised of Japanese volunteers and MoE staff, JICA works closely with the Jamaica Network of Seropositives (JN+) and the team has reached approximately 50 per cent of all schools to date to disseminate the policy, ensure understanding of its contents, and build capacity for implementation. Although still at an early stage, Jamaica has launched this process of putting the policy into practice with a strong, decentralised mechanism for outreach.

Jamaica's policy does mention workplace issues on hiring, but does not provide in-depth information on workplace policy. In conversations with the Response Team at the April meeting, participants identified other possible limitations. Even with such a good policy in place, there have been a few instances where students have been forced to leave school because it became known that they were HIV-positive. Although the students were eventually re-instated, the situation underscores the issue that policy is not law. What sanctions, then, does a policy hold? How is policy enforced?

A recent study of Jamaica's policy, funded by the UNESCO Office for the Caribbean, also points to certain areas that might be strengthened, including providing more details about 'curriculum content, teacher preparation and support, timetabling, and assessment of learning outcomes'. The report also expresses concern about the lack of high-level political support that provides 'the power of sanction and the application of resources, both human and financial to make it work'.[15]

As any MoE embarks on the important process of policy development, it is critical to build capacity for the entire process of endorsement, dissemination, implementation, and enforcement. In the early stages of development, there are a number of components a ministry must address. Figure 4.2 illustrates the following six 'Ps' of the Policy Circle[16] that flow from the central issue, stakeholders to be involved, and costs and tradeoffs, taking into consideration the political, social, cultural and economic context:

FIGURE 4.2
THE POLICY CIRCLE

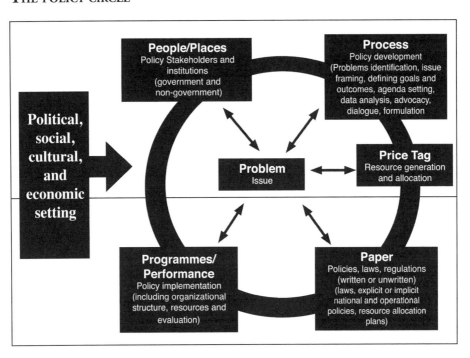

Source: *Hardee, Feranil, Boezwinkle and Clark, 2004.*

- *Problem* is the central issue that explains the need for policy attention
- *People/Places* involved (policy stakeholders and the institutions where policy gets deliberated, decided and disseminated)
- *Process* of policy-making and dissemination
- *Price tag* of the policy (the cost of policy options and how resources are allocated)
- *Paper* produced (actual laws and policies)
- *Programmes* that result from implementing policies and *Performance* in achieving policy goals and objectives

Although the Policy Circle was developed initially for use in the health sector, it is most relevant and applicable to the education sector. The framework can be used to review and analyse different levels of policy, such as national and local policies and sectoral and operational policies.

COMPREHENSIVE EDUCATION SECTOR APPROACH TO HIV AND AIDS

Across the Caribbean region, the Health and Family Life Education (HFLE) curriculum is currently the primary vehicle for imparting information and developing skills related to the prevention of HIV and AIDS. Eight countries report training teachers specifically on HIV and AIDS. Table 4.3 presents results of the survey questions about skills-based curriculum. Thirteen of the 15 respondents report that they have an HFLE policy in place. All 15 report that they have trained teachers in HFLE in some way.

For example, the Bahamas first implemented HFLE in 1991 and offers the curriculum for grades one to twelve. Although HFLE is not a core subject in the Bahamas, it is timetabled with one period per week of 30 minutes for lower primary and two periods per week of 60–70 minutes for the other grade levels. The Bahamas commits an annual budget for the procurement of materials to support the curriculum, professional development for teachers and officers, and supervision of the instructional programme. The Bahamas have also appointed a Family Life and Health Education Advisory Council, which represents a cross section of society: education, health, religion and civil society.

In the autumn of 2005, CARICOM and UNICEF led the development of the first Caribbean Regional Curriculum Framework for Health and Family Life Education for ages 9–14. EDC facilitated a process by which Caribbean experts in instructional

TABLE 4.3
FINDINGS: CURRICULUM

Question	Total (15 responses)			
	Yes	In process	No	Mixed*
Is there an HFLE policy?	13	1	1	0
Is the ministry using the HFLE Regional Framework Curriculum?	12	1	2	0
Has the ministry invested in training teachers on HFLE?	13	1	0	1
Has the ministry trained teachers to teach about HIV and AIDS?	8	4	3	0

* Mixed indicates that British and Dutch Overseas Caribbean Territories are at different stages of their responses.

development and HFLE created the product. Twelve of the 15 representatives report that they are currently using this framework.

The framework addresses four themes: (1) sexuality and sexual health, including HIV and AIDS; (2) self and interpersonal relationships; (3) appropriate eating and fitness; and (4) managing the environment. Table 4.9 (Appendix) presents a matrix of the topics, lessons titles, skills and methods addressed for themes 1 and 2 for Forms 1 and 2. HIV and AIDS are central as a critical issue for knowledge and skill development across themes. In both Forms 1 and 2 in the unit on sexuality and sexual health, eight lessons specifically address HIV and AIDS and/or risky sexual behaviour, including lessons on HIV transmission, communication, refusal skills to resist sexual pressure, and peer-to-peer advocacy for abstinence and HIV prevention. The philosophy and approach of this framework consider that a young person's emotional, sexual and physical health are interrelated.[17] Therefore, HIV and AIDS are important in the context of understanding oneself in the transition to adolescence and puberty, in developing and negotiating relationships with others, and in accepting differences. Related risk behaviours, such as using alcohol and illicit drugs, which can reduce inhibitions and responsibility, or serve as a means for transmission, are also addressed. In addition, lessons in both the Sexuality and Sexual Health Unit and the Self and Interpersonal Relationships Unit address numerous contextual factors, including low self-esteem, unhealthy relationships, negative peer pressure and economic conditions that can lead young people to engage in behaviours that put them at risk for acquiring HIV. Thus, numerous lessons for each grade level, beyond those labelled specifically as HIV and AIDS, pertain to healthy development for young people.

The framework presents learning objectives, standards for teaching, student outcomes, sample lessons and resource materials. A core curriculum, based on the framework, is being implemented and teachers are being trained to use the programme. With the curriculum in place, the emphasis is now on deeper implementation. A three-year, four-country study, Evaluating the Implementation of HFLE, is underway in Antigua and Barbuda, Barbados, Grenada and St Lucia. This study is comparing the degree of implementation and student knowledge, attitudes, skills, and reported behaviours pre- and post-intervention with comparison schools. Pre-intervention, baseline student survey data have been collected from target and comparison sites. Jamaica is conducting its own separate and independent pilot test of the HFLE framework and curriculum.

For HFLE to be successful, it is necessary to build leadership, teachers' skills and confidence, and the system support to implement these programmes at scale. As the representative from Dominica said, 'Personnel of the HFLE unit also work closely with persons from the Ministry of Health. The challenge now is to involve all schools in a sensitisation programme to target teachers and students and to prepare parents.'

HFLE is an important context for teaching about HIV and AIDS. HFLE addresses the values of the ideal Caribbean person, and the physical, social, emotional and sexual development of young people. Activities allow young people to practise skills in the classroom, with the hope they will be equipped to use them to protect themselves in real-life situations.[18] Yet, at the April meeting, Commonwealth/UNESCO Chair in Education and HIV and AIDS, Professor David Plummer, raised several important questions: Is HIV and AIDS addressed adequately with enough intensity and dosage within HFLE? Is teacher training really being implemented with the scope and reach it needs? Professor Plummer is writing a paper to respond to these and other questions for the Council for Human and Social Development (COHSOD) meeting.

Several ministry participants echoed their conviction that HIV needs to be taught in the context of HFLE, but that more staff are needed to do the job. 'I have been hired to work on HIV because it was too much work for just the HFLE person. HIV should be integrated into the HFLE curriculum. But one person with sole responsibility for it just has too much to do.'

The encouraging news is that several new curricula are about to be published. The following resources will provide teachers with additional material on HIV and AIDS that they can add to the HFLE programme.

- The forthcoming book, *Teaching about HIV/AIDS in the Caribbean*, will provide teachers with added resources to prevent the spread of the disease and equip communities to care for those who are infected and affected.[19]
- The HFLE/HIV and AIDS Project of the regional partnership in teacher education, the Joint Board of Teacher Education (JBTE), involves MoEs, teachers' colleges, teachers' unions and associations, and UWI. The JBTE project has developed a 30-hour course (HFLE-HIV and AIDS) that 'utilises the writing and experiential skills of a cross-section of lecturers from faculty in teachers' colleges.'[20]
- MoEs in Jamaica[21] and Guyana have reviewed the effectiveness of sub-Saharan African HIV and AIDS books and instructional material to inform the

adoption, adaptation or need to develop new material for the Caribbean. Although there were concerns about 'the challenges with the cultural content of the materials', reviewers suggest use of the African material with guidelines and training for teachers on adaptations. The Bahamas also report procuring African publications for their schools.

A HEALTHY PSYCHO-SOCIAL AND PHYSICAL EDUCATIONAL ENVIRONMENT

A healthy educational environment ensures that learners and educators know that they will be 'safe from harm, cared for equally and treated with respect'.[22] Furthermore, a growing body of international research documents how the psycho-social climate of the school and students' feelings of connectedness to caring adults are critical in preventing risk behaviours.[23] Other research clearly states that getting to know a person who is living with HIV and AIDS is one of the most effective strategies in overcoming stigma.[24]

In the response to HIV and AIDS, a caring and welcoming school environment that is free of stigma and discrimination against infected and affected learners and teachers is essential. Stigma is a significant barrier that stops people from seeking lifesaving testing, treatment and care.[25] Establishing clear regulations about stigma and discrimination, confidentiality, gender equity, sexual harassment, homophobia, violence and bullying are critical steps to ensure a healthy school environment.[26]

When countries were asked if they currently have a policy to develop a safe and healthy psycho-social environment at the school level, four ministries report that they do; eight report that they do not; and three report that they are in the process of developing such guidelines. Table 4.4 presents details.

When asked if they have taken steps to sensitise MoE staff to issues related to stigma towards people infected or affected by HIV and AIDS, 14 ministries report that they have begun this process. St Lucia has a zero-tolerance policy for violence and sexual harassment. Trinidad and Tobago has established a Student Support Services Division by employing additional guidance officers, school social workers and special education teachers to provide services in diagnosis, assessment and remediation.

St Vincent and the Grenadines recently identified the need for an emergency response to stigma and discrimination at the primary level. The HIV coordinator, together with several counsellors and HIV and AIDS peer educators, organised a half-day session with grades five and six. Follow-up sessions are planned with the lower school and the Parent–Teachers' Association. As part of this effort, plans are underway to establish

HIV and AIDS resource centres at seven strategically located schools. Providing counselling, as well as information about HIV and AIDS, these host schools will offer services to other schools in the vicinity.

Belize reports that ministries provide all schools with guidelines for developing a 'child friendly' school environment. Since 2004, Belize has piloted the Child Friendly/Health Promoting Schools Initiative in 16 schools country-wide.

Dominica reports that the HFLE programme is actually addressing the issue of school climate, mainly through teacher training. 'In some schools, teachers listen to and comfort children, who are known to be affected or infected. Some children are provided with safety.'

St Vincent and the Grenadines reports that, according to the 1995 Education Policy, the government regards education first and foremost as a social institution indispensable for quality production, order, progress, poverty reduction and development of individuals. The Education Sector Development Plan has outlined

TABLE 4.4
FINDINGS: PSYCHO-SOCIAL AND PHYSICAL EDUCATIONAL ENVIRONMENT

Question	Total (15 responses)			
	Yes	In process	No	Mixed*
Is there a policy to develop a safe and healthy psycho-social and physical educational environment (free from physical and sexual violence such as bullying, homophobia, sexual harassment and gender bias)?	4	3	8	0
Have there been efforts to sensitize staff in the ministry on issues related to stigma and discrimination towards people infected or affected by HIV and AIDS?	10	4	1	0
Have there been efforts to actively gain participation from persons living with HIV/AIDS in programmes addressing HIV and AIDS?	9	1	4	1

Mixed indicates that British and Dutch Overseas Caribbean Territories are at different stages of their responses.

several principles that would ensure a healthy psycho-social environment for students.

In the Bahamas, the Department of Education has coordinated training and sensitisation for school personnel and headquarters staff to address issues such as stigma and discrimination, disclosure and confidentiality. A similar training has taken place in Barbados, where 63 per cent of primary teachers and 44 per cent of secondary teachers have participated in sensitisation and training in behaviour modification strategies. Barbados reports that the ministry currently has on staff only one psychologist, an education officer for counselling, and two social workers to work with all students in primary and secondary schools.

All school staff should be familiar with universal precautions, which are 'simple standards of infection control practices' to be employed consistently and without discrimination.[27] The availability of first aid kits in schools can help educators comply with implementing universal precautions. Jamaica reports that the local office of the Pan American Health Organisation (PAHO) formally presented the Ministry of Education, Youth and Culture with 258 first aid kits to be used in schools.

Countries report that the greatest challenge in addressing these psycho-social and physical environment issues is the lack of resources, both financial and human. Coordinators also see tremendous challenges in how to enforce such policies and to actually do the work of creating healthy environments.

HIV AND AIDS SERVICES, CARE AND SUPPORT

It is impossible to overestimate the important role that MoEs can play with respect to HIV and AIDS services, care and support. Two papers published by the IATT address a range of options for the education sector to consider in the areas of treatment education, and the education, care and support of orphans and vulnerable children.[28]

In terms of other forms of youth programmes – such as peer education and youth drop-in centres – that may meet the needs of in-school and out-of-school youth, ministries can provide space and staff. Ministries and schools can educate students and staff about the nature of testing, treatment and care. Ministries and schools can provide information about how to locate services. Ministries can also provide important referrals and links to health, mental health and nutrition services, especially for sexually active youth and for children, families, and staff who are infected and affected by HIV and AIDS.

Table 4.5 presents Ministries' replies to the questionnaire about services. Participants were asked if the MoE provides access to counselling and voluntary testing. Six respondents respond that they do have a programme; eight report that they do not. Of the six who offer testing and counselling, many are partnering with the Ministry of Health to provide these services.

Developing mechanisms and protocols for partnering and collaborating with other ministries, especially Ministries of Health, NGOs and other service providers can enable the education sector to increase its capacity to provide such services. Presently, several MoEs in the Caribbean region partner with their Ministries of Health or with NGOs. However, few do so with formal agreements. Similar collaborations exist for other interventions for youth and orphans and vulnerable children.

Countries were asked what other types of youth programmes they are conducting both in and out of school, such as peer education and youth drop-in centres, which are not part of the traditional curriculum track. Testing and developing best practices for these types of interventions is part of the CARICOM Education Sector Capacity-Building Programme.

Only two countries report that they do not have programmes that target youth. Some examples follow.

- 'Kite Jen Yo Pale' in Haiti developed in partnership with UNESCO, UNAIDS, Ministry of Culture, Ministry of Health, and two NGOs (VDH and FOSREF): Students developed a popular TV show called 'Let Youth Talk'. The objectives of the programme are to equip secondary students with skills to evaluate personal risk and to develop responsible sexual behaviour. The programme engages students in understanding the principles and importance of voluntary testing and fighting against stigma and discrimination. Young people, teachers and parents learned from these students, who became stars. This is a pilot project for preventing STD and HIV and AIDS at school.

- Jamaica-based 'Ashe' Caribbean Performing Arts Ensemble and Academy has recently released a new video 'From Caterpillar to Butterfly,' produced with assistance from UNESCO.[29] The video reaches youth with HIV and AIDS prevention messages. In addition, between 1996 and 2004, Ashe partnered with ten Caribbean countries and published manuals on the methodology of 'edutainment'.[30]

In Saint Lucia, plans are underway to provide support for orphans and vulnerable children, which might be delivered through existing MoE programmes, such as the School Feeding Programme.

In Trinidad and Tobago and St Vincent and the Grenadines, care and support is one of the priority areas of the MoEs. Both countries have started programmes to train guidance counsellors and school social workers in voluntary counselling and testing. Several participants in the April meeting commented on the dearth of trained school guidance counsellors: 'The number of trained guidance counsellors and school social workers is woefully inadequate. Non-governmental organisations should be used to assist with the counselling.' Another

TABLE 4.5
FINDINGS: SERVICES

Question	Total (15 responses)			
	Yes	In process	No	Mixed*
Does the ministry provide access to counselling and voluntary testing services?	6	1	8	0
Are there youth-based strategies (such as peer education, youth drop-in centres) that address HIV and AIDS?	11	1	2	1
Are there programmes to address the needs of orphaned and vulnerable children?	8	1	6	0

Mixed indicates that British and Dutch Overseas Caribbean Territories are at different stages of their responses.

participant commented, 'Teachers can be trained to provide in-school support and care.' The demands to handle multiple tasks and the lack of clarity concerning how to integrate HIV-prevention and counselling within HLFE is illustrated in the following comment: 'I am a school guidance counsellor as well; we have not gone that far in addressing HIV. I support twenty-one schools. HIV is within HFLE, but there is not so much on HIV. So I am not so clear on how to work to bridge these two.'

There is certainly a need to strengthen all aspects of services, because they have great potential to mitigate the risks and results of HIV and AIDS in the lives of young people and staff. In addition, services can proactively address the broader physical and mental health issues in the lives of students and staff that may place them at risk. However, there are at least four major challenges facing the education sector as it aims to strengthen this component.

- There is a lack of qualified guidance counsellors in the schools, with training in HIV and AIDS. Furthermore, there is a lack of resources to train counsellors.
- Few protocols or tools exist for MoEs to plan, coordinate, and manage, or provide quality control standards for services delivered in relation to ministries and schools.
- The frameworks, vocabulary and paradigms for the health and education sectors are quite different. Each sector must acquire a basic understanding of each other, at a minimum, to ensure effective collaboration.
- Ensuring confidentiality is a key factor in enhancing care, support and services. If people do not believe their information

will be kept confidential, they will not be willing to take an HIV test. Policies that are well implemented and include rules and regulations will help to create a safe, supportive environment.

The CARICOM Capacity-Building Programme will develop protocols and a tool for the education sector to plan, coordinate and monitor the quality of services provided by NGOs and others. This tool will also consider how Ministries can align a range of services with their policies. Nevertheless, professional development for its effective use will probably be necessary.

This section presented data on efforts underway in MoEs to address the four major components of a comprehensive response to the epidemic: an overarching MoE policy (including workplace policy) on HIV and AIDS; skills-based HFLE and HIV and AIDS curriculum; a healthy psycho-social and physical educational environment; and HIV and AIDS services, care and support. It is clear that the curricular component, in almost all the countries, has been the primary means of response. However, as noted, without an overarching policy and supportive environment and services, classroom instruction is limited in what it can accomplish. Furthermore, there are still the issues of achieving adequate HIV and AIDS content in the curriculum, teacher training, and reaching children at early enough ages to make a difference.

The next section reviews and recommends capacities that MoEs might need and want to develop to enhance the response to HIV and AIDS. Such capacities will have overall benefit to strengthening the education system and academic outcomes and are not only limited to HIV and AIDS.

FINDINGS: CAPACITY DEVELOPMENT FOR MINISTRIES TO ADOPT A COMPREHENSIVE APPROACH

Capacity development involves a combination of guiding policies, knowledge, skills and competencies of decision-makers, managers and practitioners. Capacity also relies upon the existence of supportive management structures and processes, with a commitment of human and financial resources. Addressing HIV and AIDS – or any health issue – in the education sector requires some basic understanding of how to apply public health strategies within education and community settings. Capacities include having the means to:

- Access, interpret and use quality data for planning including data on prevalence, risk and protective factors, impact on systems, and human, financial, and structural resources,
- Advocate and provide leadership for a comprehensive approach,
- Meaningfully involve persons living with HIV and AIDS,
- Provide administrative structures, management capacity, staffing and dedicated budgeting to support activities,
- Develop and nurture partnerships and mechanisms for collaboration,
- Select, implement, and evaluate evidence-based approaches,
- Institutionalise and sustain efforts over time beyond support from international donors, including grant writing and fund raising,
- Design and deliver professional development and technical assistance to enhance staff knowledge and skills, and
- Track and monitor progress.

From the various sources of data collected, we detail below the knowledge and skills that HIV and AIDS coordinators report they need to fulfil their roles effectively.

ACCESS, INTERPRET AND USE QUALITY DATA FOR PLANNING

From a public health perspective, it is essential to target interventions to the populations at greatest risk, with knowledge of patterns of causes and contributing factors to the injury or disease. According to the *Education Sector Global HIV and AIDS Readiness Survey 2004*, 'a lack of data and information available to guide a response' is pervasive.[31] Currently, the lack of strong data limits a clear understanding of the extent of the epidemic, persons at greatest risk, and contributing factors, such as social and economic determinants of health. Insufficient data also hinders countries' ability to target interventions and select the right strategies and programmes, with evidence of effectiveness. Ministries of Health, PAHO and other regional agencies do have a lot of data on current patterns.[32] MoEs must have greater access to it and use it in their planning. For some issues, the education sector may have to collect its own data.

There is a critical need for MoEs to have easy access to essential data about the epidemic to use in planning programmes and services. MoEs cannot and should not duplicate data collected in the health sector. However, education ministries might need to collect specialised data about risk and protective factors for youth, schools and locales most seriously affected, and the impact on the educational system of teachers and ministry staff.

Only a few MoEs report that they are gathering data pertaining to planning for

HIV and AIDS for the year 2004 and beyond. During interviews with HIV and AIDS coordinators, they express the need for many skills related to the use of data. Making decisions about the most cost-effective ways for MoEs to have the data for the planning, tracking and monitoring they do is a very important aspect of capacity-building. As one participant noted, 'Data on both positive and negative impacts will be collected and analysed. In this way, it is hoped that a fuller, more meaningful mapping of how HIV impacts on the everyday experiences of staff and students will be generated.'

One example is a new qualitative study underway in Jamaica to identify the various positive and negative ways that HIV and AIDS affect Jamaican schools. This study was commissioned by the Ministry of Education, Youth and Culture as a component of the UNESCO HIV and AIDS work plan. Professor David Plummer, Commonwealth/ UNESCO Chair in HIV and AIDS in Education, the University of the West Indies, is overseeing the study. The study will provide a meaningful map of how HIV touches the everyday experiences of staff and students. Its findings will inform ways to improve the policy response and the selection and design of interventions. Data will consist of interviews with teachers, students and families of people infected and affected. The team includes staff from UWI, the MoEYC, and the Jamaica Network of Seropositives (JN+).

ADVOCATE AND PROVIDE LEADERSHIP FOR A COMPREHENSIVE APPROACH

Leaders at the highest level of the MoEs, their staff and leaders in other sectors who can support the education sector must advocate for a comprehensive approach.

There must be a 'sustained, informed and strategically sound personal, professional, and political commitment'.[33]

In 2005–06, UNESCO/EDC piloted an advocacy and leadership campaign in three countries: Belize, St Lucia and Trinidad and Tobago.[34] In each of these countries, eight to ten leaders across the sectors of education, business, and medicine, and parent and media groups were trained in advocacy strategies and the messages for a comprehensive approach. These trained leaders then conducted retreats with approximately 40 to 50 of the most senior level staff in the MoE of each country, which culminated in action planning. There has been strong participation by advocates from organisations that represent persons living with HIV and AIDS. Evaluations of the outcomes of the training illustrate that inclusion of persons living with HIV and AIDS was one of the most powerful components of the campaign, resulting in ministry staff having a changed view, compassion and committing to greater collaboration.

This advocacy and leadership campaign has prepared a group of about 25 leaders who will continue their advocacy efforts within the country and across the region. The campaign is expected to continue both under the CARICOM Capacity-Building Programme and under UNESCO support in four additional countries this year. Nevertheless, there is clearly a need to build this advocacy effort, because many countries still find that they need to gain support from senior-level education officials. As one country HIV coordinator stated, 'There is a lack of ownership of the issue at the higher level.'

Eleven out of 15 ministry representatives report that senior-level ministry staff have spoken publicly about HIV and AIDS in the education sector. There is a need for this public discourse to continue. HIV and AIDS managers, and the system itself, need the support of ministers of education. All senior education officials must be willing to address the issue of HIV and AIDS in the education sector. They must do so with their own staff, as well as in the many public speeches and media forums at which they are present. As one participant commented, 'Professionals of education must understand that struggle for health and the need to combat HIV and AIDS at school is their own responsibility. They must be involved.'

MEANINGFULLY INVOLVE PERSONS LIVING WITH HIV AND AIDS

The principle of Greater Involvement of Persons Living with HIV and AIDS (GIPA)[35] recognises the importance of the contribution that people living with or affected by HIV and AIDS can make in response to the epidemic. Research has shown that personal connection with persons living with HIV and AIDS (PLWHA) – either through face-to-face conversations or by hearing a testimonial from infected or affected individuals – reduces misinformation and generates empathy which, in turn, reduces stigma and prejudice.[36] A participant from the Jamaican Network of Seropostives (JN+) said at the April meeting, 'If we do not stamp out stigma and discrimination, we will have a whole generation of hungry people.'

The education sector can create opportunities for active participation of PLWHA in all aspects of the response to HIV and AIDS. Requested a representative from JN+, 'Please involve us at all stages. Do not wait until you want to offer the programme, and then say "let's include PLWHA."' Drawing on the Chiang Mai Declaration, 1997, JN+ appeals that 'our bodies are the battleground of the epidemic; it is therefore our voices that must resound the battle cry.' The Ministry of Education, Youth and Culture in Jamaica and JN+ have developed a strong working relationship to disseminate and put into action the education sector policy to address HIV and AIDS.

The Caribbean Regional Network of Persons Living with HIV and AIDS (CRN+) has gained regional and international attention in its advocacy efforts. If ministries can strengthen their collaboration with this regional network and their own country's network, there will then be tremendous potential for overcoming stigma and discrimination, for strengthening prevention efforts and for encouraging people to seek testing and counselling services.

Several barriers must be overcome to strengthen the partnership between the education sector and persons living with HIV and AIDS. An overwhelming number of ministries in the Caribbean report their inability to ensure a safe environment for PLWHA to come out publicly with their status.

JN+ has suggested numerous strategies for effectively implementing GIPA principles, especially in the education sector:

- Develop codes of ethics for all individuals working with PLWHA that make them aware of protocols and ways to behave.
- Be aware of, and sensitive to, the fact that comments from people in a workshop can have a profound effect on the life of a person who is HIV+.
- When you invite PLWHA to participate, it is a heavy responsibility – they are sharing personal information and must be treated with respect.
- Create an official partnership between the MoE response team and PLWHA networks with a Memorandum of

Understanding (MOU) to clarify roles and activities.

- Reach out to involve all levels, especially Parent Teacher Organisations (PTOs).
- Design ways that PLWHA can see how the partnership will contribute to achieving their mission and vision.
- Ask the MoE to take the lead in providing professional development activities to provide PLWHA with the requisite skills to contribute to the programme in the most effective ways.
- Involve PLWHA at all levels, from preliminary planning to the implementation stage.
- Help PLWHA reduce stigma and discrimination by having more friendly programmes and initiatives.
- Provide financial support in the form of stipends for travel, food and time. Many persons living with HIV and AIDS are very much in need of financial support.

Professor Plummer summarised the importance of involvement: 'Symbolism itself is so critical. If we do not send the message that PWLHA are part of the team, an equal partner in this journey, then we are just reinforcing stigma. Can you imagine a feminist movement without women! We do not want an AIDS movement without the frontline people, who can share valuable stories that we cannot find in any books.'

PROVIDE ADMINISTRATIVE STRUCTURES, MANAGEMENT CAPACITY, STAFFING AND DEDICATED BUDGETING

The newly appointed coordinators are in a pivotal position for capacity-building. Through interviews and focus groups, EDC learned more about their backgrounds, responsibilities and the types of structures and supports they have in place. Coordinators'

perspectives on the administrative and management issues follow.

Nine of the 15 coordinators who participated in the survey report that there is a formally appointed coordinator to address HIV and AIDS. Other coordinators have assumed the responsibility, but they have not yet been appointed officially to the title and role. Table 4.6 illustrates the administrative units within the ministries where the coordinators are based. A majority of the coordinators report that HIV and AIDS is not their only responsibility. Some also have HFLE responsibilities; others have duties related to guidance and counselling programmes. The position of coordinator reports to supervisors at different levels. Some report to the Permanent Secretary, Director of Quality Assurance, Director of National AIDS Programme or Senior Education Officer. Coordinators argue that it is beneficial for them to report to the highest-level decision-maker to be able to advocate for what is needed and to have a voice in the policy and budget allocation process.

Five of the eight coordinators who participated in telephone interviews, report that they work with a team often comprised of people from other departments. Three work alone, but might have an advisory committee. Clearly, all coordinators need to be part of a functioning and dedicated team. Acting alone is very difficult. Staff retention is low and there is little continuity if competencies are not developed in more than one person. The nature of a comprehensive approach requires a critical mass of at least three to four people with a variety of skills. Assembling a team by drawing on staff from other departments can provide the support that is necessary. *The Education Sector Global HIV and AIDS Readiness Survey 2004* states that what is needed is a 'more holistic

TABLE 4.6
LOCATION OF HIV COORDINATORS IN MINISTRY

Located within	Reports to
Curriculum Development (3)	Head of the Unit
Guidance and Counselling	Head of the Unit
Quality Assurance and Development Services	Head of the Unit
Corporate Planning	Head of the Department, Deputy Permanent Secretary, Permanent Secretary, Director of the National AIDS Programme
Headquarters	Chief Education Officer
Health Sector Development Unit	Permanent Secretary
Student Support Services	Permanent Secretary

approach to management and mitigation and the application of available funds across a more balanced agenda, including prevention, treatment, care and support; workplace issues; and management of the response.'[37]

Many of the countries currently have donor money to conduct programmes to address HIV and AIDS, with limited money coming from the national budget. Since 2001, eight countries in this sample have been part of the World Bank Multi-Country HIV and AIDS Prevention and Control Adaptable Program (MAP): Barbados, Grenada, Guyana, Jamaica, St Kitts and Nevis, Saint Lucia, St Vincent and the Grenadines, and Trinidad and Tobago.[38] As part of this programme, each country is developing a multisectoral approach to HIV that includes the MoEs. A challenge is to ensure that adequate funding from such sources is dedicated to MoEs. Beyond global funding, dedicating funds from national budgets is a necessary means to gain ownership of the issue and to institutionalise programmes in the ongoing, everyday work of the ministries. Only one coordinator reports having discretionary control over funds for HIV and AIDS programmes.

DEVELOP AND NURTURE PARTNERSHIPS AND MECHANISMS FOR COLLABORATION

All ministries report that they are currently partnering with other sectors. Collaboration is for the purpose of providing technical assistance, training and sensitisation, materials development and services. Partnerships exist with Ministries of Health, National AIDS Commissions, various United Nations Organisations and international NGOs, such as the International Red Cross.

However, there remains a need for MoEs to play more of a role in systematising these relationships and services and aligning them with their policies on HIV and AIDS.[39] Procedures for joint planning, coordination and quality control can increase the effectiveness of what is provided and reduce unnecessary duplication. It has been observed that, 'In general, ministries have neither the clarity of policy, nor the capacity to monitor NGO HIV prevention efforts.'[40] Some tools for this purpose are in development under the CARICOM Capacity-Building Programme.

SELECT, IMPLEMENT, AND EVALUATE EVIDENCE-BASED APPROACHES

It is beyond the scope of this assessment to determine the extent to which programmes underway in the Caribbean are grounded in the evidence base of effectiveness. Increasingly, for reasons of resource scarcity and the urgency to achieve results and save lives, the strategies and programme must be based on evaluation data, demonstrating effectiveness. Even so, there are many challenges. Programmes proven effective with one audience and setting might not necessarily be effective with a new audience in a different setting. Therefore, MoE staff and school leaders can benefit from some basic skills in social science and evaluation as they review and consider which programmes to select, adopt and adapt.

Figure 4.3, developed by the Substance Abuse and Mental Health Service Administration (SAMSHA) of the United States Government depicts the basic features of evidence-based programmes.[41] These programmes are well-implemented, well-evaluated programmes, meaning they have been reviewed by the National Registry of Evidence-based Programs and Practices (NREPP) according to rigorous standards of research.

As MoEs across the Caribbean region implement programmes, there is a critical need to evaluate and disseminate best practices. Many resources exist, including the following examples:

- The U.S. Centers for Disease Control and Prevention: *Compendium of HIV Prevention: Interventions with Evidence of Effectiveness* (http://www.cdc.gov)
- YouthNet: *Partners in Reproductive Health and HIV Prevention* (http://www.fhi.org/en/Youth/YouthNet/index.htm)

- Implementing research-based health promotion programs in schools: Strategies for capacity-building [42]
- UNAIDS Inter Agency Task Team on Education (http://portal.unesco.org/en/ev.php URL_ID=10967&URL_DO=DO_TOPIC&URL_SECTION=201.html)

The CARICOM Capacity-Building Programme will provide HIV coordinators in the Caribbean with guidelines to select evidence-based programmes and access to international databases that contain information about evaluated programmes. The CARICOM initiative will also evaluate the effectiveness of peer education and youth drop-in centre programmes in two Caribbean countries.

INSTITUTIONALISE AND SUSTAIN EFFORTS OVER TIME BEYOND SUPPORT FROM INTERNATIONAL DONORS, INCLUDING GRANT WRITING AND FUNDRAISING

Only a few MoEs report that the national budget funds their programmes. Across the Caribbean, several MoEs have accessed or are using major international donor funds to provide the necessary resources to support HIV and AIDS programmes. However, many more MoEs need the capacity and skills to access such resources to launch programmes. The challenge with international donor dependent programmes is that they often comprise a series of stand-alone interventions, at times driven by conflicting ideologies, and little ownership by the government. Once this international funding ends, so does the programme. Gaining commitment from the government for these programmes is critical for sustaining and mainstreaming the education sector response.

FIGURE 4.3
BASIC FEATURES OF EVIDENCE-BASED PROGRAMMES

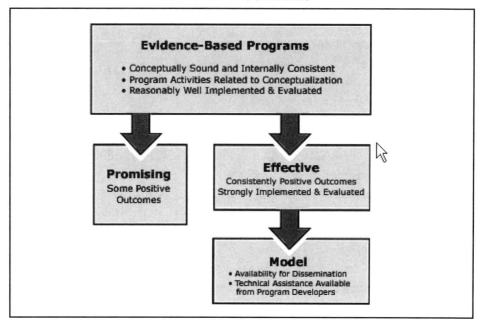

Source: *SAMSHA, 2005.*

The education sector needs support in developing the capacity to raise funds, including mastering proposal writing skills. However, even as they do so, all programmes need to think about sustainability and institutionalisation from the very beginning. If this process does not happen from the start, it is highly likely that the capacity and programmes will end when the external funding runs out.

Institutionalisation demands planning from the outset, considering what strategies are most cost effective and how they can be built into the everyday work, budget line items, position descriptions, and roles and responsibilities of staff. As one HIV coordinator stated, 'We need to eke out the school component budget from the national plan. One really needs to be crafty to get the funds. If you have a focal point person to deal with this issue, it will get more attention.'

Institutionalisation may continue to require ongoing additional funds from outside sources to complement the use of government funds, or to develop innovative, complementary features. The website http://www.promoteprevent.org offers the 'Legacy Wheel' as a conceptual model to consider the many facets of planning for institutionalisation.

DESIGN AND DELIVER PROFESSIONAL DEVELOPMENT AND TECHNICAL ASSISTANCE TO ENHANCE STAFF KNOWLEDGE AND SKILLS

The means to deliver quality professional development and ongoing coaching and technical assistance are essential to change practice. Research has shown that only five to ten per cent of what is learnt in one-time workshops is transferred to the classroom.[43]

Drawing from interviews with eight coordinators and comments gathered at the focus group in which all fourteen coordinators reviewed the titles of new HIV and AIDS training modules (developed by International Institute for Educational Planning and the University of KwaZulu-Natal), priorities for professional development include:

- HIV- and AIDS-related stigma and discrimination,
- Research with a heavy emphasis on monitoring and evaluation,
- Programme planning and implementation,
- Policy development and advocacy,
- Developing intervention ideas and procedures,
- More in-depth knowledge of HIV and AIDS: skills around treatment and counselling, and
- Curriculum development, materials production, and preparing teachers to teach HIV and HFLE.

The Caribbean region is rich with offerings of workshops on HIV and AIDS in the education sector. The challenge is to match them to the demand and provide ongoing support to ensure that schools and systems transform practices.

The CARICOM Caribbean Capacity-Building Programme, working with the Caribbean Network of Education Sector HIV Coordinators, will co-develop a menu of professional development events and ongoing coaching mechanisms through the virtual community. Under the Commonwealth/ UNESCO Chair at UWI, new courses are in development with a concentration on health promotion and HIV and AIDS. These courses will provide a range of experiences for educators in the region.

TRACK AND MONITOR PROGRESS

Tracking and monitoring progress plays a role in all the other capacities because it can inform the whole process. Tracking who was reached, with what interventions, and with what outcomes, are all key elements of information. Monitoring programmes can provide vital information to policymakers and planners, with evidence and guidance for institutionalisation and ongoing support. Documenting lessons learnt can inform programme and course correction and meaningful case studies to share in the region. Involving educators in deciding the purpose, priorities and design or selection of data collection instruments can ensure that they are feasible and can increase compliance with data collection efforts.

CONCLUSION AND RECOMMENDATIONS

This report presents a preliminary assessment of the Caribbean education sector's current response to addressing HIV and AIDS comprehensively. Data used in this paper was gathered in preparation for the first meeting of HIV Coordinators from fourteen countries and eleven British and Dutch OCTs in Jamaica, 25–28 April, 2006. EDC designed the assessment process and instruments and compiled and analysed the data, with the assistance of UNESCO and UWI, under its contract with the CARICOM Caribbean Education Sector HIV and AIDS Capacity-Building Programme.

In this chapter, we have presented our findings in two broad categories. In the first section, we discussed the importance of and need for the various ministries' current activities in the four components of a comprehensive response to HIV and AIDS. In the second section, we reported on the capacity needs identified by the HIV coordinators, and we described the additional capacities that are necessary for building the resources required to address HIV and AIDS.

KEY FINDINGS

Our analysis of the data reveals that countries across the Caribbean are at different stages of preparedness to address HIV and AIDS. Key findings from 15 country reports (one consolidated report from the OCTs, which include eleven territories):

- Ten MoEs report that no recent data has been gathered on the impact of HIV and AIDS on the education sector.
- Currently only Jamaica and Haiti have an HIV and AIDS Policy. Nine MoEs have a designated individual responsible for HIV and AIDS; however, only six have a line-item in the annual budget to respond to HIV and AIDS.
- A majority of countries report that the senior-level MoE staff have spoken publicly about the impact of HIV on the education sector. In addition most MoEs report that there have been efforts to sensitise their staff to issues related to stigma and discrimination.
- Almost all the MoEs have an HFLE Policy and are currently investing in training teachers on HFLE, which includes HIV prevention. However, only eight report that teachers have been trained to teach about HIV and AIDS.
- Most MoEs report partnering with the MoH and other NGOs to provide services (such as counselling, addressing needs of orphaned and vulnerable children, youth peer education); however, eleven report they do not have a policy to regulate NGO work. Nine MoEs report they have sought to gain participation of

PLWHA in programmes addressing HIV and AIDS, but not that much or very effectively.

Given the 'growing and generalised epidemic'[44] in the Caribbean, and the experience in many African countries, more such interventions are desperately needed. HIV and AIDS undermine 'progress towards the goal of education for all by affecting the demand, supply, and quality of education.'[45] It is imperative to provide Ministries of Education with the tools and resources they need to respond to HIV and AIDS proactively and effectively.

In this preliminary assessment, we identified five Ministry of Education capacities that must be enhanced:

1. Using data in programme planning, monitoring and evaluation,
2. Demonstrating leadership, advocacy and policy development with support at the highest level,
3. Investing in and providing professional development for the staff (HIV and AIDS coordinators and their teams, teachers, guidance counsellors and social workers),
4. Establishing sound human resources and management structures, with protocols to build partnerships (especially with support groups for PLWHA) to combat stigma and discrimination, and
5. Selecting, adapting and implementing evidence-based interventions.

It is essential to strengthen these vital and interrelated capacities to address HIV/AIDS as soon as possible. As this preliminary assessment has found, even though it has been four years since the Caribbean Ministers of Education gathered in Havana stated, 'We commit ourselves and our Ministries of Education to a heightened and concerted response to HIV and AIDS, beginning from this moment and continuing until, through education and other means, we have entered a world without AIDS',[46] there remain a number of significant gaps in the response to HIV and AIDS.

POSSIBLE APPLICATIONS OF THE FINDINGS

The findings from our preliminary assessments have some limitations. For example, we obtained information from the self-reports of Ministry staff, and the scope of our study did not allow us to secure external evaluators or conduct site visits. However, the data does provide a snapshot of the response to HIV across the Caribbean, and it has numerous applications for researchers, programme developers, educators, and policymakers. A few possible applications of the findings follow:

- Informing the development and implementation of a number of programmes across the Caribbean,
- Defining the dissemination and capacity-building agenda of the CARICOM Caribbean Education Sector HIV and AIDS Capacity-Building Programme,
- Guiding the establishment of resources, capacity and coordinating mechanisms, such as the recently formed Caribbean Network of Education Sector HIV Coordinators,
- Informing the creation and dissemination of new and targeted professional development and research tools through the newly appointed Chair for HIV at UWI and the new Masters in Education in Health Promotion, and
- Outlining priorities for using the new educational instructional material (such as the new IIEP/MTT modules on education planning and management for HIV).

RECOMMENDATIONS

- Most countries have yet to develop and implement an overarching education policy – such a policy will have many benefits to guide programming. Identifying ways to extend the CARICOM Capacity-Building Programme on policy development to more countries through the Caribbean Network of Education Sector HIV Coordinators should be a priority activity.
- MoEs should consider ways to strengthen the time and materials dedicated to HIV and AIDS within the context of HFLE and ways to train teachers and guidance counsellors in this integration process. Improving the school's psycho-social climate and instituting a policy of non-tolerance of bullying, sexual harassment and discrimination can be a part of the HFLE programme. To meet the growing demand for HIV and AIDS education, it is also important for MoEs to provide training and ongoing coaching that enhances educators' comfort with and skills in teaching these content areas. Furthermore, it is vital to increase the number of trained HIV and AIDS educators.
- Collaboration between Ministries of Education and the Caribbean Regional Network of Persons Living with HIV and AIDS (or country affiliates) has the potential to be very effective in combating stigma and discrimination. If MoEs build on and use the strategies, suggested by PLWHA in this document, these relationships and the outcomes of activities can be very effective at many levels.
- MoEs might consider dedicating more resources to hire and train guidance counsellors and social workers to provide

a range of mental health, support and HIV and AIDS counselling services to students and families. Such services can be preventive as well as supportive for those infected and affected.

- The newly appointed HIV and AIDS education coordinators are passionate and committed. To maximise what coordinators can accomplish, there can be position descriptions, with standards for the role. Rather than working alone as individuals in their ministries, placing the coordinator firmly within a supportive (perhaps cross-departmental) team will ensure that the capacity is developed to address HIV and AIDS. Having the HIV and AIDS coordinator report to a senior-level person in the Ministry of Education means that the initiative will have a voice in the policymaking process and a senior-level advocate.

- Although many ministries have an action plan, the HIV and AIDS coordinators do not necessarily have a discretionary budget or one that matches the activities of the plans they oversee. Ensuring that this function has the necessary resources to carry out the plans is a prerequisite of success.

- The newly formed Caribbean Network of Education Sector HIV Coordinators is working closely with the CARICOM Capacity-Building Programme, developing a virtual community for sharing resources and a menu of upcoming professional development activities. Developing synergy between these two entities and defining a plan of specific events, based on the needs outlined in this report, should take place in the next four to six weeks, following discussions at the COHSOD Meeting.

ACKNOWLEDGEMENTS

EDC expresses special thanks to the HIV and AIDS coordinators or ministry representatives who went to great lengths to complete country reports and questionnaires in a very short time frame and who participated in early morning focus group discussions. We acknowledge and appreciate their outstanding professional commitment.

REFERENCES

Academy for Educational Development. n.d. *HIV/AIDS Anti-Stigma Initiative*. Accessible at http://www.hivaidsstigma.org

Boler, T. and Jellema, A. 2005. *Deadly inertia: A cross-country study of educational responses to HIV/AIDS*. Brussels: Global Campaign for Education.

Brown, L., Macintyre, K., and Trujillo, L. 2003. Interventions to reduce HIV/AIDS stigma: What have we learned? *AIDS Education and Prevention* 15(1): 49–69.

Browne, D., Winkler, G., and Bodenstein, M. Forthcoming. *Teaching about HIV and AIDS in the Caribbean*.

Camara, B., and Zaidi, I. 2005. The future of the HIV/AIDS epidemic in the Caribbean. *CAREC Surveillance Report Supplement 1* June.

EDC and UNESCO. 2005. *Leading the Way in the Education Sector: Advocating for a Comprehensive Approach to HIV and AIDS in the Caribbean*. Newton, MA: Education Development Center, Inc.

EI, WHO and EDC. 2004. *WHO information series on school health: WHO teachers' exercise book for HIV prevention*. Geneva, Switserland: WHO Document Production Services.

Fixsen, D.L. and Blasé, K.A. 1993. Creating new realities: Program development and dissemination. *Journal of Applied Behavior Analysis* 26:597–615.

Fuller, M. 2006. Evaluating African HIV/AIDS Reading Material. Paper presented at the First Meeting of the HIV and AIDS Coordinators of Caribbean Ministries of Education, Jamaica.

Hardee, K., Feranil, I., Boezwinkle, B. and Clark, B. 2004. The Policy Circle: A framework for analysing the components of family planning, reproductive health, maternal health and HIV/

AIDS policies. *POLICY Working Paper Series No. 11.* Futures Group.

HoLung, J. 2006. *The Joint Board of Teacher Education's HFLE/HIV AIDS project.* Unpublished report for EDC.

IATT on Education. 2002. *HIV/AIDS & Education: A strategic approach.* New York: UNICEF.

IATT for Education. 2006. *Education Sector Global HIV & AIDS Readiness Survey 2004: Policy implications for education and development.* Paris: UNESCO.

IATT. 2004. *The role of education in the protection, care and support of orphans and vulnerable children living in a world with HIV & AIDS.* Accessible at http://unesdoc.unesco.org/images/0013/001355/ 135531e.pdf

IATT. Forthcoming. *HIV and AIDS treatment education: A critical component of efforts to ensure universal access to prevention, treatment and care.*

ILO. 2001. *An ILO code of practice on HIV/AIDS and the world of work.* Geneva, Switzerland: ILO.

ILO/UNESCO. 2006. *An HIV/AIDS Workplace Policy for the Education Sector in the Caribbean.* Geneva: ILO.

Kelly, M., and Bain, B. 2004. *Education and HIV/AIDS in the Caribbean.* Paris: UNESCO.

Kirby, D., Laris, B.A., and Rolleri, L. 2005. *Impact of sex and HIV education programs on sexual behaviors of youth in developing and developed countries.* North Carolina: Family Health International.

Ministry of Education, Youth and Culture. 2001. *National Policy for HIV/AIDS Management in Schools.* Kingston: MoEYC.

Morrissey, M. 2005. *Response of the education sector in the Commonwealth Caribbean to the HIV/AIDS epidemic: A preliminary overview.* Geneva: ILO.

PAHO. 2005. *Components of the Regional Core Health Data Initiative: PAHO Basic Indicator Database.* Accessible at http://www.paho.org/english/dd/ais/coredata.htm

SAMSHA. 2005. *SAMHSA model programs.* Accessible at http://modelprograms.samhsa.gov/template_cf.cfm?page=model_list

Skevington, S., Puitandy, M., and Birdthistle, I. 1999, 2003. *WHO information series on school health: Creating an environment for emotional and social well-being: An important responsibility of a health-promoting and child friendly school.* Geneva, Switzerland: WHO Document Production Services.

Supersad, M. 2006. *HIV/AIDS and the Education Sector: A Workplace Policy for Caribbean Education Institutions.* Paper presented at the First Meeting of the HIV and AIDS Coordinators of Caribbean Ministries of Education, Jamaica.

UNAIDS/WHO. 2005. *AIDS epidemic update. Caribbean: HIV and AIDS statistics and features in 2003 and 2005.* Accessible at http://www.unaids.org/epi/2005/doc/ EPIupdate2005_html_en/epi05_08_en.htm

UNESCO. 2000. *World Education Forum, Dakar: Final Report.* Paris: UNESCO.

UNESCO. 2005a. *The Response of the Education Sector in Jamaica to HIV and AIDS.* Draft document.

UNESCO. 2005b. *The "GIPA" principle and accelerating the response of the education sector in the Caribbean to HIV & AIDS.* Kingston: UNESCO.

Vince Whitman, C. 2004. Uniting three initiatives on behalf of Caribbean youth and educators: Health and family life education and the health promoting school in the context of PANCAP's strategic framework for HIV/AIDS. *Caribbean Quarterly* 50(1):54–82.

Vince Whitman, C. 2005. Implementing research-based health promotion programs in schools: Strategies for capacity-building. In S. Clift & B. Bruun Jensen (eds), *The health promoting school: International advances in theory, evaluation and practice*, pp. 107–136. Copenhagen: Danish University of Education Press.

Vince Whitman, C., Constantine, C., and Pulizzi, S. 2006. *Final inception report: Caribbean Education Sector HIV and AIDS Capacity-Building Programme.* Newton, MA: Education Development Center, Inc.

World Bank. 2000. *HIV/AIDS in the Caribbean: Issues and Options.* Washington DC: World Bank.

World Bank. 2002. *Education and HIV/AIDS: A Window of Hope.* Washington, DC: World Bank.

World Bank. 2005. *HIV programmes in Latin America and the Caribbean. HIV/AIDS Brief.* Accessible at http://www.worldbank.org/lacaids

NOTES

1. Convening announcement for the *Special Meeting of the Council for Human and Social Development (COHSOD) on Education and HIV/AIDS*, Trinidad and Tobago, 9–10 June 2006.
2. Vince Whitman, Constantine and Pulizzi, 2006.
3. World Bank, 2002.
4. EDC and UNESCO, 2005.
5. IATT on Education, 2002.
6. For additional information, see: http://hivaidsclearinghouse.unesco.org/ev_en.php
7. Kirby, Laris and Rolleri, 2005.
8. UNIADS/WHO, 2005.
9. Camara and Zaidi, 2005.
10. ILO/UNESCO, 2006.
11. Supersad, 2006.
12. EI, WHO and EDC. 2004.
13. Ministry of Education, Youth and Culture, 2001.
14. World Bank, 2000.
15. UNESCO, 2005a.
16. Hardee, Feranil, Boezwinkle and Clark, 2004.
17. Vince Whitman, 2004.
18. Vince Whitman, 2004.
19. Browne, Winkler and Bodenstein, forthcoming.
20. HoLung, 2006.
21. Fuller, 2006.
22. Kelly and Bain, 2004.
23. Skevington, Puitandy and Birdthistle, 1999, 2003.
24. Brown, Macintyre and Trujillo, 2003.
25. Academy for Educational Development, n.d.
26. Kelly and Bain, 2004.
27. ILO, 2001.
28. IATT, 2004 and IATT, in press.
29. DVD available from Ashe, Kingston, Jamaica.
30. Morrissey, 2005.
31. IATT, 2006: 53.
32. PAHO, 2005.
33. IATT, 2006.
34. Leadership and Advocacy website: www.caribbeanleaders.org
35. UNESCO, 2005b.
36. Brown, Macintyre and Trujillo, 2003.
37. IATT, 2006.
38. World Bank, 2005.
39. Boler and Jellema, 2005.
40. Morrissey, 2005.
41. SAMSHA, 2005.
42. Vince Whitman, 2005.
43. Fixen and Blasé, 1993.
44. Morrissey, 2005.
45. UNESCO, 2000.
46. Kelly and Bain, 2004. See pp. 280–82.

APPENDIX

TABLE 4.7
COUNTRIES, AFFILIATIONS AND STUDY INVOLVEMENT

Country	Member of CARICOM and/or OECS	Country report	Phone interview	Focus group	IIEP module
Antigua & Barbuda	CARICOM & OECS	☑	☑	☑	☑
The Bahamas	CARICOM	☑	☑	☑	☑
Barbados	CARICOM	☑		☑	
Belize	CARICOM	☑	☑		☑
Dominica	CARICOM & OECS	☑		☑	☑
Grenada	CARICOM & OECS	☑		☑	☑
Guyana	CARICOM	☑	☑		☑
Haiti	CARICOM	☑		☑	
Jamaica	CARICOM	☑	☑		
St Kitts & Nevis	CARICOM & OECS	☑		☑	
St Lucia	CARICOM & OECS	☑	☑	☑	☑
St Vincent & the Grenadines	CARICOM & OECS	☑	☑	☑	☑
Suriname	CARICOM	☑			☑
Trinidad & Tobago	CARICOM	☑	☑		☑
British & Dutch OCTs (Overseas Caribbean Territories)	British OCT: Anguilla (CARICOM associate member & OECS) British Virgin Islands (CARICOM associate member & OECS) Cayman Islands (CARICOM associate member) Montserrat (CARICOM & OECS) Turks and Caicos (CARICOM associate member) Dutch OCT: Aruba Netherlands Antilles (Curaçao, Bonaire, Saba, St Eustatius and St Maarten)	☑		☑	

TABLE 4.8
SUMMARY OF MINISTRY OF EDUCATION RESPONSE TO HIV

Question	Antigua & Barbuda	The Bahamas	Barbados	Belize	Dominica	Grenada	Guyana	Haiti	Jamaica	St Kitts & Nevis	St Lucia	St Vincent & the Grenadines	Suriname	Trinidad & Tobago	OCTs*	Yes	In Process	No	Mixed
Policy																			
Is there an HIV and AIDS policy?	N	IP	N	N	IP	N	IP	Y	Y	N	N	N	N	IP	N	2	4	9	0
Has the policy been implemented	N†	IP	N†	N	N	N†	N	Y	IP	N	N	N	N	N†	N†	1	2	12	0
Is there a workplace policy?	N	Y	N	N†	N	Y	IP	Y	IP	N	N	N	N	N	M	3	2	9	1
Curriculum																			
Is there an HFLE policy?	Y	Y	Y	Y	Y	Y	IP	Y	Y	Y	Y	Y	Y	Y	N	13	1	1	0
Is the ministry using the HFLE Regional Framework Curriculum?	Y	N	Y	Y	Y	Y	Y	Y	IP	Y	Y	Y	Y	Y	N	12	1	2	0
Has the Ministry invested in training teachers on HFLE?	Y	Y	Y	Y	Y	Y	IP	Y	Y	Y	Y	Y	Y	Y	M	13	1	0	1
Has the Ministry trained teachers to teach about HIV and AIDS? (Please quantify)	N	Y	Y	Y	Y	Y	IP	Y	IP	Y	N	Y	IP	IP	N	8	4	3	0

Y = Yes, N = No, IP = In Process, M = Mixed; * British and Dutch Overseas Caribbean Territories; † Answers to these questions were either "unknown" or left blank

TABLE 4.8 (cont.)
SUMMARY OF MINISTRY OF EDUCATION RESPONSE TO HIV

Question	Antigua & Barbuda	The Bahamas	Barbados	Belize	Dominica	Grenada	Guyana	Haiti	Jamaica	St Kitts & Nevis	St Lucia	St Vincent & the Grenadines	Suriname	Trinidad & Tobago	OCTs*	Yes	In Process	No	Mixed
Environment																			
Is there a policy to develop a safe and healthy psycho-social and physical educational environment (free from physical, sexual violence such as bullying, homophobia, sexual harassment and gender bias)?	N	IP	N	N	IP	N	N	Y	N†	Y	N	Y	N	IP	Y	4	3	8	0
Have there been efforts to sensitize staff in the Ministry on issues related to stigma and discrimination towards people infected or affected by HIV and AIDS?	Y	Y	Y	Y	Y	IP	IP	Y	Y	N	IP	Y	IP	Y	Y	10	4	1	0
Have there been efforts to actively gain participation from persons' living with HIV/AIDS in programmes addressing HIV and AIDS?	Y	N	N	N	Y	Y	IP	Y	Y	Y	N	Y	Y	Y	M	9	1	4	1

Y = Yes, N = No, IP = In Process, M = Mixed; * British and Dutch Overseas Caribbean Territories; † Answers to these questions were either "unknown" or left blank

TABLE 4.8 (cont.)
SUMMARY OF MINISTRY OF EDUCATION RESPONSE TO HIV

Question	Antigua & Barbuda	The Bahamas	Barbados	Belize	Dominica	Grenada	Guyana	Haiti	Jamaica	St Kitts & Nevis	St Lucia	St Vincent & Grenadines	Suriname	Trinidad & Tobago	OCTs*	Yes	In Process	No	Mixed
																Total			
Services																			
Does the Ministry provide access to counselling and voluntary testing services?	N	N	Y	N	N	Y	N	N	IP	Y	Y	Y	N	N	N	6	1	8	0
Are there youth-based strategies (such as peer education, youth drop-in centres) that address HIV and AIDS?	Y	Y	N	Y	Y	Y	Y	Y	Y	Y	IP	N	Y	Y	M	11	1	2	1
Are there programmes to address the needs of orphaned and vulnerable children?	N	N	Y	N	Y	Y	IP	N	N	Y	Y	Y	Y	Y	N	8	1	6	0
Capacity Needs																			
Are there current (2004 or after) data on the impact of HIV and AIDS within the education sector?	N	N	N	N	N	IP	Y	Y	IP	IP	N	N	N	N	N	2	3	10	0
Have senior-level Ministry staff spoken publicly about the impact of HIV and AIDS on the education sector?	N	Y	Y	Y	N	Y	Y	Y	Y	Y	Y	Y	N	Y	M	11	0	3	1
Is there a designated line-item in the annual budget to respond to HIV and AIDS?	N	N	Y	N	Y	N	N	N	Y	N	Y	Y	N	Y	N	6	1	8	0
Is there policy to regulate NGO work?	N	Y	N	N	N	N	N	IP	N†	N	N	IP	Y	N	N	2	2	11	0

Y = Yes, N = No, IP = In Process, M = Mixed; * British and Dutch Overseas Caribbean Territories; † Answers to these questions were either "unknown" or left blank

Table 4.9
Caribbean regional curriculum framework for Health and Family Life Education for ages 9–14

Form 1 – Self and interpersonal relationships

	Lessons	Topic	Skills	Activity
1.	Self-concept	Factors that Influence Self-Concept	Self awareness	Small group discussion Large Group discussion
2.	Being Assertive	Assertive Communication	Assertive communication	Small group Role play
3.	How Peer Pressured are You?	Negative and Positive Peer Pressure	Critical thinking	Scenarios
4.	Dealing with Peer Pressure	Resisting Peer Pressure	Assertive communication	Video – ASHE
5.	A & B Healthy Relationships	Healthy and Unhealthy Relationships	Self-management	Small group work Posters
6.	Impact of Alcohol on decision making	Risks of Alcohol	Decision making	Video – Brandon's Story
7.	Managing Anger	Anger Management	Self-management anger management	Small group work
8.	Resolving/Managing Conflict	Conflict Management	Interpersonal skills	Role play
9.	Coping with Domestic Violence	Domestic Violence	Coping skills	Group Discussion

Form 1 – Sexuality and Sexual Health

	Lessons	Topic	Skills	Activity
1.	Puberty	Pubertal Changes	Coping skills	Small/large group discussion
2.	Now What's Happening to Me	Dealing with Pubertal Changes	Healthy self-management Problem Solving Skills	Video – "Now What's Happening To Me"
3.	Gender Roles	Gender Roles	Critical-thinking skills	Large group discussion
4. & 5.	Gender Role Stereotyping	Gender Role Stereotyping	Critical-thinking skills	Scenario Role Play
6.	Sexuality	Human Sexuality	Critical-thinking skills	Large group activity Tree/leaves
7.	Risky Behaviours	Factors Influencing Risky Sexual Behaviour	Critical-thinking skills	Scenario's
8.	Minimizing the risks of HIV and AIDS	HIV Transmission	Critical-thinking skills	Video "HIV and AIDS :Staying Safe: Game
9-10.	Choosing Abstinence	Peer Pressure to Engage in Sexual Behaviour	Communication skills Refusal skills	Story-telling Role play

TABLE 4.9
CARIBBEAN REGIONAL CURRICULUM FRAMEWORK FOR HEALTH AND FAMILY
LIFE EDUCATION FOR AGES 9–14

FORM 2 – SELF AND INTERPERSONAL RELATIONSHIPS

	Title and number	Subject	Skill
1.	I Look In The Mirror And What Do I See?	Positive self-concept	Self-awareness skills
2 & 3.	Impact of Media Influence	Media influence on decisions	Critical-thinking skills
4 &5.	What Everyone Needs To Know About DRUGS	Drug use	Critical-thinking skills
6.	Could It Happen To Me?	Consequences of drug use	Decision-making skills
7.	Drugs And Sports -Pressure To Achieve	Performance-enhancing drugs and sports	Critical-thinking skills
8.	Refusal Skills: What Do I say Now	Peer pressure to engage in drug use	Communication and refusal skills
9 &10.	Embracing Diversity	Prejudice and tolerance	Interpersonal skills

FORM 2 – SEXUALITY AND SEXUAL HEALTH

	Title and number	Subject	Skill
1.	Healthy Relationships	Healthy relationships with friends of the same and opposite sex	Interpersonal skills
2.	Expressing Sexuality	Different aspects of human sexuality	Critical-thinking skills
3.	Healthy Dating Choices	Peer pressure to date	Decision-making skills
4 & 5.	Choosing to Protect Myself	Peer pressure to engage in sex	Communication and Refusal skills
6.	How HIV is spread	HIV transmission	Critical-thinking skills Empathy skills
7.	Preventing The Spread Of HIV/AIDS Through Advocacy	Peer advocacy for abstinence and HIV testing	Advocacy skills Creative-thinking skills
8.	Is It Worth It?	Poverty and HIV risk	Problem-solving skills Help-seeking skills
9.	Mia's Letter	Child Abuse	Coping skills Help-seeking skills
10.	Aftershock: Coping with Grief and Loss	Grief and Loss	Coping skills

5

ASSESSING THE EDUCATION SECTOR RESPONSE TO HIV & AIDS IN JAMAICA

DAVID J. CLARKE

Few countries have undertaken comprehensive assessments of their education sector response to HIV and AIDS. Jamaica is one of the first. This is a summary of the rapid assessment which included both a situation and a response analysis. Given the rapidity of the process, there are clearly limitations. The results are a snapshot of the situation at the time of the assessment and provide a rough baseline against which progress can be measured.

The main findings are presented. Jamaica, with high quality support from its development partners, has taken some of the essential steps to respond to HIV and AIDS in the education sector. The Ministry of Education and Youth has shown leadership in addressing HIV and AIDS, which is reflected in Jamaica being the first country in the Caribbean region to have put in place a comprehensive policy and organise a country-wide dissemination process. It has built technical capacity to institutionalise the response and decentralise it to all education districts through the establishment of the HIV and AIDS Response Team. The next step is to develop a comprehensive strategic plan for the sector for the next five years as a contribution to the next National AIDS Strategic Plan. A revised Health and Family Life (HFLE) curriculum for HIV prevention education is being piloted. This is a particularly important intervention and the results from the pilot process will be of relevance not only to Jamaica but to the Caribbean region as a whole.

The Government of Jamaica is embarking on a process of education reform to address the disappointing performance of the education system particularly with regard to learning outcomes. This provides a potentially favourable opportunity to harness the system for HIV prevention education and to address social issues which have a bearing on the HIV epidemic such as gender inequality, drug abuse and violence. While issues concerning the quality of education, including its relevance to young people, need to be addressed, the high levels of participation in primary and junior secondary education make the school a promising vehicle for HIV prevention education.

INTRODUCTION

A study to assess the education sector response to HIV and AIDS was funded by the UNESCO Office for the Caribbean and undertaken in August 2005 as a contribution to supporting capacity building of the education sector in Jamaica to implement an effective response to HIV and AIDS. It aimed to undertake a rapid assessment of the state of Jamaica's current and planned response, highlighting strengths and identifying areas where more investment is required. It made recommendations for consideration by the Ministry of Education and Youth and development partners to be considered as inputs into the development of a strategic plan on HIV and AIDS for the sector.

METHODOLOGY

On the basis of existing frameworks and checklists for assessing the education sector response to HIV and AIDS an analytical framework was constructed to guide the collection, organisation and analysis of data. Of particular importance in this regard were:

- 'Rapid Appraisal Framework for HIV/ AIDS and Education' (M. Kelly and B. Bain. 2003. *Education and HIV/AIDS in the Caribbean*);
- 'Mapping Matrix (draft)'. EDUCAIDS. UNESCO, Paris.
- 'HIV/AIDS and Education. A Toolkit for Ministries of Education' (UNESCO. Bangkok, 2003);
- 'Guidelines for the Assessment and Endorsement of the Primary Education Component of an Education Sector Plan' (EFA FTI Secretariat. 2005); and
- 'Global Readiness Survey Report'. (UNAIDS IATT on Education and MTT 2004) .

Four key parameters in the education response were identified. Each of the four headings below is broken down into sub-components in the analytical framework. (See appendix).

These were:

- Policy, strategic planning and institutional capacity;
- HIV prevention;
- Impact mitigation; and
- Leadership.

The assessment was based on data obtained through a review of documents, key stakeholder interviews and field visits in Kingston, Browns Town and Ocho Rios. In line with UNAIDS (2000) guidance for strategic planning the review attempted to identify what was working well and should be continued or expanded, what was not yet working but should be continued, what was not working and needs a new strategic approach and what was not relevant and should be dropped.

THE CHALLENGE OF HIV IN JAMAICA

Jamaica is the third largest island in the Caribbean with a population of approximately 2.6 million (2002). Tourism is the country's main source of income, followed by bauxite mining/processing, agriculture and light manufacturing. Tourism and mining are sectors often associated with social factors which drive HIV epidemics and at the same time they are vulnerable to their impacts. A macro-economic AIDS impact assessment (Nichols et al. 2000) projected that HIV and AIDS would result in a substantial impact on employment and labour supply in Jamaica. It was estimated that AIDS would reduce employment in the agriculture sector by 5%, by 4% in manufacturing and by 8% in services. Assuming a prevalence of

1.5% among Jamaicans between 15 and 49, the IFC (2003) estimated that there would already be 16,500 people living with HIV and AIDS in the national workforce.

Jamaica has an estimated national HIV prevalence of 1.5% in the age range 15–49, (UNAIDS 2006) which places it among those countries in the category of a generalised epidemic, one in which HIV is established in the general population (UNAIDS 2005a). With an estimated 25,000 people living with HIV and AIDS (UNAIDS op cit.), it has one of the largest populations of people living with HIV and AIDS in the Caribbean. Jamaica has the fourteenth highest prevalence outside Africa (DFID et al. 2005).

HIV transmission in Jamaica is predominantly through heterosexual sex, while vulnerability to HIV is conditioned by social marginalisation and gender inequality. Men who have sex with men are severely stigmatised (Human Rights Watch). HIV presents a significant challenge to the health of Jamaican people and to the long-term development of the country. UNAIDS (op cit.) highlights the importance of intensifying HIV prevention and this applies pertinently to Jamaica.

Young people, particularly females, constitute a vulnerable group to HIV and at the same time are disproportionately affected by the impact of AIDS on the family. In 2003, AIDS was the second leading cause of death in children aged 1–4 and there were an estimated 5,125 children under the age of 15 that had lost a mother or both parents to AIDS. The number of children orphaned is set to rise to 5% of all children by 2010. (UNAIDS, UNICEF and USAID. 2004). Adolescent females aged 10–14 and 15–19 had twice and three times respectively the risk of HIV infection as boys of the same age groups. This is ascribed to social factors whereby adolescent girls are having sex with HIV-infected older men. While young Jamaicans have high rates of early and unplanned pregnancy and sexually transmitted infections (STIs), those at greatest risk of HIV infection are male youth who have sex with men and all youth who engage in transactional sex (USAID 2004).

THE NATIONAL RESPONSE TO HIV AND AIDS

The national response is set out in the *Jamaica HIV/AIDS/STI National Strategic Plan* (JHANSP) for 2002–2006 (Ministry of Health 2002). This recognises the gravity of the HIV epidemic and its negative consequences for development in both the nation and the region. HIV and AIDS are identified as a high government priority within government. Alleviating the effects of stigma and discrimination is one of several broad policy issues that are identified to be addressed. The goals of the JHANSP are:

- To build an effective multi-sectoral response to HIV and AIDS;
- To mitigate the socio-economic and health effects of HIV and AIDS;
- To decrease individual vulnerability to HIV infection;
- To reduce the transmission of HIV infection; and
- To improve care, support and treatment services of People Living with HIV and AIDS.

The JHANSP was reviewed in 2005 and steps were being taken to develop the next 5-year strategic plan. A National Policy on HIV and AIDS is in the process of being endorsed by the government.

THE EDUCATION SECTOR RESPONSE TO HIV AND AIDS

Developing the education sector response as part of the national multi-sectoral approach is the responsibility of the Ministry of Education and Youth (MOEY, formerly the Ministry of Education, Youth and Culture or MOEYC). Its contribution to reduced individual vulnerability to HIV infection in the JHANSP was through *revision of the Health and Family Life Education (HFLE) curriculum to include HIV prevention and awareness and messages.* This formed a sub-component of the Behaviour Change Intervention and Communication (BCIC) component and with development and dissemination of sectoral HIV and AIDS policy, these represented clear responsibilities for the education sector during the plan period. The strong emphasis on prevention was appropriate and arguably the first priority for the education sector, though at the same time potentially the most difficult to achieve because of the multiple levels of intervention and long-term investment that are required for eventual effectiveness. This was recognised by MOEYC and reflected in its draft work plan, which was provided within the JHANSP.

Four priority objectives were set. These were to:

i) regain momentum on the HIV/AIDS/STI component of the HFLE programme (see section on HFLE);

ii) produce appropriate teaching and learning materials to generate awareness (see HFLE);

iii) provide training for teachers in order to develop competence in the delivery of the HIV/AIDS/STI education programme including the development of peer educators (see section on teacher training); and

iv) increase awareness by the Ministry's personnel and stakeholders of the need for greater responsibility for adopting programmes and workplace policies relating to HIV/AIDS/STI (see section on policy dissemination).

A number of key gaps and constraints were identified that would have to be overcome to achieve these objectives. These were:

- Lack of adequate support materials for teachers and students;
- Inability to sustain a high level HFLE programme due to budgetary constraints;
- Inadequate resources (human and financial);
- Inadequate knowledge base of MOEYC personnel; and
- Insufficient appreciation of the connection between irresponsible behaviour and the consequence in contracting HIV/AIDS/STI –combined with denial and cultural myths.

The core barriers related to resources, human and financial. They argue implicitly for a capacity building approach involving the recruitment of technically capable staff specifically for the HIV and AIDS response which would leverage greater sums of money from both government and development partners for programme activities to provide support for teachers and learners.

EDUCATION IN JAMAICA

The education response to HIV and AIDS needs to be contextualised in terms of the strengths and weaknesses of the sector. This in turn will provide insights into the ability of the sector to carry out the roles it has assigned to it within the national HIV and AIDS response.

Universal Primary Education (UPE) was achieved in Jamaica more than decade ago. The Net Primary Enrolment Rate in 2001 was 97.8% (MOEYC Statistics Unit). However, the survival rate to grade 5 is in decline having fallen from 96.5% in 1999/2000 to 87.6% in 2001/2. This is attributed by the World Bank (2004) to the 1998 policy prohibiting automatic promotion to grade 5 with promotion being performance-based in the National Grade 4 Literacy Test.

High levels of participation in primary education and lower secondary education as found in Jamaica are likely to be a strong contributory factor towards reducing the vulnerability of young people to HIV transmission. A growing body of international evidence suggests that children who are out of primary school are exposed to greater life risks including sexual risks than those who are in school. At the same time the widespread primary schooling in Jamaica means that the majority of young children can be easily reached through the school for HIV prevention education through HFLE rather than through more costly and difficult to implement outreach programmes.

Despite the achievement of UPE the education system faces profound challenges. The Task Force on Educational Reform reported (2004) that after substantial financial investment in education – Jamaica spends an average of 6% of GDP on education, more than most countries, although slightly below the Caribbean average of 6.5% (World Bank 2005) – the outcomes are cause for concern. Attendance is low, averaging 78% at primary level. Learning outcomes are poor; about 30–40% of grade 6 leavers are functionally illiterate. The expansion of the education system and the achievement of UPE arguably came at the cost of quality and poor education outcomes. While the

high level of expenditure on education attests to the commitment of government, the investment needs to be more efficiently managed and translated more effectively into educational outcomes. Recurrent funding is largely devoted to the payment of salaries (94%) which leaves few resources available for teaching and learning materials including textbooks which are essential for learning (World Bank op cit).

Education system performance is uneven. The quality of schools is variable. The number of classroom hours is low by regional standards, partly because crime and civil disturbances force schools to close (World Bank op cit). Poor students have less educational opportunity. They enrol into lower quality schools and difficult home circumstances can undermine their education. Generally, children of the poor end up with less education and this perpetuates a vicious cycle of poverty. The World Bank (op. cit.) recommends an increased focus on early learning to raise grade 6 functional literacy to 100% through teacher training, setting standards of service, providing educational materials to improve overall education outcomes. It also recommends that Government of Jamaica improve incentives and facilities for below average schools and make school results public. These issues resonate with the shortcomings already identified with regard to HFLE within the JHANSP.

Implementing HFLE in this context, without investing in improving the performance of the education system, is likely to provide sub-optimal results. Improving the quality of education processes and outcomes therefore is an agenda that is fully congruent with addressing HIV and AIDS, while HFLE needs to be fully considered as a contribution to improving the quality of education on offer. HFLE therefore needs to be considered as integral to educational reform in Jamaica.

The *Task Force on Educational Reform Final Report* included a short-term plan to March 2005 to establish a Transformation Team to lead the recommended restructuring and transformation of the education system together with a Medium Term Plan to March 2007 for the transformation of education in terms of:

- Institutional arrangements;
- Accountability for performance;
- Terms and conditions of principals and teachers;
- Chronic underachievement of the education system;
- Anti-social behaviour;
- Curriculum development and implementation;
- Student assessment;
- Management of teaching staff;
- Access to schools;
- School capacity and physical plant;
- Special needs education;
- Role of students; and
- Stakeholder partnerships.

This is quite a comprehensive list, but the *Task Force on Educational Reform Final Report* did not address HIV and AIDS education in any of its thematic area assessments apart from remarking that as a cross-cutting curriculum issue it is not always given the prominence necessary for the holistic development of the child.

The Government of Jamaica is responding to the issue of poor attendance and the need for pro-poor policies by linking social safety net support through the *Programme of Advancement through Health and Education* (PATH) to families to promote regular school attendance. Other support programmes include a school feeding programme in all primary schools and the free provision of primary textbooks

to all children. These programmes have the potential to provide support for children affected by HIV and AIDS, the orphans and vulnerable children (OVCs).

Gender inequality is a significant issue in education. Progress towards eliminating gender disparity in primary and secondary education has been assessed as 'lagging' (Government of Jamaica, 2004). In contrast to the prevailing situation in much of the world, it is boys not girls who are missing out on education. Males are under-represented at upper secondary and tertiary education. A significant gender disparity is to be found in learning outcomes. Male students are underperforming in relation to girls in reading in particular. Some 45% of male students assessed passed the grade 4 literacy test in contrast with 70% of the girls. Large numbers of those who are functionally illiterate at grade 9 and unable to either read or write are boys. Motivation has been identified as a critical factor (op cit). This signals the high priority that should be given to gender analysis and sensitivity in reforming Jamaican education and at the same time developing the response to HIV and AIDS at school.

Perhaps significantly, males are also underrepresented in the teaching force. The majority of teachers at primary and secondary levels are female: over 17,200 out of a total of 22,363 in 2004 (op. cit). This means a shortage of male role models at school and may contribute to the alienation of boys.

To conclude, the Jamaican education system faces a difficult and long-term challenge in improving the quality of education delivery and learning outcomes. It will require a strategic approach covering the entire sector. Addressing HIV and AIDS should be seen as integral to these efforts. It is an area of educational development that involves making the curriculum more relevant to the lives of the learner, teacher education to equip teachers with better skills for participatory learning and to be more responsive to the psycho-social needs of the learner. HIV and AIDS education is an area of some sensitivity in that it deals with gender relationships, life skills and sexuality which will require mobilising school staff and communities to support its introduction. It is at the sharp end of educational reform.

ASSESSMENT OF THE EDUCATION SECTOR RESPONSE TO HIV AND AIDS. KEY FINDINGS

WHAT IS WORKING WELL AND NEEDS TO BE CONTINUED?

Policy on HIV and AIDS

The development of comprehensive policy is essential to guide the education sector response to HIV and AIDS (Kelly 2003). Such policy is additional to developing the National AIDS Policy, because the latter being a broad enabling document would lack attention to the detailed needs of education institutions and processes (MTT 2004).

There is a lack of international consensus on the key dimensions of policy: content, process and power (Walt 1994), for the education sector regarding HIV and AIDS. Current appraisal toolkits for assessing the education response to HIV and AIDS tend to take a binary approach (UNESCO 2003; UNAIDS IATT on Education and MTT 2004; Kelly and Bain 2003); either there is a policy in place or there is not. The former indicates achievement, the latter a deficit. There is little guidance available to Ministries of Education on policy content apart from the checklist provided by the World Bank (2005). The ILO Code of Practice on HIV/ AIDS and the World of Work (2001), has been adapted for the education sector in the

Caribbean (ILO and UNESCO 2006) and will be a useful resource to policymakers in the region.

Arguably the most significant step taken by the Jamaican Government in supporting an education sector response was to approve a national policy for HIV and AIDS in schools. Technical and financial support were provided by UNICEF and CIDA. Although drafted in 2001, it took until 2004 to be endorsed suggesting a cautious approach to the issues to be addressed. That the government now has an official set of positions on prevention and non-discrimination provides it with a platform for initiating comprehensive action in early childhood, primary and secondary education in public and private schools. HIV and AIDS policies for higher education fall outside the policy framework for schools with the risk that this may bring about a disconnect between the two sub-sectors.

ANALYSIS OF POLICY CONTENT

The *National Policy for HIV/AIDS Management in Schools* covers a range of issues, many of which could be considered as workplace issues (see table 5.1 below). These include non-discrimination, HIV testing in relation to admission and appointment, attendance of children living with HIV, disclosure and confidentiality and HIV prevention through education in the school setting. It is, reportedly, the first comprehensive national HIV and AIDS policy for education in the Caribbean region. Jamaica is now in a position to implement a policy-based approach, which is necessary for a scaled up response in the sector.

There are gaps in the policy and some areas, which could benefit from further definitional detail. There is a lack of explicit attention to the impact of AIDS on education whether on the staff or students especially orphans and vulnerable children (OVCs). There is no mention of gender issues or access to treatment, care and services. The policy on HIV education could be usefully augmented with details about curriculum content, teacher preparation and support, timetabling and assessment of learning outcomes. Responsibilities at all levels of the system for implementing the policy could be made more explicit.

POLICY DISSEMINATION

MOEYC embarked on an active programme of policy dissemination in school year 2004–05 with support from UNICEF and CIDA which greatly raised the profile of the HIV and AIDS response. The approach involved a programme of workshops targeted at school level stakeholders implemented through the 6 Regional Education Offices.

People living with HIV and AIDS PLWHA through the Jamaican Network of Seropositives (JN+) were involved in workshop delivery, in line with international best practice on Greater Involvement of People Living with HIV and AIDS (GIPA). Anecdotal evidence suggested that this was a very effective approach.

This decentralised approach enabled some 1,570 representatives from 440 schools out of a total of around 1,000 to be oriented to the new policy at the time of the assessment. All junior high schools had been covered and the programme was proceeding to cover all the remaining primary schools and early childhood programmes. Policy dissemination thus represented work in progress. Issues about the quality of and consistency of the programme and the level of stakeholder participation in the process had been raised.

CAPACITY BUILDING THROUGH THE ESTABLISHMENT OF THE HIV AND AIDS RESPONSE TEAM (HRT) TO OPERATIONALISE POLICIES AND PLANS

The importance of institutionalising the response to HIV and AIDS is clearly made by Carr Hill et al. (2002). In this regard, the setting up of the HRT in 2004 was a significant practical achievement by MOEYC. It offers a model of good practice in capacity building for the education sector at central and decentralised levels. As a result, there is now dedicated full time institutional capacity on HIV and AIDS at MOEYC headquarters in the Guidance and Counselling Unit. In addition, there is health promotion expertise in all 6 Regional Education Offices. The HRT team comprising 16 persons, including Japanese volunteers, is now responsible for disseminating and subsequently supporting the implementation of the MOEYC policy on HIV and AIDS. It represents a key strategic advance without which dissemination and implementation of policy would have been very much more problematic. Support for this initiative was provided by UNESCO, UNICEF, JICA and the World Bank.

The HRT had already been formatively evaluated with UNESCO support (Chambers 2005). The findings of the evaluation process were generally positive resulting in an endorsement for a continuation of the approach. The Global Fund to Fight AIDS, Tuberculosis and Malaria (GFATM) support together with that of Japan International Cooperation Agency (JICA) through the financing of Japan Overseas Cooperation Volunteers (JOCV) will help to sustain the HRT in the short run. In the longer run MOEY would need to determine whether it wishes to sustain the HRT and if so at what level of human resources. At the time of the assessment only one member of the team was being funded by the Government of Jamaica.

UNIVERSITY POLICIES ON HIV AND AIDS

Policies on HIV and AIDS have been formulated and approved by the University of the West Indies (UWI, 2004), which has a campus in Jamaica (Mona) and University of Technology, Jamaica (2003). The former is a regional institution, the latter Jamaican. Higher education policies lie outside the framework established by MOEY policy, which as its title suggests is for schools only. Achieving consistency and complementarity between the two levels of policy is a challenge for the national Jamaican HIV and AIDS response, especially as UWI is a regional entity.

TABLE 5.1:
NATIONAL POLICY FOR HIV/AIDS MANAGEMENT IN SCHOOLS. POLICY CONTENT SUMMARY

Policy Content Area	Finding
Statement of political endorsement by the Minister of Education.	No statement.
Guiding principles and definitions.	No guiding principles and definitions.
Scope of application	Applies to all educational institutions that enrol students in one or more grades and at all levels
HIV Prevention	a) Health and Family Life Education (HFLE) which must be implemented through integration in the curriculum at all school and institutions for all students (in pre-primary, primary and secondary schools) and school personnel. b) Adoption of universal precautions at school.
Children infected and affected by HIV and AIDS	Mention only of children living with HIV (see below)
Workplace policies.	The following are included: • Non-discrimination and equality; • HIV testing, admission and appointment; • Attendance at institutions by students with HIV and AIDS; • Disclosure and confidentiality • A safe institutional environment; • Prevention measures related to play and sport. Refusal to study with or teach a student with HIV or AIDS or work with or be taught by an educator with HIV or AIDS.
Access to treatment, care and support	No mention
Gender equality, sexual harassment and abuse	No mention

As with MOEYC policy the two policies have their strengths and weaknesses. Neither policy is as comprehensive as it might be. Both can serve as a vehicle for mobilising the institution to support the response to HIV and AIDS through addressing them through the core functions of university in teaching, learning and research. Both address stigma and discrimination. There are striking differences between the two in terms of their content and coverage of potential issues. Both are light in terms of the details of the prevention education to be available to students and responsibilities for policy implementation. Further work is needed in developing a wider coverage of workplace issues. Fostering active student participation in policy formulation and implementation appears to be a key challenge for UWI in particular. Both universities could develop more effective policy dissemination strategies as well as ensuring that HIV and AIDS policy implementation is appropriately included in university strategic plans.

CAPACITY BUILDING FOR HIV AND AIDS IN HIGHER EDUCATION

An innovative capacity building programme on HIV and AIDS has been implemented at UWI. This is the UWI HIV/AIDS Response Programme (UWI HARP) which has been supported by the European Commission (EC). New professional staff members have been taken on in health economics, communication, behavioural sciences, medicine and public health. While multi-sectoral in remit, there was the perception that the programme is health-biased as it is based in the Medical Faculty. UWI HARP supported the integration of HIV and AIDS in more than 20 courses and 17 new courses were developed (Crewe and Maritz 2006).

At the time of the assessment there appeared to have been very limited added-value for the education sector response in Jamaica or elsewhere. The challenge for UWI then is to broaden the scope of capacity building to include other disciplines such as law and education. The latter will be catered for in large measure by the establishment of the Commonwealth/UNESCO Chair in Education and HIV and AIDS. This represents a key innovation in the region. The Chair can help accelerate the regional response to HIV and AIDS and support national efforts by addressing key areas such as educational debate, research, capacity building in key areas such as life skills education, gender analysis, monitoring and evaluation, and documenting best practice.

There was concern about UWI HARP's reliance on donor funding which was coming to a close. UWI needs to allocate its own finances to consolidate the gains made by UWI HARP and institutionalise them.

RESEARCH

There has been some relevant good quality research on young people carried out during the last 5–10 years by academics and NGOs through various initiatives which should be familiar to education policy makers. Some has been focused on HIV and AIDS, some on issues with are relevant to vulnerability and risk in young people's lives. In aggregate, they provide a reasonably good knowledge base for policymakers and practitioners to plan a comprehensive response to meet their needs. However, research on what young people say they want or need in relation to HIV prevention education is conspicuously missing.

Among the key sources of information are the *National Knowledge, Attitudes, Behaviour and Practices* (KABP) Survey carried out under the aegis of the JHANSP and the *Knowledge, Values, Attitudes and Practice* (KVAP) survey (JAMR, 2005) among adolescents with disability supported with UNFPA funding. Additional qualitative research is needed among young people to complement these. A study of adolescent reproductive health and survivability (Gayle et al., 2004) in urban St Catherine yields many insights into the constellation of risk and vulnerability that young people face in their daily lives. This includes, hunger, fear of violence, physical abuse by parents, teachers and others, sexual abuse and prejudice against them. HIV and AIDS interventions need to take these contextual factors into account in a multi-factorial approach. Similarly the insights into gender and masculinity in particular that are provided by Chevannes (2001) need further exploration and programmatic responses to address male under-performance at school. UNICEF and UNFPA have published research (2002) on meeting adolescent development and participation rights which includes factors which shape the initiation of early sexual behaviour.

Research is particularly needed in relation to:

- Implementation of HFLE;
- Preventing and responding to HIV and AIDS-related stigma and discrimination at school; and
- Gender and masculinity in education.

LEADERSHIP

MOEYC has shown leadership by developing policy on HIV and AIDS and building institutional capacity to implement it. The Guidance and Counselling Unit has played a significant role in this. The Minister of Education has given prominence to HIV and AIDS on World AIDS Day and on other occasions. However, leadership at all levels in the sector could be further strengthened with the implementation of the HIV and AIDS policy. This particularly applies to school principals and Regional Education Directors. Commitment should be visible, continuous and consistent. Development of a sector strategic plan on HIV and AIDS would provide an opportunity to mobilise and support educational leadership throughout the system.

DEVELOPMENT ASSISTANCE

The support provided by Jamaica's development partners has been key in achieving outcomes to date and for providing the platforms for further action. It appears to have been relatively well co-ordinated, strategic with some important innovative developments being supported. Much of the financing and technical support for the education sector so far has come from development partner assistance. Such assistance needs to be continued but with a longer planning time frame and an increased commitment from the Government of Jamaica. There is room for greater harmonisation of development partner procedures. The development of a strategic plan for HIV and AIDS in the education sector could support this process.

WHAT IS NOT YET WORKING, BUT SHOULD BE CONTINUED?

HIV Prevention Education. Health and Family Life Education (HFLE)

HFLE has been identified as the main vehicle for HIV prevention education in all Jamaican schools (MOEYC 2001). HIV and AIDS constitute one of 4 themes. It is also considered as a way to reduce demand for drugs, a means of promoting wellbeing and addressing violence. It is a regionally developed curriculum, originating from an initiative supported by PAHO/WHO, UNICEF and the CARICOM Secretariat in the early 1980s and targeted at lower secondary grades 7–9 (Morrissey 2005).

HFLE is defined as a comprehensive life skills programme (Whitman 2004. CARICOM and UNICEF 2001). It is based on research undertaken on the social and health profile of Caribbean children and youth (PAHO 1998; UWI-Cave Hill 1998; UNICEF and CARICOM 1997 and the Commonwealth Youth project. 1997).

HFLE is a CARICOM multi-agency programme but the HFLE curriculum has been slow to be translated into classroom practice (Morrissey 2005). The implementation problems identified in 2001 (CARICOM and UNICEF 2001) highlight the problems encountered and to be addressed. In summary, these include:

- Poor vision and strategic planning;
- Multiple and overloaded curricula;
- Focus on content not behavioural change;
- The benefits not forcibly presented;
- Lack of broad-based stakeholder involvement and ownership;
- Inadequate teacher training, materials development, monitoring and evaluation;
- No sustained political will; and
- Inadequate collaboration among support agencies.

This adds up to a comprehensive list of shortcomings to be addressed. To these could be added that HFLE is not part of the core and examinable curriculum.

Despite these, in 2002, there was a renewal of commitment to HFLE by the regional CARICOM Council for Human and Social Development (COHSD) which resulted in the development of a new curriculum framework and prototype lessons

for the four HFLE themes (Morrissey op cit). The revised detailed curriculum was completed in early 2005.

An important regional programme is the CARICOM/IDB/UNESCO *Caribbean Education Sector HIV/AIDS Response Capacity Building Programme.* The IDB and UNESCO have supported the development of the *Caribbean HIV/AIDS Training Package for Teachers: Advocacy and Instructional Materials for Teacher Training institutions.* The Joint Programme Identification Study (JPIS) for the above-mentioned project undertaken in 2003 identified a number of critical weaknesses in the HFLE programme. These include:

- **Content.** HFLE is broad in content; HIV and AIDS do not appear to be sufficiently prominent; sexuality is not discussed openly enough;
- **Curriculum status.** The subject has low priority because it is not an examination/ qualification subject;
- **Teaching skills**. Life skills requires skills in participatory teaching and learning; teacher preparation has been inadequate; teachers are not comfortable with teaching some of the content;
- **Stakeholder support.** There is some opposition from the church and parents;
- **Young people**. Youth have not been directly involved in the content, planning; and
- **Delivery of HIV and AIDS and sexuality components.** Many would like teachers from outside the school;

These shortcomings are significant and will need to be addressed if HFLE is to be an effective means of HIV prevention. There is widespread perception that behaviour change is not taking place.

Implementation of HIV and AIDS prevention education within HFLE represents arguably the greatest challenge and highest priority for MOEYC in achieving its policy objectives. HFLE has been identified in MOEYC policy as the main vehicle for HIV prevention education and which 'must be implemented through integration in the curriculum for all students and school personnel'. Currently it is unclear to what extent HFLE is being implemented in schools. It has a low status in the curriculum because it is not a core subject and not examined.

Currently it is planned that a strategy and tools for the monitoring and evaluation of HFLE delivery will be developed. An HFLE co-ordinator has been identified to coordinate the activities of the CARICOM/ UNICEF HFLE project with consultants and stakeholders. UNICEF is to provide technical and financial support to strengthen MOEYC capacity to monitor and evaluate. To support this the following steps will be taken:

- A policy environment survey based on the National Policy for the Management of HIV/AIDS in Schools within 6 months of policy dissemination. This should give better data on the extent of HFLE implementation in schools;
- A rapid assessment of HFLE and existing M&E structures and mechanisms at all levels in the education system. This will recommend strategies for strengthening M&E of the delivery of HFLE in schools; and
- Development of an overall performance framework for M&E of process and impact of MOEYC's programmatic response.

Outside of the HFLE project, a curriculum scope and sequence for the early childhood level has been recently developed and approved. It is aligned to the CARICOM regional framework.

Currently MOEYC is attempting to build stakeholder support in schools through its policy dissemination workshops. This needs to continue. The piloting of the revised HFLE curricula was about to take place in 24 schools in 2005 with a plan to scale up to 200 in 2006. This is an important and complex intervention, which will require the development of a robust monitoring and evaluation framework to measure progress towards objectives and outcomes.

In preparing for the HFLE pilot and ensuring it works effectively in supporting behaviour change, lessons can be learned from international experience in introducing skills based health education as a means of HIV prevention education. The *UNAIDS Benchmarks* (World Bank, 2004) provide pointers towards good practice in this field. Some of the issues to be faced include:

- **Time on task.** HFLE is broad in content and this limits time available for teaching and learning about HIV and AIDS;
- **Teacher preparation.** Teachers need adequate training preparation to teach the new content and to use participatory methods effectively. In the short run, in-service training at the project level can be used to kick start the approach, but in the longer run investments must be made in pre-service or initial teacher training and in developing a national programme of in-service training and professional support. Capacity to undertake teacher training on HIV and AIDS will need to be developed. This is being developed in a separate project. HFLE is to be piloted in 4 teachers' colleges as part of initial training in what should be a linked initiative with the HFLE schools' pilot;
- **Participation of young people.** It is unclear to what extent young people have

participated in the revision of the HFLE curriculum. The new curriculum must motivate the students, both boys and girls, and feel that it is relevant to their lives, and is not simply messages being broadcast to them. The introduction of good quality peer education may assist this. Jamaica Red Cross (JRC) are to pilot a peer education approach in a separate initiative;

- **Teaching and learning materials**. Materials need to be developed to support both teaching and learning. This could include textbooks, teachers' guides and readers. Currently no materials are available apart from IEC pamphlets although readers developed for Africa will be piloted this school year through Jamaica Library Service Mobile Bus in a separate initiative and a **Lesson for Life Activity Pack** has been prepared for World AIDS Day in another separate initiative;

- **Building community level support**. Attention needs to be paid to building stakeholder support at community level by working with the church, faith based organisations and parents;

- **Linkages with youth friendly services**. This is lacking in the MOEYC Policy, yet it is critical to success in relation to HIV prevention.

INITIAL TEACHER TRAINING ON HIV AND AIDS

Effective HIV and AIDS education programmes require that educators are being professionally developed. Teacher educators need to be professionally trained in HIV and AIDS issues and in curriculum implementation. School teachers need to be adequately prepared through pre-service and in-service training to teach a skills-based approach to HIV prevention.

To date, teacher education has been a neglected area in the education response to HIV and AIDS. This needs to be set in the context of the Jamaican education system in which the majority of teachers (63%) have a teaching diploma, but no subject specific qualification. Only 20% of teachers in the public system were graduate-trained. There is no requirement for teachers to continue to improve their professional learning once they have received their teaching qualifications. Where there were specific projects, however the MOEYC offered professional development throughout the year (Task Force Report 2004).

The challenge is twofold:

- First, to ensure that that all teachers who take a professional teaching qualification receive appropriate training on HIV and AIDS for working in schools in a world with HIV and AIDS;

- Second, to develop a comprehensive project to establish continuous professional teaching skills development especially in relation to the implementation of HFLE. The MOEYC Policy is silent on what is intended for teacher preparation on HIV and AIDS.

It is particularly important that HIV and AIDS are being given appropriate priority in initial teacher education. HIV and AIDS and life-skills should be integral components in the curriculum for the professional preparation of all new teachers. Materials for teacher education need to be developed. It is worth considering the setting up of small resource centres for HIV and AIDS education for staff and student use in Teacher Training Colleges.

The Joint Board of Teacher Education (JBTE) is embarking on a project, funded by GFATM, to pilot in 4 Teacher's Colleges, for the period 2005–2008, the implementation and institutionalisation of an HFLE/HIV and AIDS curriculum. JBTE is under the aegis of the Institute of Education (IOE) at UWI which will be the source of professional direction of the project. The project will train lecturers in behaviour change, education values and other strategies.

The project will deliver the following outputs:

- A 2 credit HFLE / HIV and AIDS 30 hour curriculum in 4 teacher's colleges for all student teachers as part of their personal development programme;
- Handbooks and other teaching and learning resources;
- Networks within colleges and the community;
- Research on HFLE;
- Graduate level HFLE/HIV and AIDS course at UWI; and
- HFLE/HIV and AIDS for teacher training.

TEACHING AND LEARNING MATERIALS

An effective HIV education programme requires good quality teaching and learning materials to have been developed and in use at all levels in the education system. Such materials should be professionally developed and piloted before their final adoption. Provision needs to be made so that sufficient quantities of materials are distributed to all institutions and their use is monitored. Every teacher and learner should have access to appropriate teaching and learning materials.

Browne (2005), in reporting on a UNESCO-funded evaluation of HIV and AIDS textbooks stated that as yet no instructional materials have been put out by MOEYC. This represents a major impediment to effective teaching and learning about HIV and AIDS. How HFLE can be implemented consistently without there being accompanying teaching and learning materials is difficult to imagine. The absence of materials puts an additional preparation burden on the teacher which often results in a didactic approach in the classroom. Materials are needed to support participatory activities.

HEALTH ADVISORY COUNCILS (HACS)

The MOEYC Policy specifies that each institution, including schools, should establish its own HAC and develop action plans to give operational effect to the policy. This is as yet untested. There is currently no detailed guidance available and no resources for HACs to use. Setting up HACs might best be approached in a pilot project approach on a limited scale so that lessons can be learned through formative monitoring and evaluation about what makes for an effective HAC and these can then inform subsequent scaling up.

HIV PREVENTION IN CO-CURRICULAR EDUCATION

Although the MOEYC policy usefully encourages the integration of HIV and AIDS education in sport and work has begun in implementation, further exploration is needed in relation to making good use of co-curricular opportunities for prevention education. Staff involved in sport will need specific training and guidance/resource materials to undertake their new work effectively. Peer education programmes could also be supported. This issue needs to be incorporated in any strategic planning exercise on HIV and AIDS for the sector.

HIV PREVENTION IN SPECIAL EDUCATION

Mention has been made already of the KVAP survey (JAMR 2005) among adolescents with disabilities. They represent a vulnerable group with special needs. This needs to be recognised in policy and practice. A strategic approach to HIV and special education needs to be taken.

WHAT IS NOT WORKING AND NEEDS A NEW STRATEGIC APPROACH?

Addressing Stigma and Discrimination

The persistence of stigmatisation of children living with HIV and AIDS is a reality in Jamaica and results in children facing exclusion from education despite unambiguous MOEYC policy. Unless addressed effectively it will tend to undermine prevention efforts. A more comprehensive approach to preventing stigma and discrimination is needed in schools. It is unclear at the moment whether the revised HFLE has the potential to achieve any impact in this field, but this is an obvious area of application. Consideration needs to be given to fostering the development of innovative activities in this field. It may be an area of policy implementation that the HAC will want to take on.

How can education comprehensively tackle stigma and discrimination? Kelly and Bain (2003) advocate a multiple response involving the following set of actions:

- Establishing a clear regulatory framework which is rights-based and including a manual for use by school boards and parent teacher associations;
- Ensuring that every educational institution manifests a welcoming approach for infected and affected children and staff with zero tolerance for discriminatory behaviour;
- Ensuring that every pupil has sufficient knowledge of HIV and AIDS to dispel common myths about HIV transmission and prejudices about and intolerance towards those infected with HIV or affected by AIDS;
- Including education on ethics, values and human rights. Aggleton and Parker (2003) recommend the promotion of human rights generally and in particular of PLWHA as well as the implementation of lifeskills education.

IMPACT MITIGATION

In many contexts it has become standard practice for the Ministry of Education to commission an AIDS impact study. In addition to assessing the current impact of AIDS, projections can be made of the impact of AIDS on likely enrolments and teacher requirements at various levels of the system over the next 5–10 years. The study may be widely disseminated and used to inform sector policy development and strategic planning in relation to managing the supply and ensuring the quality of education on offer.

In Jamaica, no comprehensive assessment of the current or future impact of HIV and AIDS on the demand for and the supply of education has yet been undertaken. A study investigating the impact of AIDS on the supply of educators and the demand for education (Bailey and McCaw-Binns 2004a), funded by UNESCO, found no evidence of significant mortality among teachers due to AIDS. It was hypothesised that Jamaica teachers may be a relatively low risk group as they are not very mobile, many are married and many are female. In the same study, discriminatory attitudes and practices towards children affected by HIV and AIDS were evident, including negative attitudes of some school personnel. It is therefore not altogether surprising that actions are not being taken to mitigate the impact of AIDS on the education system. Steps have not been taken to improve and accelerate teacher recruitment; review teacher education and training; develop teacher substitution policies or ensure access to treatment and care.

The impact of AIDS on the education sector is omitted from the MOEYC policy. While attention is paid to protecting the rights of children living with HIV and AIDS, there is no mention of orphans and vulnerable children (OVCs).

The situation of orphans and vulnerable children does not appear to be monitored by MOEYC. A comprehensive situational assessment has not been conducted on orphans and vulnerable children including their access to education.

A rapid assessment of the situation of orphans and other children living in households affected by HIV and AIDS was undertaken in 2002 (National AIDS Committee 2003). With regard to education concern was expressed about irregular attendance, particularly among children from poor families. About a third of all secondary school children were reported as taking advantage of government school fees, while two thirds of children participate in school feeding programmes. Impediments to accessing financial relief were reported as in need of study and action.

Ramsey et al. (2004) report that children known to be affected by the virus are greatly disadvantaged as a result of stigma, increasing poverty and social disruption.

A study on the barriers to the integration of HIV and AIDS infected and affected children into the school, system (Bailey and

Bailey 2004b), identified the following issues:

- Negative effects of disclosure due to strong stigmatisation;
- Decline in school performance;
- Increased financial burden of the disease leading to poor diets and irregular attendance at school;
- Orphans being taken into institutional care where there is no provision of education;
- Fears of teachers who were unwilling to share space with affected children;
- Basic school teachers were sometimes poorly informed about HIV and AIDS; and
- Majority view that children living with HIV should be not be taught with the healthy.

There is a lack of a national policy framework to respond to the special needs of increasing numbers of orphaned and other vulnerable children. There is a National Plan for Orphans and Vulnerable Children. The National Plan of Action for Orphans and Other Children Made Vulnerable by HIV and AIDS was developed for the period 2003–2006 (Child Development Agency, MoH). A national Steering Committee on orphans and other children made vulnerable by HIV and AIDS has been established. There is a national OVC focal point within the Child Development Agency, but there is no OVC focal point within MOEYC. It is not clear if there has been a mid-term review of this plan.

Quantitative data on OVCs appear to be lacking in relation to education, possibly a consequence of fear or stigmatisation. Qualitative research provides evidence for OVCs suffering significant disadvantage as a result of stigma, deepening poverty and social disruption. Attention needs to be given to developing a policy-based response to the educational disadvantage being faced by OVCs. The strategies for the education sector in the National Plan of Action for Orphans and Other Children Made Vulnerable by HIV and AIDS were developed prior to the approval of the MOEYC Policy on HIV and AIDS and need to be revisited and updated/revised.

GENDER RESPONSIVENESS

Addressing gender inequalities is going to be critical not only for developing an effective response to HIV and AIDS, but also for the future of educational reform in Jamaica. The MOEYC Policy currently does not explicitly address gender issues. Gender needs to mainstreamed throughout the MOEYC HIV and AIDS response at all levels including HFLE. Institutional capacity needs to be created within the HRT to enable it to undertake gender analysis and monitor programmes from a gender perspective.

MONITORING AND EVALUATION

The need for monitoring and evaluation capacity is a theme throughout this report. Currently this is an area where capacity is conspicuously lacking. It is particularly needed for assessing the effectiveness of HFLE and HIV prevention efforts in general. What is needed is a monitoring and evaluation framework for policy implementation and HRT staff trained in M&E. This would be best addressed through a strategic planning exercise which would identify SMART indicators and institutional capacity needs for the medium term sector programme.

STRATEGIC PLANNING

Implementation of comprehensive policy on HIV and AIDS requires a strategic planning approach for what will be a multi-component set of interventions. In many countries the National AIDS Strategic Plan has preceded the formulation of education sector policy and has contributed to its development. Jamaica is in the mainstream in this regard. The Jamaica HIV/AIDS/STI National Strategic Plan (JHANSP) was developed for the period 2002–2006. It provides the basis for the education sector response.

The lack of a detailed and comprehensive strategic plan for the sector is a major impediment to building a scaled up response. There are numerous initiatives on HIV and AIDS being planned for or already under way in the education sector. These need to be included within a single strategic sector plan for HIV and AIDS to enable co-ordination of effort, coherence of implementation, adequate resource mobilisation, sustainable capacity building and effective monitoring and evaluation.

WHAT IS NOT RELEVANT TO CURRENT NEEDS AND SHOULD BE DROPPED?

No evidence was found of redundant or irrelevant programmes.

AFTERWORD

This is one of the first rapid assessments of the education sector response to HIV and AIDS. Other countries in the Caribbean and elsewhere will undertake their own assessments. It would be useful to enable countries to share experiences including in methodology to strengthen the response at all levels, but particularly in terms of policy, strategic planning, capacity building and monitoring and evaluation.

ANNEX: ANALYTICAL FRAMEWORK

A. POLICY, STRATEGIC PLANNING AND INSTITUTIONAL CAPACITY BUILDING

1. POLICY

1.1 **There is an agreed and publicly disseminated policy framework for HIV and AIDS for the education sector.** The policy has been adopted by the government, is comprehensive and covers the entire education sector. The policy includes issues such as non-discrimination, gender, prevention, orphans and vulnerable children, HIV and AIDS as a workplace issue, HIV prevention education, universal precautions etc. Mechanisms are in place for implementation including accountability structures.

1.2 **The education sector policy on HIV and AIDS is explicitly linked to the National AIDS policy.** The National AIDS Policy has been adopted by the government and includes education in a multi-sectoral approach.

1.3 **There is a workplace policy developed and in use for HIV and AIDS in the education sector compliant with ILO guidance** (ILO 2001). The workplace policy includes HIV and AIDS awareness programmes for all employees at national, district and institution levels. It addresses issues such as stigma and discrimination, sick leave and absenteeism, care and treatment of staff and enforcement of codes of practice. Existing rules, codes of conduct and regulations of the Ministry/Institution have been reviewed and where necessary revised in the light of HIV and AIDS.

2. STRATEGIC PLANNING

2.1 **The Education sector response is a key component of the multi-sectoral National AIDS Plan.** The priority components of the education sector response are fully included in the National AIDS Plan.

2.2 **There is an education action plan/ action framework for addressing HIV and AIDS.** It is linked to policy, detailed, fully costed and included in annual education budgets. It covers the whole education sector. SMART performance indicators have been selected for monitoring implementation.

3. INSTITUTIONAL CAPACITY

3.1 **The HIV and AIDS response is being institutionalised.** At the national level, there is a dedicated committee or management unit that is responsible for co-ordinating the education response to HIV and AIDS. The leadership of the unit is of sufficient seniority to ensure that action takes place. An assessment of the capacity building needs of the unit/Ministry to implement policy and programmes has been undertaken and a training plan developed.

3.2 **The management of the education sector response to HIV and AIDS is being decentralised.** Comprehensive capacity building is taking place and resources are being made available so that the management of the HIV and AIDS response is effectively decentralised.

3.3   Management is data driven and supported. Information about HIV and AIDS in the education sector is being collected, analysed, stored and disseminated. The educational management information (EMIS) system has been adjusted to incorporate HIV and AIDS perspectives and data. It includes HIV and AIDS specific indicators e.g. teacher mortality and attrition data and teacher absenteeism data.

3.4   The HIV and AIDS response is being effectively coordinated throughout the education sector and across sectors. A full time HIV and AIDS focal point, dealing only with HIV and AIDS and related issues, has been appointed in the Ministry of Education and appropriately resourced. Roles and responsibilities have been sufficiently well defined. NAC coordination mechanisms effectively support multi-sectoral action.

4.   RESEARCH AND KNOWLEDGE MANAGEMENT

4.1   Commissioning action/operational research on HIV and AIDS and the education sector is a priority. There is an agreed HIV and AIDS research agenda for the education sector. Research capacity is being developed in universities. Knowledge generated by research informs policy and programme development.

5.   PARTNERSHIPS

5.1   There is a collaborative relationship between the Ministry of Education and International Development partners. Sufficient external funding is available for capacity building and technical assistance. The sources of external funding and technical assistance are clearly mapped out. Coordination among IDPs is effective.

5.2   Civil society partnerships are included in the sectoral response framework. NGOs and CSOs are considered to be important partners. There is partnership with networks of PLHIVs. Funds may be channelled to NGOs, faith-based organisations and other partners outside government.

5.3   Effective linkages have been made with the provision of health services. These services are considered to be 'youth friendly.' Treatment and care are available to education personnel and children.

B. EDUCATION FOR HIV PREVENTION

1.   EVIDENCE OF RISK AND VULNERABILITY

1.1   There is a knowledge base on HIV-related vulnerability and risk of children and young people. Comprehensive knowledge is available and used in planning and for policy formulation. Such knowledge has been subject to rigorous gender analysis. Research been commissioned to inform the education sector response where gaps in knowledge have been identified.

2. VULNERABILITY REDUCTION

2.1   Efforts are being made to maximise participation in good quality education for young people. The achievement of education for all (EFA) is linked to HIV prevention in policy and programmes.

2.2   Efforts are being made to address gender inequality in the education sector. A comprehensive gender analysis of the education sector has taken place. Policies and programmes have been developed to address gender inequalities. Gender is mainstreamed in policy and practice.

2.3   **Efforts are being made to address the vulnerability of education personnel to HIV.** Human resource policies have been reviewed and amended to minimise vulnerability to HIV.

2.4   **Efforts are being made to ensure that schools are safe and healthy places.** Policies and programmes address gender-based harassment and violence. Schools are health promoting.

2.5   **Efforts are being taken to reduce the vulnerability of out-of-school children/youth through non-formal education programmes.** Second chance education opportunities are being offered. Outreach programmes are targeted at highly vulnerable out-of-school children and youth.

3. CURRICULUM DEVELOPMENT

3.1   **Learners are being guided through an appropriate skills-based curriculum on HIV and AIDS at primary, secondary and tertiary levels.** HIV and AIDS are integrated into a wider skills-based health programme. The curriculum content includes safe sex and appropriate behaviours and attitudes to people living with HIV and AIDS. It addresses gender power issues and stigma and discrimination. Life skills and peer education are promoted. An appropriate gender-sensitive curriculum has been developed for all learners and is a required component.

3.2   **The HIV prevention curriculum is consistent with the UNAIDS benchmarks for skills-based health education and the characteristics of effective HIV prevention programmes.** There is a strong emphasis on M&E to assess programme effectiveness.

3.3   **There has been appropriate stakeholder participation in curriculum development (planning, implementation, evaluation and redesign).** There has been an orientation process for parents and community leaders. Young people and PLWHA been directly and consistently involved in the curriculum development process. Partnerships have been developed between the school and the community.

3.4   **The Ministry of Education promotes the use of edutainment for HIV and AIDS education.** The use of media including theatre for development feature in curricular and co-curricular activities.

3.5   **HIV and AIDS are integrated into co-curricular activities.** Co-curricular activities such as sports are used for HIV and AIDS education including prevention and stigma prevention. School clubs include HIV and AIDS related activities including peer education. There are 'Anti AIDS Clubs'.

3.6   **An appropriate HIV and AIDS curriculum has been developed for out-of-school children/youth and is being implemented.** Capacity has been developed for Non Formal Education (NFE) curriculum development, resources are available for materials printing and programme implementation. There is an M&E framework.

4.   TEACHING AND LEARNING MATERIALS

4.1   **Good quality teaching and learning materials have been developed and are in use at all levels in the education system.** Materials suitable for learners in schools and post school institutions been professionally developed. Sufficient materials been distributed to all institutions and their use is monitored. Every teacher and learner has access to these materials.

4.2   Good quality non-formal education materials have been developed and are in use. Teaching and learning materials for HIV and AIDS are provided to out-of-school children/youth. The coverage of these programmes is comprehensive. HIV and AIDS have been incorporated into literacy materials for young people and adults.

5.   TEACHER PREPARATION

5.1   Effective HIV and AIDS educators are being developed. Teacher educators been professionally trained in HIV/AIDS issues and curriculum implementation. School teachers are being adequately prepared through pre-service and in-service training to teach a skills-based approach to HIV prevention.

5.2   HIV and AIDS are being given appropriate priority in initial teacher education. HIV and AIDS and life-skills are integral components in the curriculum for the professional preparation of all new teachers. Materials for teacher education have been developed. Resource centres for HIV and AIDS education are in use in Teacher Training Colleges.

5.3   Guidance on HIV and AIDS is available for all teachers. Guidelines for teachers on HIV and AIDS in schools and all education institutions have been prepared, disseminated and are being implemented. Teachers guides are available to support the implementation of the curriculum

5.4   Teachers are provided with professional support for HIV prevention education. Teacher performance in implementation is supported within the school and by the inspectorate and school principals. Performance is monitored/quality assured.

6.   PARTNERSHIPS

6.1   A multi-sectoral partnership for prevention has been developed. The Ministry of Education is supported by other partners in government such as the Ministry of Health. There is access to 'youth-friendly' health services including for the treatment of sexually transmitted infections (STIs). There are partnerships with civil society to support HIV prevention efforts including faith-based organisations, the private sector and networks of PLHIVs.

C.   MITIGATING THE IMPACT OF AIDS ON THE EDUCATION SECTOR

1.   IMPACT ASSESSMENT AND RESPONSE

1.1   The Ministry of Education has undertaken an AIDS impact study. An assessment been conducted on the likely impact of AIDS on the education sector. Projections have been made of the impact of AIDS on likely enrolments and teacher requirements at various levels of the system over the next 5–10 years. The study has been widely disseminated and used to inform sector policy development and strategic planning in relation to managing the supply and ensuring the quality of education on offer.

1.2   Actions are taken to mitigate the impact of AIDS on the education system. Steps have been taken to improve and accelerate teacher recruitment; review teacher education and training; address stigma and discrimination; develop teacher substitution policies; ensure teachers access to treatment and care.

2. CHILDREN INFECTED WITH HIV AND AFFECTED BY AIDS, ORPHANS AND VULNERABLE CHILDREN

2.1. The situation of orphans and vulnerable children is being monitored. A comprehensive situational assessment has been conducted on orphans and vulnerable children including their access to education.

2.2 There is a national policy framework and plan to respond to the special needs of increasing numbers of orphaned and other vulnerable children. The national plan for orphans and vulnerable children is aligned with the national education sector plan.

2.3 Policies and programmes are being developed to ensure access to education for all, including orphans and vulnerable children. Cost barriers, direct and indirect, to education are being removed. The education system helps maintain attendance at school through cash/food transfers and school health programmes.

2.4 The role of schools to provide care and support to orphans and vulnerable children is being expanded. Children who are affected and infected are being provided with a caring environment/culture of care. Learners who are affected by AIDS find help/counselling from their teachers or from persons other than teachers. Teachers who are dealing with the trauma of children affected by AIDS are getting training and support to cope.

2.5 Schools have adopted policies and practice to protect orphans and other children made vulnerable by HIV and AIDS. Policies and practices have been introduced to address stigma and

discrimination as well as sexual abuse and exploitation.

D. STRONG LEADERSHIP AND COMMITMENT TO ACTION

1.1 There is visible political and professional leadership at all levels to support the education response to HIV/AIDS. Leaders at all levels are knowledgeable and committed to action.

1.2 The Ministry of Education shows leadership and actively communicates that HIV and AIDS is a part of its core business. Ministry publications carry articles on HIV and AIDS. The Ministry/University websites have an appropriate HIV and AIDS webpage. All policy documents include HIV and AIDS.

REFERENCES

Aggleton, P and Parker, R. 2002. A Conceptual Framework and Basis for Action. HIV/AIDS Stigma and Discrimination. UNAIDS. Geneva.

Aggleton, P. Parker, R. Maluwa, M. 2003. Stigma, Discrimination and HIV/AIDS in Latin America and the Caribbean. Sustainable Development Department Technical Papers Series. IDB. Washington. DC.

Bailey, W and McCaw-Binns 2004b. Barriers to integration of HIV/AIDS infected/affected children into the Jamaican School system. University of the West Indies. Mona, Kingston

Bailey, W and McCaw-Binns. 2004a. Is the HIV epidemic affecting the supply of educators and the demand for education in Jamaica? University of the West Indies. Mona, Kingston

Bain. B, 2004. The UWI HIV/AIDS Response Programme. *Caribbean Quarterly*. Vol. 50. No 1. March 2004. pp. 11–14.

Browne, D. 2005. Final report on the HIV/AIDS Textbooks Evaluation. UNESCO/Ministry of Education, Youth and Culture.

CARICOM. 2001. Health and Family Life Education. Empowering Young People with Skills for Healthy Living. UNICEF. Barbados.

Carr-Hill, R. Katabaro, K.J. Katahoire, A.R. and Oulai, D. 2002 The Impact of HIV/AIDS on Education and Institutionalising Preventive Education. UNESCO.IIEP. Paris.

Chambers. C. 2005. The MOEYC HIV/AIDS Team. Preliminary Evaluation of Effectiveness. Final Report.

Chevannes. B. 2001. Learning to Be a Man. Culture, Socialisation and Gender Identity in Five Caribbean Communities. UWI. Mona.

Child Development Agency. 2003. National Plan of Action for Orphans and Other Children made Vulnerable by HIV and AIDS. Kingston.

Commonwealth Youth Project. 1997. Situation Analysis of Caribbean Youth.

Crewe. M and Maritz. J. 2006. Review of the University of the West Indies HIV and AIDS response. In 'Expanding the Field of Enquiry. A Cross Country Study of Higher Education Institutions' Responses to HIV and AIDS'. 2006. UNESCO. Paris.

DFID, WHO/PAHO, GFATM, UNAIDS and World Bank. 2005. HIV/AIDS in the Caribbean Region: A Multi-Organisation Review.

Gayle. H, et al. 2004. The Adolescents of Urban St Catherine. A study of their Reproductive Health and Survivability. UWI. Mona.

Government of Jamaica. 2004. Millennium Development Goals.

Human Rights Watch. 2004. Homophobia, Violence and Jamaica's HIV/AIDS Epidemic. November 2004. Vol.16, No 6 (b)

IFC. 2003. IFC Against AIDS-Partnerships List: Jamaica.

ILO and UNESCO. 2006. An HIV/AIDS Workplace Policy for the Education Sector in the Caribbean. Port of Spain.

ILO. 2001. The ILO Code of Practice on HIV/ AIDS and the World of Work. ILO. Geneva.

Jamaican Association on Mental Retardation (JAMR). 2005. Study of the Knowledge, Values, attitudes and Practice (KVAP) Among Adolescents with Disabilities and their Parents. KVAP Interim Report. EC and UNFPA.

Kelly. M.J and Bain. B. 2003. *Education and HIV/AIDS in the Caribbean*. UNESCO: International Institute for Educational Planning. Paris; Kingston: Ian Randle Publishers.

Ministry of Education, Youth and Culture. 2001. National Policy for HIV/AIDS Management in Schools. Kingston.

Ministry of Health. 2002. Jamaica HIV/AIDS/ STI National Strategic Plan. 2002-2006. Time to Care. Time to Act. Kingston.

Ministry of Health. 2005. National HIV/AIDS Policy. Jamaica. MOH/GFATM. Kingston.

Morrissey. M. 2005. Response of the Education Sector in the Commonwealth Caribbean to the HIV/AIDS Epidemic: A Preliminary overview. ILO. Sector Notes. Geneva.

National AIDS Committee. 2003. A Rapid Assessment of the Situation of Orphans and Other Children Living in Households Affected by HIV and AIDS in Jamaica. Kingston.

Nicholls. S, Mc Lean. R, Theodore. K, Camara. B and team. 2000. Modelling the macroeconomic impact of HIV/AIDS in the English speaking Caribbean: The case of Trinidad, Tobago and Jamaica. CAREC, UWI, PAHO/WHO.

PAHO. 1998. Caribbean Adolescent Health Survey.

Schenker, I. 2004. Caribbean HIV/AIDS Training Package for Teachers. IDB. Kingston.

Task Force on Educational Reform. 2004. Jamaica. A Transformed Education System. Kingston.

UNAIDS IATT and on Education and MTT. 2005. Global HIV/AIDS Readiness Survey. UNESCO/HEARD. Paris.

UNAIDS IATT on Education. 2002. HIV/AIDS and Education. A Strategic Approach.

UNAIDS IATT on Education. 2004. The role of education in the protection, care and support of orphans and vulnerable children living in a world with HIV and AIDS. UNESCO IIEP. Paris.

UNAIDS, UNICEF and USAID. 2004. Children on the Brink. A Joint Report of New Orphan Estimates and a Framework for Action. UNAIDS .Geneva.

UNAIDS. 2000. Guide to the Strategic Planning Process for a national Response to HIV/AIDS. Geneva.

UNAIDS. 2005. Intensifying HIV Prevention. UNAIDS policy position paper.

UNAIDS. 2006. Report on the Global AIDS Epidemic. UNAIDS. Geneva.

UNESCO. 2003. HIV/AIDS and Education. A Toolkit for Ministries of Education. UNESCO Bangkok.

UNICEF and CARICOM. 1997. Children and Youth in the Eastern Caribbean.

UNICEF and UNFPA 2002. Meeting Adolescent Development and Participation Needs. The Findings of Five Research Studies on Adolescents in Jamaica. Kingston.

University of Technology, Jamaica. 2003. HIV/AIDS Policies. Kingston.

USAID. 2004. Jamaica. Country Profile.

UWI. 1998. HFLE Needs Assessment. UWI. Cave Hill.

UWI. 2004. University of the West Indies Policy HIV/AIDS. August 2004.

UWI-HARP. 2004. HIV/AIDS Manual. A Caribbean Perspective. UWI.

Walt, G. 1994. *Health Policy. An Introduction to Process and Power.* Zed Press. London.

Whitman. C.V. 2004. Uniting Three Initiatives on Behalf of Caribbean Youth and Educators: Health and Family Life Education and the Health Promoting School in the Context of PANCAP's Strategic Framework for HIV/AIDS. *Caribbean Quarterly.* Vol. 50. No 1. March 2004. pp 54-83.

World Bank, 2005. Accelerating the Education Sector Response to HIV/AIDS in Africa: A Review of World bank Assistance.

World Bank. 2004. A Sourcebook of HIV/AIDS Prevention Programmes. Washington DC.

World Bank. 2004. The Road to Sustained Growth in Jamaica. Washington. DC.

World Bank. 2005. Country Assistance Strategy. Washington. DC

6

JAMAICA'S NATIONAL POLICY FOR HIV/AIDS MANAGEMENT IN SCHOOLS: A CASE STUDY

PAULINE A. RUSSELL-BROWN

CONSULTANT, UNIVERSITY OF THE WEST INDIES
HIV/AIDS RESPONSE PROGRAMME[1]

Jamaica was the first country in the Caribbean region to develop and approve a policy for the management of HIV and AIDS in schools. The policy, titled National Policy for HIV/AIDS Management in Schools *represents at least three years of effort by the then Ministry of Education, Youth and Culture[2] to provide a framework for school managers, principals, teachers and students to respond to the epidemic in their immediate environment. The process of developing and implementing the policy provides important lessons and insights from which others charged with addressing similar concerns in the education sector can benefit.*

INTRODUCTION

This case study reviews the policy development and implementation processes. Arguably, this case study is premature. Experience suggests that ten years or more is an ideal period for completing at least one cycle of formulation, implementation, and reformulation and to obtain a reasonably accurate portrait of programme success and failure (Sabatier and Jenkins-Smith 1993). This case study is being conducted a mere two years after the policy was approved. It is expected, therefore, that this study will only provide a snapshot of the early years in the life of the policy. But many lessons are yet to be learned.

PROPOSED FRAMEWORK FOR ANALYSIS

Several frameworks and models are available for describing and analysing policy development and implementation. The one selected for this case study is the six 'Ps' of the Policy Circle.[3] The Policy Circle framework was developed for use in the health sector but can be applied in other sectors. Apart from its application to describing the policy process, the Policy Circle framework can also be used to analyse different levels of policy, including national and local policies, and sectoral and operational policies.

Why use this framework and not some other? The Policy Circle framework has at least three advantages. First, it considers the policy process as cyclic rather than linear. The advantage of this conceptualisation is that the analysis process then becomes dynamic, not static, with on-going opportunity for feedback and adjustments. The second advantage of the Policy Circle framework is that it acknowledges the critical role of the political, social, cultural and economic environment and factors in the policy process. The third advantage is that it brings together all the key components and factors that should be considered in policy making. Figure 6.1 depicts the components and seven themes of the policy analysis framework:

- the **Problems** that arise requiring policy attention
- the **Process** of policy making and dissemination
- the **People/Places** involved (policy stakeholders and the institutions where policy gets deliberated and decided and disseminated)
- the **Price Tag** of the policy (the cost of policy options and how resources are allocated)
- the **Paper** produced (actual laws and policies)
- the **Programmes** that result from implementing policies
- their **Performance** in achieving policy goals and objectives.

SOURCE OF DATA FOR THE CASE STUDY

Two sources of data were used for this case study: qualitative interviews with key informants and a review of related research and evaluation reports. Qualitative interviews with a sample of 9 key informants were the main source of data. A copy of the interview guide is attached (Annex). All but two of the interviews were face-to-face interviews.

A key informant was defined as an individual that makes a difference or that can affect or be affected by the achievement of the objectives of the policy. Key informants were selected from the Ministry of Education, Youth and Culture (MoEYC) head office and field staff, the Japanese International Cooperation Agency (JICA), and the donor and technical assistance communities namely, UNESCO, UNICEF and the National HIV/STI Control and Prevention Programme (NHSCPP). Individuals from the NHSCPP

FIGURE **6.1**
THE POLICY CIRCLE

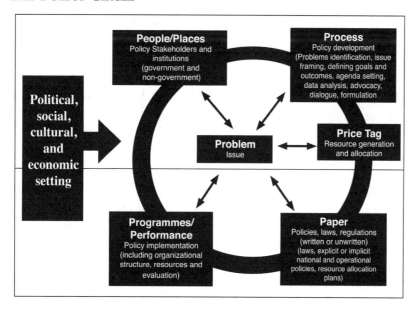

were competent to provide information from the perspectives of the World Bank and Global Fund supported activities.[4]

In addition to the data collected through stakeholder interviews, information was abstracted from two recent studies of the policy process commissioned by the MoEYC and UNESCO. They are:

1. David Clark, 2005. The Response of the Education Sector in Jamaica to HIV and AIDS. Final Report. UNESCO
2. Claudia Chambers, 2005. The MOEYC HIV/AIDS Team. Preliminary Evaluation of Effectiveness. Final Report. UNESCO

THE CASE STUDY

I.   PROBLEM IDENTIFICATION

The first case of AIDS in Jamaica was identified in 1982. Review of the epidemiology of HIV and AIDS indicates that in 2001, when the problem that the policy was designed to address surfaced, an estimated 1.5% of the adult population in Jamaica were living with HIV or AIDS and between 10,000 and 20,000 children were already at risk of losing one or both parents to AIDS. The national HIV/STI Control and Prevention Programme (NHSCPP) of the Ministry of Health reported the following at the end of June 2001.[5]

- HIV/AIDS and Sexually Transmitted Infections (STI) are the second leading cause of death for both men and women in the age group 30–34 years in Jamaica.
- Ten per cent (10%) of all newly reported AIDS cases in Jamaica are in the age group 20–29 years indicating that infection is taking place during early adolescence.
- All 14 parishes are affected by the epidemic, however, St James, Kingston and St Andrew, three of the most urbanised parishes, recorded the highest

number cases of HIV and AIDS. Parishes such as St Catherine (with large urban centres) and St Ann and Hanover (more rural parishes but which contribute significantly to tourism sector activities) showed a very rapid increase in the number of cases of HIV and AIDS in the last year compared to the previous year.

The number of newly reported HIV cases in female adolescents and youth in the age group 15–24 years then was three times higher than for males in the same age group.

These data were cause for concern in both the health and education sectors. Yet, the epidemiology of HIV was not the trigger for the policy process in the Ministry of Education. A school principal faced with the decision whether to deny, or not, entry of a student into school set off the chain of events that resulted in the development of the policy named *National Policy for HIV/ AIDS Management in Schools.*

As a former Deputy Chief Education Officer tells it, action to develop a policy for managing HIV in public schools was predicated on an urgent telephone call she received from a Roman Catholic priest (a school board chairman) in Montego Bay. The problem he faced at the start of the school year 2001 was whether to admit a child with HIV to the institution given the reaction of parents to the rumour that the child's mother had died of an AIDS-related illness.

Given the epidemiological data on HIV, and the knowledge that the trend was for the number of HIV infected children of school-age to increase, the case presented by the school board chairman provided clear evidence of the need for a policy on how to manage HIV in the education sector. Such a policy needed to address, if nothing else, how to manage children with HIV attempting to enter the system as well as students already enrolled in the system. The nature and timing of the request triggered action by the Ministry. Senior managers had the sense that this situation was likely to surface in many more schools in the near future and there needed to be clear guidelines for school administrators.

II. POLICY DEVELOPMENT - SATISFYING THE TECHNICAL AND LEGAL REQUIREMENTS OF THREE SECTORS

Policy formulation can be a lengthy and difficult process. The formulation of the *National Policy for HIV/ AIDS Management in Schools* was no exception. Once the Ministry of Education had decided that a policy for managing HIV in the education sector had to be formulated, a committee was formed to guide and direct the process. The committee comprised individuals from technical, administrative and policy units of the MOEYC as well as individuals from the National HIV/ STI Control and Prevention Programme, the Planning Institute of Jamaica (PIOJ) and the National Family Planning Board (NFPB). The Committee recommended hiring a consultant to develop a first draft of the policy. The fact that the consultant was someone who had worked in the HIV policy arena and was very familiar with the issues in education served to expedite matters. It was also advantageous that the consultant would accept a stipend rather than a consulting fee as there was no specific allocation in the Ministry's budget for the development of an HIV policy.

That done, the Guidance and Counselling Unit of the MoEYC took over responsibility for the process. The head of that unit, who later became the deputy Chief Education Officer, guided the draft policy through a long and 'torturous' review and revision process in the Ministry of Health and the NHSCPP. The most contentious

issues in that phase of the process were (i) how to address requirements for universal precautions in a school setting so as not to draw attention to, stigmatise or appear to discriminate against the student with HIV and (ii) how 'communicable' was to be defined.

Other critical reviews and consultations of the draft policy were conducted with the office of the Attorney General to ensure that, legally, the policy was consistent with the Education Code and other national laws and policies including the Public Health Act. One key informant notes that 'one of the significant challenges of the process at this stage was how to change a technical, essentially medical document, to a legal document with appropriate language and context'.

> A significant challenge of the policy development process: changing a technical, essentially medical document, to a legal document with appropriate language and context.

As shown in Figure 6.2, a revised draft policy document was then submitted to the Senior Management Group in the MoEYC and later to the Education Policy Group for sign off. The MoEYC then prepared a Cabinet Submission and the Chief Parliamentary Counsel was consulted in order to ensure that the main principles were adequately covered. This is consistent with Jamaican legal practice. Laws, national policies and ministerial policies are promulgated at different levels of government. Laws must be passed through the legislature (Parliament) and have legal sanctions for not being followed (Hardee and Subaran 2001). National level policies, such as the *National Policy for HIV/ AIDS Management in Schools*, while promulgated by government Ministries, also go through

FIGURE 6.2
ACTIVITIES AND TIME LINE FOR POLICY DEVELOPMENT: NATIONAL POLICY
FOR HIV/AIDS MANAGEMENT IN SCHOOLS, JAMAICA

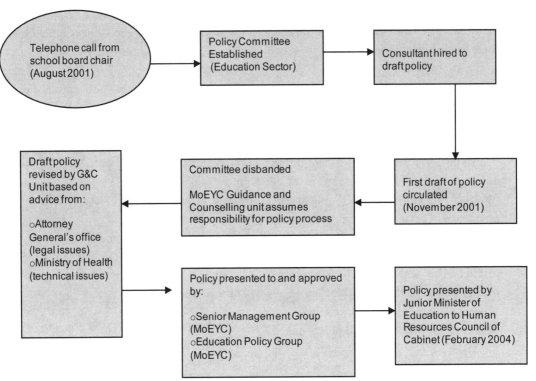

the Cabinet, but do not have the same legal status as laws. They provide the broad vision and framework for the action of the government.

In February 2004, the Junior Minister of Education,[6] presented the draft policy to the Human Resources Council of the Cabinet for its approval. At that stage, a period of some 30 months had elapsed between the problem surfacing and approval of the policy.

While this timeline may appear to be long, in the view of MoEYC key informants the time line for this policy was considerably shorter than for other policies developed by the MoEYC. One key informant attributed the shorter time line to the 'sense of urgency on the part of education to get this done'. This urgency, it was felt, is linked to the need for the ministry to preserve its image as a responsible and responsive agency.

> The shorter than usual interval between development and approval of the policy is attributed to a 'sense of urgency on the part of education to get this done' (Female, Key informant, MoEYC).

III. POLICY STAKEHOLDERS AND INSTITUTIONS

The Policy Circle framework recommends that 'once the problem has been identified, it is vital to understand the people (or stakeholders) who participate in the process of policymaking, the places inside and outside the government that they represent in policymaking ....." (Hardee et al. 2004).

The primary stakeholder institutions engaged in the policy process were the MoEYC, the National HIV/STI Control and Prevention Programme (NHSCPP) in the Ministry of Health, UNESCO, UNICEF, and the Japanese International Cooperation Agency (JICA).

Within the MoEYC, the Guidance and Counselling Unit assumed responsibility for policy formulation and revision and all the steps leading to final approval of the policy by Cabinet. Other key groups of persons in the MoEYC that supported the policy process were the Senior Management Group and the Education Policy Group. This latter group includes senior managers from the education ministry and the Ministers.[7] The NHSCPP provided oversight and guidance in the drafting of the policy and in approving funding from available sources (World Bank and Global Fund) for the development and

implementation of the policy.

At the formulation stage of the *National Policy for HIV/AIDS Management in Schools*, the key stakeholders were individuals from the MoEYC and the NHSCPP. At the MoEYC, the process was guided by the Deputy Chief Education Officer. A senior officer in the Planning Unit of the MoEYC was also a staunch ally. Key stakeholders from the NHSCPP were the Director, and the Policy Technical Officer. There was high level of commitment to the formulation of a policy from MoEYC and NHSCPP personnel. Any delays experienced in the policy formulation and revision processes were not attributed to lack of desire to have a policy in place but rather to differences of opinion on issues like the introduction of universal precaution requirements originally developed for medical settings to an education (school) setting.

FIGURE 6.3
LAWS, NATIONAL POLICIES AND OPERATIONAL POLICIES AND LEVEL OF GOVERNMENT PROMULGATION

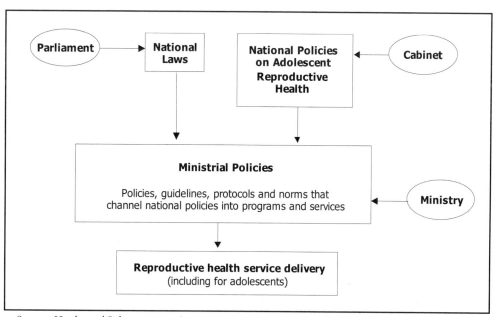

Source: *Hardee and Subaran. 2001. Steps in Passing Laws and Policies in Jamaica.*

Key stakeholders at the policy implementation stage were also affiliated with the MoEYC and included the Association of Secondary School Principals and the Jamaica Teachers Association. Other stakeholders were UNESCO, UNICEF and the Japan Overseas Cooperation Volunteer programme (JOCV) and Jamaica Network of seropositives (JN+). The donor and technical assistance groups were critical to assisting the MoEYC to organise and maintain the HIV/AIDS Response Team (HRT). JN+ was a very supportive partner in the sensitisation workshops conducted for school administrators.

The 8-member HRT is the group of members of staff of the MoEYC dedicated to implementing the policy. As originally conceptualised, the team would comprise a Coordinator, a Public Relations Specialist and six Health Promotion Specialists. The HRT Coordinator's role is to accelerate awareness of schools and ensure schools work to increase HIV awareness and awareness of the policy among teachers and students. Health Promotion Specialists (HPS) are expected to:[8]

- Assist in ensuring adequate and appropriate response and implementation to the HIV/ AIDS reality, coordinating delivery of HFLE with the HIV/ AIDS component in schools, and HFLE implementation and evaluation;
- Liaise with schools and related personnel and other relevant institutions; and
- Provide advice /recommendations on improved delivery of HFLE at classroom level and best practice for field-level implementation.

The importance of stakeholders in the policy process can not be overestimated. In the case of Jamaica, the stakeholders affiliated with the donor and technical assistance organisations shared the desire of the MoEYC and the NHSCPP to develop a *National Policy for HIV/AIDS Management in Schools*. In fact, there was a suggestion at one stage that the MoEYC develop two separate policies – one that addressed the school as a system, another for the school as workplace. Ultimately one policy was developed.

This shared vision and expectation helped to reduce obstacles to policy development. In addition, in the opinion of a key informant from the MoEYC, 'successful policy development and implementation requires persons with integrity, with a vision and drive, a passion and commitment to what is being done, experience with working with the health sector on issues, and a passion for the youth and youth development'.

> ...Successful policy development and implementation requires persons with integrity, with a vision and drive, a passion and commitment to what is being done, experience with working with the health sector and health issues, and a passion for the youth and youth development. (key informant, MoEYC)

IV. THE POLICY

The *National Policy for HIV/AIDS Management in Schools* was approved in November 2004, close to three years after the process was initiated. The goal of the policy, as stated, is to promote effective prevention and care within the context of the educational system. In addition to the six objectives of the policy, the document includes seven Statements of Intent that cover a range of issues – for the child with HIV as well as the teacher with HIV. These Statements are:

1. Non-discrimination and Equality
2. HIV/AIDS Testing, Admission and Appointment
3. Attendance at Institutions by Students with HIV/AIDS
4. Disclosure and Confidentiality
5. Education on HIV/AIDS
6. A Safe Environment
7. Prevention Measures Related to Play and Sport
8. Refusal to Study with or Teach a Student with HIV/AIDS or to Work with or be Taught by an Educator with HIV/AIDS

All these are presented in the context of the legal and policy frameworks.

The strength/ benefit of having the policy is that it provides, for the first time, a written statement of intent and for professional behaviour of teachers regarding the management of HIV in schools. School managers and teachers have something to guide school management behaviours. It also provides or helps create a structure within which to increase awareness of HIV and AIDS and ensure that staff and students are guided to become engaged in discussions about stigma and discrimination.

The view expressed by one of the key informants from the MoEYC is that the policy challenges public schools to:

• Ensure the inclusion of HFLE in the curriculum;
• Address fears and ignorance of the school management;
• Positively influence community attitudes; and
• Manage competing demands for time (100 days are available in the school year).

At the same time, the challenge to the independent schools is to balance the rights of the HIV-positive student to education and the need of the institution to survive financially.

The policy has been criticised by some for not being sufficiently comprehensive. Among the shortcomings identified are that it does not address / provide penalties for individuals who discriminate against or stigmatise persons living with HIV. Other criticisms are that the policy does not accommodate the treatment of students and teachers living with HIV nor does it explicitly address the issue of homosexuality.

One major limitation of the policy acknowledged by all key informants from the MoEYC is that it is limited to government-run and controlled schools. Independent schools are not required to apply the policy. Under the existing education policy, the MoEYC can use persuasion to get independent schools to apply the policy. What actions have been taken to address this limitation? Through the efforts of the policy advocate in the National HIV/STI Control and Prevention Programme, resources have been allocated to conduct parallel interventions in and with independent schools to enable them to get on board with the policy. These interventions include sensitisation and training for school administrators and dissemination of the policy.

Hindsight is fifty-fifty. The timing of the development of the policy and the nature of the problem that triggered its development influenced the focus given to the problem. That focus was on public primary and higher educational institutions. It was not focused on early childhood educational institutions. In essence, the policy had not adequately taken account of the fact that even as prevention of Mother-to-Child Transmission (MTCT) programmes and antiretroviral (ARV) treatment programmes become institutionalised, the number of HIV infected children surviving will increase creating a new challenge for the early childhood institutions.[9]

Another perceived gap in the policy relates to sanctions for non-compliance. There are those who feel that the policy needs to be explicit regarding sanctions for those who do not implement the policy. One key informant questioned whether this is the role of policies and indicated that the MoEYC stakeholders remind implementers that the policy is not an isolated document and the process is not an isolated initiative. Rather, the policy and its implementation are linked to an existing legal instrument – the Education Code – under which education services are provided in Jamaica. It is within that code that sanctions can be imposed on public educational institutions that do not implement the new management of HIV in school policy. The situation for the independent schools is different. The legal instrument within which the new policy could be located is the Independent School's Act.

The matter of confidentiality is another gap identified in the policy. The current policy speaks to the 'best interest of the child'. Within that framework the parent would disclose to the Principal and at least one other person who works directly with the child. The Guidance Counsellor or teacher should be provided with the parent's telephone number. This language 'best interest of the child' is consistent with the Child Care and Protection Act (2004) which emphasises that the interest of the child should always be taken into account. The Act in section 2 (2) provides guidance on what is 'the best interests of the child' (The Child Care and Protection Act 2004). The following are six of the eight factors that the professionals should take into account in determining the child's best interest:

- the safety of the child;
- the child's physical and emotional needs

and level of development;
- the importance of continuity of care;
- the child's religious and spiritual views;
- the child's level of education and educational requirements; and
- the effect on the child of a delay in making a decision.

Even as this case study is being written, there is talk of revising the policy. The MoEYC key informants point to the section of the policy that states 'It will be reviewed within a five year period to take into account....'

What is driving the call for revision? First is the changing health scene. Between 2001 when the need for the policy was identified and the present, the medical management of HIV has changed. In addition, issues not evident at that time are now central to the response to HIV. Two of these medical/ health issues are ARV treatment and voluntary counselling and testing (VCT). The second factor driving the call for policy revision is the need to address issues critical to HIV prevention. It is felt, for example, that a new policy may:

- Force the MoEYC to take a position on condom distribution in schools. In this matter the MoEYC has to be guided by the Attorney General
- Further strengthen the implementation of HFLE through specific guidance given to the deployment of teachers and time tabling
- Provide clearer direction to the implementation of HFLE especially at the early childhood level
- Address the management of HIV and AIDS in early childhood educational institutions.

v. POLICY IMPLEMENTATION

The *Programmes* that result from

implementing policies and their *Performance* in achieving policy goals and objectives represent implementation of the policy.

National level policies, such as the *National Policy for HIV/ AIDS Management in Schools*, while promulgated by government Ministries, do not have the same legal status as a law. They merely provide the broad vision and framework for the action of governments. To succeed, the national policies that do not become law must be translated into programmes to achieve the goals set out at the national level. Moving from national policies to local programmes requires the design and implementation of ministerial policies, guidelines, and protocols that channel national laws and policies into programmes and services.

The MoEYC, through a series of internal consultations in combination with imperatives of funding agencies, devised a plan to implement the *National Policy for HIV/ AIDS Management in Schools*. The plan revolved around three components: (1) Sensitisation of school managers and managements; (2) Development of a 'Plan of Action' by individual schools; and (3) Implementation of that 'Plan of Action'. Funding support for the ministry's plan came from multiple sources: The World Bank project in Jamaica, UNESCO and the Global Fund to fight AIDS, Tuberculosis and Malaria, the last through Jamaica's Country Co-ordinating Mechanism for HIV/AIDS Response.

Responsibility for policy implementation was assigned to the HIV/AIDS Response Team (HRT). The team was introduced in September 2003. The size of the team at that time was one Coordinator and four Health Promotion Specialists (HPS). In the period since 2003, the size and composition of the team has changed. A Public Relations Specialist was added to the team and two additional HPS are on board to bring that total to eight persons.

The HRT was further supported by six JICA/JOVC volunteers in the policy implementation effort. Volunteers are assigned to work with the HPS. Their specific roles are to provide administrative and technological support to the HPS and to the policy implementation programme generally. It was observed by two of the key informants that the volunteers could have been more involved in the technical aspects of policy implementation. Language difficulties may have limited the extent to which volunteers were used in the programme.

OPERATIONALISING THE IMPLEMENTATION PLAN

1) SENSITISATION OF SCHOOL MANAGERS AND MANAGEMENTS

The HRT organised a series of one-day sensitisation workshops in all six regions served by the MoEYC. The purpose of the workshops was two-fold:

- Sensitise and increase awareness about HIV and AIDS and related issues; and
- Increase awareness about the new policy – the interpretation, meaning, implementation, principles, and how the policy affects individuals.

Secondary schools were primary targets for the first workshops. Primary schools were targeted in a second tier. Ten schools were invited to participate in each workshop. Persons invited to the workshops included the principal, school board chairs, guidance counsellors and school nurses, teachers and representatives of parent teachers' associations.

HRT members used a range of methodologies to achieve the workshop objectives. Formal presentations with discussions were combined with role and real play and dramatisation of scenarios likely to be encountered in the school situation. Each workshop was supported by print material – the policy, posters and other special information, education and communication (IEC) materials.

2) DEVELOPMENT OF A PLAN OF ACTION BY INDIVIDUAL SCHOOL SYSTEMS

Following a workshop, the Health Promotion Specialist (HPS) for the respective region would get commitment from the individual school to form a health advisory committee. This committee is a representative body that includes the Principal, PTA representative, a person with HIV, school nurse or guidance counsellor. This group is tasked with developing an action plan for the school to achieve three strategic objectives: (1) implementation of a life skills-based HFLE programme (2) sensitisation of the school community around HIV in general and the policy in particular (3) universal precautions.

The rate of developing Plans of Action for schools has been uneven. It is observed that where principals are well-informed about HIV and have experience with the issue in other contexts (for example through their churches or community organisations, etc.) the action plan development process progresses reasonably quickly. On the other hand, in schools where the level of awareness about HIV and AIDS among the principal, especially, is low, the HPS needs to spend a longer time doing the sensitisation and awareness raising. The Plan of Action development in those situations moves less quickly.

3) IMPLEMENTATION OF PLANS OF

ACTION

Information on the implementation of Plans of Action by schools is spotty. Recongising the need for monitoring and evaluation (M&E) of the policy and its implementation, the MoEYC has hired an M&E expert. The evaluator is responsible to design M&E indicators, methods and a plan to measure the process, degree and quality of change after implementation of life skills-based HFLE. The evaluator works closely with the HRT to develop the plan and reports to the Chair of the CARICOM HFLE advisory Committee within the MoEYC.

EFFECTS OF THE IMPLEMENTATION PLAN

It is too early in the policy implementation process for the MoEYC to evaluate whether the policy goals and objectives have been achieved. As indicated, the evaluator is on board and in the process of designing and implementing the monitoring and evaluation plan. There is evidence, however, of successes in implementing the sensitisation and awareness programme. As reported by key informants, to date:

- 80% of primary and secondary schools have been reached by the HRT sensitisation efforts. At the time of reporting, this represented 1000 public sector primary and secondary schools. Schools have embraced the policy.[10]

- Independent schools are now on board and important alliances have been formed between MoEYC and the independent schools. How did this happen? Through the intervention of the Advocacy Specialist in the NHSCPP in the MoH, support and funding were made available through the Global Fund to reach out to independent schools. In addition, through the Pan American Health Organisation (PAHO), 250 independent schools have been provided with first aid kits.

Several of the key informants interviewed are of the view that 'Leadership' is the reason for success in implementation, where it is observed. They report too that, where the school principal has an interest in HIV and related issues, there is an increased likelihood that the school will attend the workshop and will prepare and implement an action plan. Where the school already has an existing related programme, the chance of successful policy implementation is enhanced.

Strong leadership, especially among principals, is the key to successful policy implementation.

Not all principals attended the workshops when invited. Principals were not interviewed in this study, but reports from the HRT are that principals have other demands on their time. They are therefore not always available to attend activities that are not mandatory. They will, however, send an alternate who could be the vice-principal or a senior teacher. Given the importance of principals to the success of implementing the *National Policy for HIV/AIDS Management in Schools*, the MoEYC should make special focused efforts to engage those who do not or are unable to attend workshops. Principals could be reached at meetings of their professional organisations or through their peers to ensure that they all buy into the policy and the MoEYC's plans to implement it.

There is a standard implementation model that schools are encouraged to follow – namely develop and implement plans of action. However, each school is different. They are managed differently and a standard implementation model may not be appropriate for all schools. Further, having a

standard implementation model may not be appropriate because schools are at different stages on the HIV awareness and response continuum. In this context, greater success may be achieved if each school in given the autonomy to decide how to implement its plan of action. Adopting this open approach to policy implementation will challenge the Ministry's ability to supervise the process and it may make evaluation of the process of implementing the policy difficult. However, in the long term it may enable better results.

The process adopted by Jamaica to support policy implementation through creating awareness among schools has had its share of challenges. Analysis of the key informant data suggests that the challenges include:

- Difficulty managing the post-workshop process. Schools require ongoing visits and support to develop and implement their action plans. Schools need assistance and often turn to the MoEYC and MoH for resource persons. Six HPS is not enough to efficiently and effectively reach all schools in the public sector. The MoEYC is challenged to find creative and cost effective ways of solving this problem.
- Schools do not always cooperate in as timely a manner as required. They prepare their action plans but do not take it to the next level. The guidance counsellor who in many cases is the person responsible for implementing the plan of action is not always able or capable to move the process.
- The structure and composition of the HRT does not lend itself to easy coordination with the establishment – for example, coordination between HPS and MoEYC officers, guidance officers at parish and regional level. Special efforts are required to ensure that the parish and

region are aware of the inputs of HPS and vice versa.

- Getting the commitment from administrators (principals) is one of the greatest challenges. The issue of HIV is not always internalised and without a principal's support it is not possible to assure that implementation will take place. One needs to use the Principals association as an entry point – using the venue to conduct workshops and use the policy to work through the issues. The presence of this challenge raises the question of whether principals and their association should have been engaged earlier in the policy process. That may have created another set of stakeholders – individuals who could make a positive difference to the implementation process.

VI. RESOURCE ALLOCATION

The *Price Tag* of the policy - that is the cost of policy options and how resources are allocated.

'Without access to the resources we have had, the Ministry could have developed the policy but its implementation may have been handled differently and may have been less successful' (Female informant, MoEYC).

It was not possible to get a complete costing of the policy development and implementation process. What is clear, however, is that the MoEYC benefited from financial and human resource support that enabled the drafting, finalising, printing and dissemination of the policy document. There was also financial and other support for the development and implementation of the national programme to sensitise school managers, teachers and communities about HIV and the policy and ease implementation of the policy. Support from UNICEF and

UNESCO, and from the World Bank and Global Fund was critical in these areas.

Initially, salary support for the Coordinator of the HRT was provided through the UNICEF country programme. The MoEYC has subsequently picked up this position. The HPS were initially supported through UNESCO. The World Bank and Global Fund have also provided salary support. UNESCO funds have been committed to training, building capacity and material development, in supporting policy implementation at the field level through the JICA, and in convening management retreats designed to bring the hierarchy of the MoEYC on board. Negotiations are continuing with UNESCO and the UNESCO Japanese funds should soon be starting a new implementation phase.

As sector partner in the national HIV/AIDS response team, the MoEYC is a beneficiary and recipient of funds under the Global Fund. Through the Fund, support was available to the Ministry to develop a HFLE curriculum for early childhood institutions, and to revise the HFLE primary and secondary scope and sequence and curricula. At the time of writing, the new early childhood and secondary curricula and the primary scope and sequence have been pilot tested. A report on the pilot is being prepared. Modification of the curricula and scope of sequence is the next stage and should be completed in 2007.

Parallel support for the sensitisation of principals and functionaries in the independent schools system, thought to be outside of the direct control of the policy, was contributed by the NHSCPP.

Development and implementation of the *National Policy for HIV/AIDS Management in Schools* took place in a relatively resource rich environment. As resources become limited, MoEYC will need to find ways of maintaining/institutionalising the mechanism in place for implementing the policy. As indicated, the MoEYC has absorbed the post of the Coordinator of the HRT. However, the HPS posts are paid from special project funds. Conversations are now in train with the NHSCPP to negotiate salaries for the HPS. It is likely that the NHSCPP will support three of the six posts. The other three positions may be re-classified in the Education officer scale and aligned as Guidance Officers.

VII. THE POLITICAL, SOCIAL, CULTURAL AND ECONOMIC CONTEXT

Policymaking takes place within greatly varying settings. Countries have different political systems and forms of government, in addition to various economic systems and levels of development. In Jamaica, policy development linked to HIV and AIDS is identified as a priority area for the National Strategic Plan (NSP). A sub-objective of the plan is 'to foster the development of a policy and legal framework protective of the human rights of persons living with and affected by the HIV epidemic'.[11] Policy development is the responsibility of the partners identified in the NSP. Five key public sector ministries (line ministries), selected private sector organisations (including the Private Sector Organisation of Jamaica) and several NGOs have been involved in drafting policies and policy guidelines since 2002. The NHSCPP in the MoH provides technical and material support[12] for policy implementation in the line ministries.

In a 2005 review of the national programme,[13] it was observed that some 20 large private organisations, 11 government ministries and 50 educational institutions were in the process of either adopting or implementing policies to address HIV/AIDS (Russell-Brown 2005).

This is the environment in which the *National Policy for HIV/AIDS Management in Schools*, approved in January 2004 by the MoEYC was developed. The evidence that the drafting of policies has proceeded apace since 2002 is compelling. See Box 6.1 for a list of selected policies approved in Jamaica 2002–2004.

In the wider society, the policy is benefiting from a growing recognition of HIV as an education issue and not only a health issue. The adoption of a multi-sectoral response to HIV by the Government of Jamaica and the participation of the Ministry of Education as a key partner in the implementation of the NSP (2002–2006) have contributed to this shift. In the interim, with important financial and stakeholder support, the thrust for introducing Health and Family Life Education (HFLE) into primary and secondary schools has gained momentum. It is now proposed to make HFLE an examinable subject in the regional Caribbean Examination Council (CXC). It is argued that the fact that HFLE is not examinable has contributed to it not being taught or not being taught well.

The donor community is also very supportive, as evidenced in funding for the implementation of the policy, as is the University of the West Indies. The Joint Board of Teacher Education at the UWI, Mona campus, is supporting HIV at the teacher college/ training institutions. Since 2000 the University of the West Indies (UWI) has made tangible strides to strengthen the university's response to HIV and AIDS. The UWI, in 2001, established a focal point for UWI's liaison with CARICOM for implementing their response. Out of this initiative came the UWI HIV/AIDS Response Programme (UWI HARP) which operates on the three campuses of the university (Russell-Brown

2005). More recently, with support from UNESCO, UWI has established a Chair for HIV on the St. Augustine campus.

Compared to the early years of the epidemic, the HIV/ AIDS Response in Jamaica is currently well-resourced. Data from the MoH indicate that in 2003, funding for the NSP was at an all time high with HIV/AIDS funding constituting more than 80% of the GOJ's health projects budget. The majority of funding comes from 3 sources: a loan (2002–2007) from the World Bank, a grant (2004–2008) from the Global Fund to Fight AIDS, TB and Malaria (GFATM) and US$5 million in support (1999–2003) from USAID. A proportion of the US$8 million budget of the Jamaica Adolescent Reproductive Health project (USAID) was also directed to HIV/AIDS education, services and research with adolescents. USAID recently finalised a new HIV/AIDS strategy for the period 2005-2009 with an expected budget of US$6.5 million. In addition to funds available through the NHSCPP, some line ministries, like the MoEYC, receive funding from other sources like CIDA, UNESCO and UNICEF.

Financial and technical resources are being applied to policy development, as well as to policy implementation where stronger and visible advocacy is required. To support the process, a policy officer position has been established within the NHSCPP that is now geared to measure performance of its advocacy and policy efforts using the AIDS Program Effort Index (API). The

Box 6.1
Selected HIV/AIDS Policies formulated and approved in Jamaica 2002-2004

- o Guidelines to improve access to contraceptives to minors approved by Cabinet in September 2003. (Policy Working Group (PWG) convened by the Youth.now project).
- o *National Policy for HIV/AIDS Management in Schools* approved in January 2004. (Ministry of Education, Youth and Culture)
- o National HIV/AIDS Policy – approved by Human Resources Council (HRC) in October 2004 and is awaiting Cabinet approval. (Ministry of Health)
- o National Workplace Policy on HIV/AIDS – was reviewed by Human Resources Council in October 2004 and is awaiting final approval pending revisions requested by the HRC. (Ministry of Labour and Social Security).
- o Tourism Policy Guidelines on HIV/AIDS, 2002. (Ministry of Tourism)
- o Draft HIV/AIDS Policy of the Ministry of National Security regarding HIV/AIDS in the Workplace, 2003. (Ministry of National Security).
- o Draft of the Workplace Policy Document on HIV/AIDS, 2004. (Ministry of Local Government, Community Development and Sports.
- o Draft guidelines for the treatment of STIs and HIV/AIDS for adolescents prepared. (Policy Working Group (PWG) convened by the Youth.now project).
- o Several sector policies and workplace policies which have been drafted; a national policy on HIV/AIDS has been prepared and accepted by Cabinet for submission to Parliament.

methodology for this effort is for periodic (every 2 years) collection of data from a defined sample of knowledgeable individuals from all sectors associated with the NSP. The key informants will be asked opinions about progress in several areas of HIV and AIDS programming. This index is the average score given to the national programme, and its components, by a defined group of knowledgeable individuals.

One expects that the education sector and its response to HIV and AIDS will be one of the areas of programming that will be included in these periodic surveys. The API is one way of validating monitoring and evaluation data collected by the M&E officer. The MoEY, therefore, is well placed to benefit from and contribute to the process.

One observes that the social environment in 2004 when the policy was approved was significantly less hostile on the issue of HIV and persons with HIV. The process of community education about HIV and AIDS that had been undertaken first by the MoH and NGOs, and in more recent years by all sectors, including MoEYC, is serving to increase knowledge about HIV and AIDS and reduce negative attitudes towards persons with HIV. The 2004 KABP survey found that 60% of men surveyed and 66% of women would agree to have a teacher with HIV continue teaching. Some 60% of respondents in that same survey would not want a family member's HIV status to be kept a secret (Hope Enterprises 2005). In this social environment, the current policy should have a better chance of success than if it were implemented 10 years earlier.

LESSONS LEARNED

The interval between approval of the *National Policy for HIV/ AIDS Management in Schools* and this case study is a mere 4

years and six months. It is too early in the process, therefore, to support or refute Stover and Johnston's (1999) conclusion that, 'A supportive policy environment is crucial to the implementation of successful programs that prevent the spread of HIV, deliver care to those infected, and mitigate the impacts of the epidemic.' Interviews with key informants for this review provide evidence of important lessons that can be learned from the Jamaica experience.

- The *National Policy for HIV/ AIDS Management in Schools* is not a perfect document. The key players in the MoEYC are aware that it has gaps and that it does not address some important issues. However, making changes to an existing policy at this time is not the best approach. In the opinion of many of the key informants one should allow the process to continue a while longer before modifying the policy.

- Successful policy formulation requires having 'persons of integrity, with a vision and drive, a passion and commitment for what is being done, experience with working with MoH and health issues, and a passion for young persons'. These are the thoughts of one of the key informants. The MoEYC was fortunate to have more than one person with these qualities.

- Access to financial and human resources can facilitate the process of policy implementation. There is no question that the relatively resource-rich environment of the first five years of the new century (2000–2005) significantly enhance the Ministry's chances to develop and implement the policy. The MoEYC was enabled during the period to also develop and test new HFLE curricula that can be introduced by schools to fulfil the requirement under their plans of action.

- It is important to identify one committed, credible, senior individual within the organisation who is knowledgeable about the policy approval system as the person responsible for moving the policy forward. The former Deputy Chief Education Officer played that role.

- Committed stakeholders in the donor and technical assistance communities/ organisations who share the vision of the organisation and understand its goals are a vital factor to accessing the resources needed to implement the policy. In the case of Jamaica, as the MoEYC was moving forward with developing the policy, the NSP for Jamaica's response to HIV and AIDS was being introduced. The NSP called for a multisectoral response to HIV and AIDS and for the first time shifted the responsibility for responding to the epidemic from the health sector to other sectors. Education was one of the key sectors named in the NSP.

- While a broad and comprehensive consultative process may be important to assuring that the policy addresses all the issues, it also is time and labour intensive. One of the key stakeholders – principals and principals associations – was not engaged in the policy formulation process. Implementation of the policy may have been made significantly easier if principals were engaged earlier in the process. The trade off is the increased time needed to get the policy through to approval.

ANNEX: INTERVIEW GUIDE - HIV POLICY IN SCHOOL - JAMAICA CASE STUDY

Name:

Position:

Role in the policy process?

Factor(s) delaying, enabling, maintaining the policy process? One key factor? Other factors?

Phases of Policy Making	Start date	End Date	Opinion on time: Longer than expected, shorter than expected, about the time expected
Conceptualisation			
Drafting			
Revisions Approval			
Approval			
Dissemination			
Implementation			
Evaluation			

Most difficult aspect of the process? Reasons?

Aspect of the process that was easiest? Reasons?

Most challenging aspect of your work on the policy? What made it challenging?

Perceived benefit(s) of the policy? For whom?

Perceived gaps in the policy? Are there gaps? What are they? How should gaps be addressed?

Resources needed to move the process? Source of resources?

REFERENCES

Ainsworth, M, Beyrer C, and Soucat A. 2003. AIDS and Public Policy: The Lessons and Challenges of "success" in Thailand" Health Policy 64(1): 13–37.

Chambers, Claudia. 2005. The MOEYC HIV/AIDS Team. Preliminary Evaluation of Effectiveness. Final Report. UNESCO.

Clark, David. 2005. The Response of the Education Sector in Jamaica to HIV and AIDS. Final Report. UNESCO

Government of Jamaica. The Child Care and Protection Act (2004). Child Development Agency. Ministry of Health.

Hardee, Karen and Subaran. Sonia. 2001. Steps to passing laws and policies in Jamaica. Kingston. Jamaica: Youth.now ARH Project, Futures Group.

Hope Enterprises. 2005. HIV /AIDS Knowledge, Attitudes, Beliefs and Practices Survey. Ministry of Health. Kingston.

ILO/ UNESCO. 2006. An HIV/ AIDS Workplace policy for the education sector in the Caribbean. International Labour Organization.

Ministry of Education, Youth and Culture. 2001. National HIV/AIDS Management in Schools, November 2001.

Ministry of Health. 2005. National HIV/AIDS Policy, Jamaica. May 2005.

Russell-Brown, PA. 2005. An Assessment. The National HIV/STI Control and Prevention Programme (Jamaica). Prepared for Caribbean Health Research Council under the Project: "Strengthening the Institutional Response to HIV/AIDS/ STIs in the Caribbean (SIRHASC). Project Managed by CARICOM. European Union.

Russell-Brown, Pauline A. 2005. Cric? Crac! UWI HARP .... The Story: Based on documentary evidence, reflections of key programme personnel and interviews with students at Mona. UWI HIV/AIDS Response Programme: Mona.

Stover, John and Johnson, N. 1999. The art of policy formulation: Experiences from Africa in developing national HIV/AIDS policies. POLICY Occasional paper No 3. Washington, DC: POLICY Project.

Sabatier, P. and Jenkins-Smith, H. 1993. Policy Change and Learning: An Advocacy Coalition Approach. Boulder, CO: Westview Press, Inc.

NOTES

1. UWI HARP is implementing partner, with Education Development Centre, for the CARICOM Caribbean Education Sector HIV and AIDS Capacity-Building Programme.

2. The change of leadership in 2006 led to the reassignment of the Culture portfolio. The Ministry is now Ministry of Education and Youth. This change is not likely to influence the policy implementation process in any way.

3. The Policy Circle: A framework for analyzing the components of family planning, reproductive health, maternal health and HIV/AIDS policies was developed by Futures Group in collaboration with Research Triangle Institute, the Centre for Development and Population Activities under the POLICY Project.

4. Key Informants Interviewed : Ms Jenelle Babb, Public Relations Specialist, HRT, MoEYC., Ms Gillian Bernard, Sector and Community Response HIV Prevention Coordinator (Global Fund Support), Ms Lovette Byfield, MoH NHSCPP (World Bank Support), Dr. Deloris Brissett, Deputy Chief Education Officer. Curriculum and Support Services (ret), Ms Faith Hamer, Policy Technical Officer, NHSCPP (Global Fund Support), Ms Penny Campbell, Programme Officer, UNICEF, Mr Christopher Graham, Coordinator, HIV/AIDS Response Team, Ms Mavis Fuller, Ministry of Education, NSP, and Mr Michael Morrissey, Consultant, UNESCO.

5. National HIV/STD Control and Prevention Program Facts and Figures January-June 2001. Ministry of Health.

6. The Ministry of Education is assigned two parliamentary representatives.

7. Two Ministers are assigned to the MoEYC. Both are members of the Education Policy Group.

8. Summary of Health Promotion Specialists' Terms of Reference.

9. In January–June 2004, there were 40 children under the age of ten years newly reported with AIDS compared to 22 children in the previous year. However there were fewer Paediatric AIDS death (18) compared

to 29 AIDS death from the previous year. This is also attributable to the improvement in care and treatment for HIV-positive children and decrease in Mother to Child Transmission of HIV.

10. Personal communication, July 8, 2006.

11. Jamaica HIV/AIDS/STI National Strategic Plan 2002–2006, pg. 19.

12. National AIDS Committee. HIV/ AIDS Workplace Policy Toolkit.

13. An Assessment. The National HIV/ STI Control and Prevention Programme (Jamaica) Prepared for Caribbean Health Research Council. Prepared under the Project: 'Strengthening the Institutional Response to HIV/AIDS/ STIs in the Caribbean (SIRHASC)'. Project Managed by CARICOM.

7

Barriers to Integration of HIV and AIDS infected/affected Children into the Jamaican School System

**Wilma Bailey and
Affette McCaw-Binns**

University of the West Indies, Mona

Programmes aimed at secondary prevention of HIV/AIDS will increase the population of persons living with HIV/AIDS. Information, through focus group discussions with teachers, community members and parents, was gathered in 2004 on the readiness of the education sector to accept children affected by the epidemic – those who were either infected with the virus as well as the healthy offspring of HIV-positive parents. Parents and guardians of HIV affected children expressed reluctance to disclose their status (if the parent was HIV positive) or that of the child (if the child was infected) for fear of stigma, even to close relatives, as ignorance regarding the disease was still the order of the day. This was supported by the views expressed by some teachers that 'they should be quarantined.' In communities exposed to persons living with HIV/AIDS, both school personnel and community members were more supportive and positive toward having the HIV affected child in the classroom. Where this experience was lacking however, there were very negative attitudes and an unwillingness to share the same space. Parents reported that non-infected offspring were denied an education when teachers knew of the parents' status, necessitating the move of children to other schools. Financial constraints were also significant as the cost of medication and special diets conflicted with the needs of other family members for simple things such as bus fare and lunch money. The mental health of these children was also compromised as they knew something was wrong, but often they were not told what the problem was, and parents felt that this affected their academic performance. Parents also felt that the disease affected the academic performance of infected children.

INTRODUCTION

At the end of 2003, it was estimated that there were between 410,000 and 720,000 adults living with HIV/AIDS in the Caribbean and prevalence ranged from just over 1 per cent to almost 6 per cent in the region (UNAIDS 2004). Jamaica was estimated to have a rate of less than 2 per cent. This prevalence made the Caribbean the second most affected region after sub-Saharan Africa. The majority of those affected were adults between the ages of 15 and 45 years but the disease is taking an increasing toll on young children. Roughly 22,000 children were estimated to be infected in 2003 (UNAIDS). However, as the epidemic begins to claim more young adult women in the Caribbean and assume the pattern that now obtains in sub-Saharan Africa, it is expected that more children will be affected, with some becoming infected and others made vulnerable through orphaning and the social and economic impoverishment of AIDS-affected households.

At the same time, although the numbers are still quite small, an increasing number of HIV-positive children in Jamaica are having access to antiretroviral therapy. This means that the children are going to live longer and many will live to school age. Public schools must, therefore be prepared for the enrolment of increasing numbers of HIV-positive children as well as those living in households affected by the virus. The society must also be sensitised to those factors operating within HIV/AIDS affected households that may rob these children of the basic right to education and the means of ensuring a productive future.

This study investigates the barriers to the integration of HIV/AIDS infected/affected children into the Jamaican school system. Specifically, it examines the problems encountered by parents and guardians in their efforts to secure places for their children in the public school system and the readiness of the education sector to accept these children into the learning environment.

BACKGROUND

In a policy statement, the Committee on Pediatrics of the American Academy of Pediatrics, stated that asymptomatic children with HIV virus infection cannot be distinguished from those without and should have the same educational opportunities (Pediatrics 2000). They should neither be excluded nor isolated within the school setting. There are no documented instances of the spread of the infection in schools and no basis for the fears of such an occurrence by school personnel. If infected children are to be integrated into the school system efforts must be made to allay these fears by the appropriate education and create a receptive environment. The right of all children to a primary education is upheld by the United Nations Convention on the Rights of Children and reaffirmed at the Millennium Summit in 2000. By creating opportunities and choices, education provides opportunities and this is particularly important for those children who find themselves in difficult circumstances. The education sector must be in the forefront of those offering support and services to the affected.

The Ministry of Education, Youth and Culture in Jamaica has responded to the need for clear guidelines for schools to develop and institute HIV/AIDS action plans (Ministry of Education 2004) and, in the main, the National Policy echoes the sentiments of the international community. HIV-positive students are expected to attend classes as long as they are able and disclosure of status is not compulsory. Policy statements of this sort become necessary because there is a widespread perception that children known to be affected by the virus are greatly disadvantaged as a result of stigma, increasing poverty and social disruption. (Ramsay et al., 2004). These factors are creating barriers to education and therefore to the development of the full potential of persons living with HIV and AIDS (PLWHA). These barriers need to be understood if HIV affected children are to be fully integrated into the education system.

METHODOLOGY

Two groups of children are affected by the HIV/AIDS epidemic. There are the relatively small numbers who are infected with the HIV virus, and there are the HIV-negative children of infected parents. In both groups some are orphans, already having lost one or both parents.

Group interviews were employed to gather data from the two groups of parents and guardians. The study design envisaged the selection of purposive samples comprising nine parents/guardians of infected children and nine infected parents. However, in spite of the assistance of The Centre for HIV/AIDS Research, Education and Services (CHARES) an organisation which provides care and support to persons living with and affected by HIV, and despite assurances of anonymity, the target was not met. The sample comprised four parents and guardians of infected children and eight HIV-positive parents. Audio-taped interviews were conducted in the seminar room of CHARES where privacy was assured with the Moderator and Note taker in attendance. The interviews probed the socio-economic situation of the parents/guardians, support systems, coping mechanisms, experience with the school system and the attitude/behaviour of the children. Ethical approval for the interviews was obtained from the Ethics Committee of the Faculty of Medicine of the University of the West Indies.

Group discussions were also held with teachers and guidance counsellors in Basic, Primary and Secondary Schools in two parishes in the island. The purpose of these interviews was to gain an understanding of the teachers' perception and knowledge of the epidemic and their attitude to the inclusion of HIV affected children in the class rooms. An Infant/Primary school was selected in a community in the Kingston Metropolitan Area (KMA) in which previous research had revealed a pocket of infected adults and a number of deaths from the disease. The schools served the local community and occurrences were known to members of the small community. A Primary and High

School were also randomly selected from outside of the KMA for group discussions. The investigation had the full support of the Ministry of Education. In addition, in depth interviews were conducted with the directors of the two institutions that look after HIV-positive orphans.

RESULTS

PARENTS/GUARDIANS

Of the parents/guardians of the infected children, two were males and two females. They ranged in age from 30 to 52. One of the male participants was the guardian of two infected children aged 7 and 12 who lived with him and whom he was in the process of formally adopting. The older boy had lived on the street for a while. The mother of the seven-year old was currently in the hospital dying of an AIDS related illness. The other male participant was a father who had recently taken his affected son from the child's maternal grandmother who had taken care of him following the death from AIDS of his mother. The infected child, a boy of five years, was currently living with his paternal grandmother in a household comprising six other relatives. The father reported that he had taken the child from his maternal grandmother because he was being ill-treated. Both fathers were employed.

One of the female participants was the aunt of a 13-year-old boy, one of twins orphaned by the death of her sister. Since the death of their mother from AIDS, they had lived with guardians, whom, the participant said, had been neglecting them. She had taken one of them to live with her and had only recently learned of his status. She was in the process of making arrangements for his twin who still lived with a guardian to be tested for the virus. The participant lived with her boyfriend and their two children, aged 13 and 6, and she seemed to be torn between a desire to keep her nephew and send him to a home. She could not accommodate him fully in her small apartment and so he slept with her parents and his grandparents who lived close by. The other female participant was a mother of six children. Her oldest, a boy of 14 was a haemophiliac who had contracted HIV at the age of seven after a blood transfusion. He was now extremely ill, had developed brain tumours and was receiving both anti-retroviral and anti psychotic drugs.

The infected parents in the sample were all women between the ages of 20 and 58 and those who were willing to share their experiences had remarkably similar stories to tell of being infected by a boyfriend/husband; of being deserted and/or widowed. One had an infected five year old. The eight mothers had 25 children among them ranging in age from nine months to 21 years. Some had had themselves tested on learning of their partners' condition. Other participants had found out about their condition in the process of preparing to migrate; on becoming pregnant or in seeking treatment for repeated yeast infections.

There were 35 HIV-positive orphans in care in two homes in the island. Twenty-three were in a home designed for infants and all but three were between the ages of two and five. These children were infected as a result of mother to child transmission and had been abandoned and found living under desperate conditions. Most were being treated with anti retroviral drugs. The others at this home were three teenagers about to be transferred to a smaller facility which housed 12 children aged ten to fifteen. The teenagers were infected through sexual encounters.

DISCLOSURE

In a society in which there are preconceived stereotypes regarding HIV/AIDS the diagnosis immediately induces the fear of negative moral judgements; of being rejected and abandoned; of being subject to isolation and even violence. There was little doubt that among all the participating parents the psychosocial outweighed the physiological implications of the disease:

> It is me alone. I need a job. I come here (CHARES) and the Jamaica AIDS Support. I have been begging all around and can't get a job. Sometimes I say to myself "Look what I have come to! That is what bothers me."

The fear of rejection induces secrecy and the need to keep the secret leads to feelings of isolation. The overwhelming impression gained from the discussions with the parents was that they were alone and that they had no option than to rely on their own resources. For most, disclosing their status was out of the question and much of the discussion revolved around the effect disclosure would have on their lives and the lives of their children. If their lives were to assume a semblance of normality and if their children were to be accepted in schools, their status had to be kept a secret.

HIV/AIDS has created a crisis in family life. It was interesting that the only instance in which a voluntary decision was taken by a parent either to reveal the child's status to the child in question or the parents' status to their children, was in the case of the child who had been infected through a blood transfusion. Disclosure may reveal information about a parent's sexual orientation, drug use or marital infidelity. It therefore reflected on the entire family. There may also be guilt about transmission. However, when the virus was transmitted through a blood transfusion the family was absolved of blame and the stigma that is associated with sexual transmission (Herek and Capitanio 1999). Therefore the entire community could be told of the status of this young boy and what was remarkable in the context of the Jamaican society was that the community was reported to be protective of him. It was not that the community had a liberal position on the issue. This young boy occupied a special place:

> If you come to (Community) and ask for him, they have to find out why you want him and if you have bad intentions they will kill you.

To disclose the child's status in this case was to make a statement of the state of health care in the island. In every other case, participants feared community and/or family rejection. The two male parents of infected children were, at the time of the discussions, struggling with the problem of how and when to inform the children of their status. In one case, in order to explain the visits to the clinic and the use of the medication, the child as well as other members of the family had been told that he had cancer. This was not an illness that could reflect on the family. The social issues associated with the diagnosis of HIV/AIDS made disclosure a far more complex issue. The deception met with the approval of other parents, for the affected children as well as other children in the family had to be spared the problems consequent upon disclosure.

Infected parents had a similar problem with disclosure. There was no instance in which the diagnosis was discussed with a child because the parent was ready to share the information. In one case, the child, at the age of four, had been present when the doctor revealed the diagnosis to the parent and even at that age, demanded an explanation of what it was since it meant that they could not migrate. In every other instance where the parents' status was known, disclosure was forced by the actions of others. For the most part, participants were taking great pains to keep their status a secret from their children, many of them teenagers. In the case where the mother had passed on the virus to her five year old, the child's status was also a secret. The secrecy involved attempts to hide medication, side effects and, in one case, the frequent doctor's appointments. They gave several explanations for their behaviour. To one parent, the timing was a critical element:

> When I decided to tell my son, he was doing his GSAT (primary level examinations). Now my daughter is doing CXC (secondary level examinations).

Others seem to be approaching disclosure as a process in which, initially, they test their children's reaction to a hypothetical situation. So far, they had not been encouraged by the responses to these advances or by comments which suggested that their children had adopted the attitudes of the society:

> I can't tell him because I hear him talking some things.

> Sometimes I want to tell him but he says some things. I've tried to tell him but it doesn't work.

Above all, parents could not disclose because they had difficulty coping with their own illness and the felt need to keep their status a secret robbed them of the mechanisms that would make coping easier. They could not share their secret with their friends and members of their families. In some cases there was an absolute lack of trust in the ability of family members to respect confidentiality.

"Not even my mother"
"Me neither. I don't trust her"
"My mother doesn't know. It is between me and my God."

This attitude was strengthened by the experiences of those who had shared their secret. The 'closeness' which formerly existed within the family had disappeared. The family, one participant said, doesn't 'use it against me' only because they were afraid that it would become known to the community and that they too would be affected. The mother of one woman had found out but behaved as if she didn't know. The decision to hide the problem that had reshaped and overshadowed their lives protected them from the pain of rejection but, as with women in similar circumstances elsewhere (Crandall and Coleman 1992), it led to isolation and robbed them of the support networks that had the capacity to assist them in working through their feelings of fear. One of the infected participants acknowledged support from an aunt and her three sisters.

However, it was apparent from the discussions that it was difficult to hide such a devastating illness from older children and that the attempt itself could create unexpected tensions. All the participants were convinced that the withdrawal and depression of a 17-year-old girl, her declining performance in school were explained by the anxiety experienced because she knew that her father had died of AIDS and suspected that her mother and infant brother were infected, as indeed they were. She did not have and was probably hesitant to seek the information that would have allowed her

to make sense of the situation. In addition, there was always the possibility that the right to make the decision as to how and when the child should receive the information could be taken from the parent and the child receive the information in a non-supportive manner. One of the eight infected parents was forced to disclose her status to her children when the cause of her husband's death was revealed to her son. One of the twins was told of his status by an angry and probably grieving grandfather:

'He told him that his mother had AIDS and died and that he has it and will die too … He didn't want him there … I noticed that he looked withdrawn … and I explained it fully. I told him he doesn't have AIDS but HIV which doesn't have to develop into AIDS…"

'I told my brother that I was positive and he told a friend…The information get into the primary school and my children were abused. I couldn't walk on the street. I was so ashamed of myself.'

Even then this mother could not admit the truth:

'All I told them was that everyone was going to die. Even me.'

THE EFFECTS OF DISCLOSURE

The very strong support among participants for keeping the infection a secret sprang from their own experiences and the impact disclosure had had on their lives and the lives of their children. The National Policy advises that while a parent may choose not to disclose the status of a child to the school, it might be in the interest of the child to do so to a responsible person. However, the fear of discrimination and loss of privacy outweighed the potential benefits of disclosure. An education for their children in the public school system was only possible if their HIV status remained a secret. The adoptive parent had this to say:

> I told the Principal (about the child's illness) and he gave me the run around. The argument was that I was late with registration…I called the Ministry of Education…which intervened….For two and a half hours (the Principal) had me waiting…He made me complete a medical form and put on it that he is positive…The teachers were told. I went to (a Private School) and told the Principal. She told me that she had to speak to the Board and came back and told me 'yes'.

The children in question did not know of their illness or of the negotiations that were taking place over their entry into the school system. In this sense they were more fortunate than the affected children. The haemophiliac boy had been withdrawn from the school system because the brain tumours were affecting his behaviour. He, however, had siblings in school:

> I made the mistake of telling the Vice Principal and my other son was beaten …by students and ill treated by the teacher….That made him fail GSAT. He was told "Your brother has AIDS and you must have it too. I don't want any AIDS victim here." I was so upset…I reported it to the Principal but nothing was done….I had to move him.

The effect on the girl who had been told of her mother's condition at the age of four was interesting. The participant felt that she had to prepare her daughter to be stronger than she was, to have the self-esteem that would enable her to avoid the mistakes her mother had made. She had to be able to look after herself. So that by the age of five, the participant said, her daughter was able to cook and wash and to make positive decisions. Today, at the age of 14, the roles are reversed. The daughter has become the parent and it is she who insists on secrecy.

> …it is feeding back on me now. She questions everything…I can't tell her to do anything. Not only me. She is the same at school…

The child has had to assume an adult role and this has taken its toll. At the time of the discussions the child was receiving professional counselling

SCHOOL PERFORMANCE

Most of the parents believed that their children were not performing well in school and this held for both the infected and affected. To the parents, the work of the affected 'fluctuated'; the children 'did not appear to have much interest' in school; they were depressed and withdrawn:

> '…she was bright but everything is going down….She goes to school but her mind is not there. If I had money, I would send her to a professional.'

> 'Recently, my son was in a corner by himself. He doesn't talk about it. I know he is bleeding inside.'

> 'Now, all my daughter's marks are low. I wonder if I did the right thing in telling her that her father died from it. It's worrying me a lot.'

The parents of the infected were almost unanimous in their belief that their children were not coping academically:

> '…he goes to a slow learning school.'

'We have been taking them to Mico Teachers' College (for special education). Both are slow learners.'

'I notice that he is not learning anything...he doesn't know all the letters of the alphabet....I went to the school and they asked him to repeat Seventh Grade.'

Evidence suggests that the virus can interrupt in-utero brain development, cause a decrease in cognitive function and a resulting decline in academic performance (Nozyce et al. 1995; Gay, Armstrong and Cohen, 1995). But poor school performance was reported by parents of those children who were not infected by the virus and it may be that the young children were depressed by knowledge of their parents' condition or by uncertainty of their parents' status. One parent placed the blame on the shortcomings of the public school system rather than the virus. For, removed to a private school, his adopted son who was formerly labelled slow:

...'now excels. He is one of 12 students and two teachers...'

POVERTY ALSO EXCLUDES

There was also the problem of the financial burden of the disease. Many were unemployed and even those who were employed had difficulties in meeting the cost of the subsidised drugs and the type of food which were essential to their health and that of the infected children. Luckily, the parents were not in need of antiretroviral drugs and looked extremely healthy. The health problems mentioned by a few were unrelated to the virus. But they all found the cost of the food which, they said, were responsible for their appearance, extremely burdensome.

The mother of the haemophiliac child spoke at length of the problems associated with living on her husband's earnings of J$7,000 (~US$115) a fortnight, meeting the needs of six children; purchasing the special food needed by the child as well as the anti retroviral and anti psychotic drugs. She also had to pay the cost of the damage he inflicted on property in the community. When the drugs are to be purchased, she said, the rest of the family must go without proper food. The financial problems experienced by most parents affected attendance at school. Choices had to be made and the medication for the infected was given priority:

'I have bills, three children to school... daughter's bus fare, son's bus fare. I wonder how I do it. Sometimes there is no food.'

'If they go to school this week, they can't go next week.'

'Meeting expenses is more stressful than the sickness itself.'

Irregular attendance at school, poor diets and the general poverty of the socio-economic environment are other conditions that must be factored into the explanation of poor school performances.

ORPHANS IN CARE

Parents/guardians had the option of keeping the status of their children a secret but this was more difficult in situations where children were living in institutions devoted to the care of HIV-positive orphans. At the moment, the youngest children are being schooled on site. However, the Director of the institution freely acknowledged that the children were simply being kept occupied and no real education was taking place. There was a need for them to enter the public system. The dilemma is that a very protective Director would like to arrange for their education in a manner that would not force disclosure. She rejected the Primary school nearby on the grounds that it would be impossible to hide the status of the children. In spite of the protective wall that has been built around these children, they are already asking questions about their status.

The teenagers who lived in the home were in schools where their status was not known. They lived with self stigma, in fear of disclosure and rejection and for these reasons, had made no friends at school and hid from visitors to the home. The secrecy protected them from rejection but not from the stress of isolation. The twelve children who lived in the home for teenagers were not in school at the time of the interview and the institution had no means of providing an education for them and in the prevailing climate saw no immediate solution.

THE SCHOOL ENVIRONMENT

A. THE KINGSTON METROPOLITAN AREA

The community in which group interviews were conducted among Basic and Primary School teachers was a low-income community in which more than a half of the householders lived in informal housing and unemployment was in excess of 60 per cent. This community had been targeted for intervention in an early study conducted by researchers at the University of the West Indies (UWI) and it became known that there was a pocket of HIV-positive persons. The Headmaster of the Primary school was an enlightened individual who had been involved in Jamaica Teachers' Association workshops on the issue and, in informal discussions, he expressed a strong belief that

that the children of the affected had a right to an education and to be educated with the healthy. Probably because of this attitude, he described a relationship with the community in which HIV-positive parents were able to inform him of their condition and to give him the assurance that their children would be frequently tested for the virus.

Some of the HIV-positive parents were known to the teachers. In some cases the parents themselves had informed the teachers. In other cases, the teachers said that they just knew:

'I met a parent who said she was infected. Her child is in Grade 2.'

'When I was teaching in the Infants' Department there was a child whose father died of AIDS and the mother has it.'

'…her children are tested regularly.'

They explained that an epidemic of this sort should be expected in the community because of the pervasive poverty. Mothers do not work and are dependent on men. They do not have control over their lives. Moreover, they suspected that some of the children in the school were also infected and there was a long discussion among themselves during which they calculated the time of death of the parents and the ages of the children of those parents.

'I was wondering if one in my class is infected because she is four. Her father died a couple of years ago. Her mother has it and she was born during that period.'

They discussed the fact that several of the children – in one case, five – were brothers and sisters but did not share both parents and that in some cases, the parents had died of AIDS.

The suspicion and knowledge, they said, made no difference to the manner in which they interacted with the parents and the children:

'…She comes to pay for the children's lunch. To me she looks well, and I treat her the same.'

They described what they referred to as an 'understanding spirit' in the school which explained why parents were not 'intimidated' and why they were able to disclose the nature of the illness. HIV-positive children just needed 'more attention and more love.' They attributed this spirit to the attitude of the school Principal.

DISCLOSURE

The teachers were disturbed, however, that they had to guess at the status of the children. They felt that they ought to be told and their position was based on two factors, one of which was clearly articulated. They felt that at any one time there were large numbers of children in the schools with cuts and bruises and that in poor environments, these took a long time to heal.

'Some of the parents don't pay attention and so they get infected. Some have to wear slippers to school when they get a cut because it won't get better….'

The children were involved in contact sports and under these circumstances; they felt, there was an increased risk of transmission. It was not that they should be barred from involvement in contact sports but they needed to be carefully supervised. In the same way, they needed to be carefully monitored in the class room where they could be cut by sharp edges and nails. Generally,

there was a fear of coming in contact with infected blood. But the HIV-positive children also needed to be protected from the healthy:

'If I sneeze on somebody who has AIDS, they could die of a cold because their immune system is being eaten away everyday.'

'It was for this reason that they needed "more love and more attention."'

But there was another reason that was more implied that actually stated. The fact that they suspected that there were HIV-positive children in the school did not affect their attitude to them. Familiarity with the condition had brought with it a measure of acceptance. One teacher actually said that just as they had been informed of the presence of a child with juvenile diabetes, they ought to be informed of the presence of the HIV-positive child. It was ignorance of the fact that put them at risk.

There was a concerted effort to transmit this positive attitude to the student body. Guidance classes formed a part of the curriculum for Grades 2 through 6 and this was the medium for exposing the children to the issues surrounding HIV/AIDS and other sexually transmitted diseases. There was satisfaction with the impact of the programme on the attitude of the children who benefited from the programme:

'Some began to draw pictures to express how they feel after class and one boy wrote, "Corey is my friend. He has AIDS. I would still hug Corey and he would still be my friend."'

However, the Guidance Counsellor felt that it was a pity that guidance time did not cover all grades and that so little time was devoted to the subject. There were, she felt, some unhealthy tendencies among the children which could be addressed in the class room:

> 'Sometimes the children tease children whose parents had died of AIDS. I've had to call in more than one of them and explain, and talk to them. So I would say that education is an ongoing process.'

The biggest challenge they had to face was the attitude of the parents of healthy children. The teachers were sure that there would be complaints about the presence of infected children in the class room. But even this, they felt, could be overcome with the right approach. Parents are young. They go to dances; listen to songs; they put DJs on pedestals and they saw this as the best medium for putting positive ideas on HIV/AIDS across to the population.

In the meantime they all felt that they could benefit from more information especially on how to take care of HIV-positive children while avoiding infection.

BASIC SCHOOLS

Basic school teachers are not at all informed and the lively discussions which characterised other sessions were absent. The problem stemmed from a huge knowledge gap:

> 'Can you get it from mosquitoes?'

Attitudes were expressed verbally and in a body language which suggested that some attention must be paid to what for many children, is the first level of entry to the school system. The teachers did not live in the area and did not know the community. They appeared to be disturbed over questions and issues that they were forced to consider for the first time:

> 'This makes me think …that they (the children) need to get check ups. I could have one and don't know.'

They were not prepared to teach infected children and they gave no response when asked whether they were unprepared in the sense that they were unwilling or lacked the knowledge. It was clear, however, that they needed very basic information on transmission – assurance that mosquitoes are not vectors and that the virus cannot be absorbed through unbroken skin, for example.

RURAL PARISH

Group sessions were held with teachers in one Primary and one High School outside the KMA. The groups comprised ten teachers each and, in the High School the teachers were drawn from a range of subject areas – English Language, Literature, Drama, Home Economics, French, Spanish and the sciences. In both schools, the Guidance Counsellors were included.

TEACHERS' FEARS

Teachers had very strongly held ideas which they did not hesitate to express and at times it required a tremendous effort on the part of the Moderator to keep the discussion on track. The attitude in both schools to the disease was essentially the same but some of the strongest views were expressed by teachers in the secondary system. For the most part, they were unwilling to share space with affected children:

> 'I believe that Cuba has set a good precedent. We should build a large compound, nice and spacious with cute little cottages, and once they have it, they must go there.'

'…it may not be fair, but a compound would be a loving environment where there would be people around who understand what it is like to have the disease. Almost like group counselling.'

'Quarantine! We can't allow sympathy to override an issue like this…'

'And let us not be like the Americans who say, well, they have rights so we must embrace them…It is a burden that they have to walk about with the hope that nobody finds out. If they are quarantined they will be with people who they can relate to. This is absolutely the best thing you can do for them.'

'Mental retards are separated. So what is the difference!'

'We should have a place where these people can go…They would be considered heroes.'

The teachers were fearful for themselves, for the children in their charge and concerned about the effects of negative attitudes on the infected children. In the session in the high school there was frequent reference to the uniqueness of the disease. Even for a dreaded disease such as cancer, there was some hope for a cure, they said, but not for HIV/AIDS and since they were all sexually active, they were all at risk.

'I am so afraid that I would not go for a test'.

'Even the doctors are afraid. Some of them don't want to take blood.'

They were not simply afraid of the ravages of the disease. Heap and Simpson (2004) comment on the capacity of the epidemic to create metaphors of a society's 'dis-ease' with itself. Its early association with homosexuals in an homophobic society has created a situation in which men felt the need to distance themselves from the affected and in which the diagnosis of HIV/AIDS raised questions about sexual preferences. In this context also, a clear distinction was made between cancer which, like AIDS had the potential to cause loss of life and HIV/AIDS which stigmatised.

'When someone has it, the first question you hear is, how did you get it? If it is cancer, we do not ask that.'

'When a man has AIDS…most people feel that he was involved in some homosexual activity.'

HIV/AIDS therefore, provoked a type of irrational fear to the extent, they said, that an affected person standing nearby compromised their manhood. 'That is the fear.'

They also expressed concern for the safety of the unaffected children and they introduced one aspect that was not discussed in the focus groups in the KMA and that was, the problems of controlling sexual activity in the school. The primary school teachers said that they had to keep a careful watch on the children in grades 4 and 5 and this observation sparked an interesting debate over the need to know who is infected, an issue that was also keenly debated in the high school. Is the teacher who knows in a better position to protect the student who may not know? What does a teacher do if he sees a student known to be HIV-positive 'checking' a girl who doesn't know? Can they trust the infected to be careful or to reveal his status to a partner? Wouldn't everyone be safer if there is full disclosure? There was some anxiety here also for the HIV-positive child in an unaccepting school environment.

The teachers were anxious to avoid giving the impression that they were heartless and uncaring. They cared but:

'We are just afraid. When we watch these programmes we cry. But we still will not go and shake the hands of someone with it…'

'It is like being beside a man-eating lion and somebody telling you it won't eat you.'

SCHOOLING THE INFECTED

The overwhelming majority believed that the children deserved an education but that they should not be taught with the healthy. They suggested home schooling. A few found themselves in position in which they were uncomfortable with both inclusion and exclusion if only because only those known to be HIV-positive would be excluded. One primary school teacher initially recommended segregation but confessed that during the discussion she had become increasingly uncomfortable with that view. If there were a code regulating the kind of physical contact that could take place between teachers and students, she said, then both infected and healthy could be treated in the same way. Her problem was that she wanted no physical contact with the affected but did not want them to feel that they were being treated differently. Two teachers said that they would accept infected children into the school without reservation. Those who recommended home schooling said that their attitude would be the same if their children were infected. Their presence in school would put others at risk and the stigmatisation would be bad for their psychological health. But one teacher could not see the point of home schooling when the children did not have long to live anyway.

When asked for their reaction, as parents if one of their children's class mates was known to have the infection, they said that they would request immediate transfer for their children. Further, there would be a mass exodus from the schools should parents learn of the presence of an infected child. However, in both types of schools the attitude of the teachers to the possibility of having to work with an infected peer or to have an infected teacher teach their children was markedly different. A majority could see no problem and felt that it would be important to give that teacher their full support. Only a few were ambivalent. That difference was explained by the fact that they saw teachers as responsible adults who, knowing that they were infected would take the necessary precautions. They had no objections to eating or sharing a bathroom with them. Those who were ambivalent related tales of vindictiveness and deliberate attempts to spread the infection. One high school teacher, however, accused his fellow participants of hypocrisy. He reminded them of the teacher who was suspected of having AIDS and had died during the previous year.

'…there is a bed that he used to rest on and nobody will go near it.'

Participants were asked whether more information and education would allay their fears. Most of the teachers felt that they had enough information on the subject but there was a great deal of skepticism among Primary school teachers about the reliability of the information that they received. They were careful to explain that in saying that they did not trust the information received from the Ministry of Health, they were not criticising the Ministry but making a statement about medical knowledge. HIV/AIDS was first presented to them as a 'gay' disease. Today, it is affecting heterosexuals. They feared that in time they may be told that they could 'get it through their pores.'

If formal education gave an advantage then the level of accommodation should have been highest in the High School where most of the teachers had University Degrees. Instead, the views of a segment of this group were among the most intransigent. There was one instance in which information seemed to have made a difference. One of the Guidance Counsellors at the High School felt that she had to make a deliberate effort to overcome her prejudice if she were to perform efficiently:

'As a Guidance Counsellor, I had to do reading on HIV/AIDS and its management....This research was also influenced by an experience I had when I was hugged by someone with the disease and I itched for months. I said to myself that it cannot be like this. I need to be able to reach a point where I can counsel somebody with it. So, I had to read.'

She did not say whether she had overcome her fears but she was able to counsel.

PUTTING A HUMAN FACE ON HIV/AIDS

What seemed to have made a real difference is contact with people with HIV/AIDS. Those teachers who had met persons with HIV/AIDS held the more liberal views.

'I met someone with AIDS....He came to a function to give a talk and when he finished, he said that he had the disease. I hugged him, and in my mind I was worried because he was sweating a lot. Overcoming that fear has helped me because the main problem is fear.'

'I have had the opportunity to share with people who are living with AIDS. Some have died....With drugs they are living longer. They want to be loved just like everybody else.'

This is what accounts for the marked difference between the attitudes of the Primary School teachers in the high prevalence area in the KMA and their more highly educated counterparts in the High School. They had survived contact.

CONCLUSIONS AND RECOMMENDATIONS

With medication children with HIV/AIDS will live longer and must be given tools to lead a productive life. They should be educated alongside healthy children. But the challenges to the instilling of non-discriminatory attitudes as outlined in the National Policy are tremendous. To avoid stigmatisation and discrimination, many parents opt for non-disclosure. They hide their status and that of their children. They hide their status from their children and the children's HIV status from the infected and affected children.

Disclosing a diagnosis is not an easy task and parents need emotional support. They do not feel that they could trust members of their own family, the institution that traditionally was relied on to perform this function. Therefore they are cut off from the most important sources of social support. Some of the children in the study were teenagers and secrecy becomes increasingly difficult as children age. Although there can be no set rules as to what age a child should be told of his or a parent's status, the study has shown that there are risks associated with continuing secrecy. Disclosure is necessary if only for long-term planning and to increase the likelihood of success of the plans.

Some are not given the choice between disclosing and not disclosing. The death of parents will increase the number of affected orphans in care and these children will have to enter the school system. While legal protection must form an essential component of a country's response to discrimination and stigma, discrimination can and does occur in spite of protective legislation. Efforts must be made to create more positive attitudes to those affected by the disease and ultimately, the goal must be the creation of a safe, informed, caring school environment. This is still a distant goal. This study suggests that putting a human face on HIV/AIDS can dispel misinformation and generate empathy. Those in the study who reported contact with people with HIV/AIDS had more favourable attitudes and no objections to interacting with them in a classroom situation. Opportunities must be created in which the public can interact either directly or vicariously with the affected. Experience elsewhere has shown that this can reduce stigma and prejudice (Brown et al. 2003).

But stigma is double edged. Children living with HIV/AIDS must cope with being stigmatised by the community. They must also learn to overcome the shame felt in response to the reaction of others to their plight or the self stigma. There is a loss of confidence and esteem and a tendency to separate themselves from society, reinforcing their social exclusion. The affected children also can benefit if more adults living with AIDS become involved in the public education programme; if they are exposed to the diversity of the epidemic. Beyond this a special attempt must be made to develop intervention programmes to deal with self stigma among children with HIV.

REFERENCES

Brown, L. et al., (2003) 'Interventions to reduce HIV/AIDS stigma; what have we learned.' *AIDS Education and Prevention* 15 (1): 1, 49–69.

Ministry of Education. Youth and Culture, Jamaica (2004) National Policy for HIV/AIDS management in schools.

Gay, C.L. F.D. Armstrong and D. Cohen (1995). The effects of HIV on cognitive and motor development in children born to HIV-seropositive women with no reported drug use: birth to 24 months. *Pediatrics* 95; 1078–1082.

Heap, Brian and Tony Simpson (2004). 'When you have AIDS people laugh at you' A process drama approach to stigma with pupils in Zambia. *Caribbean Quarterly* 50 (1): 83–98.

Nozyce, M, J. Hittelman, L. Muenz, S. Durako. M. Fischer and A. Willoughby (1994). Effect of perinatally acquired HIV on neurodevelopmental growth in children in the first two years of life *Pediatrics,* 94:883–891.

Herek, G.M. and J. Capitanio (1997). AIDS stigma and contact with persons with AIDS: effect of direct and vicarious contact. *Journal of Applied Social Psychology* 271: 1–36.

UNAIDS (2003, 2004). Report on the global AIDS epidemic.

American Academy of Pediatrics (2000). Policy Statement. *Pediatrics* 105: 1358–1360

Ramsay, H, S. Williams, J. Brown and S. Bhardwaj (2004). Young children, a neglected group in the HIV epidemic: perspectives from Jamaica. *Caribbean Quarterly* 50 (1): 39–53.

ACKNOWLEDGEMENT

Preparation of this report was supported by a grant from UNESCO. We are grateful for the cooperation of the Ministries of Health and Education and acknowledge the assistance of The Centre for HIV/AIDS Research, Education and Services (CHARES).

8

Assessment of the Response of Four Caribbean Universities

Marie Jose N'Zengou-Tayo, Mary Crewe,
Johan Maritz, Lydia Emerencia, Esthela Loyo
and Justine Sass

UNESCO organised a cross country study of Higher Education Institutions' response to HIV and AIDS in 2005 and published the result, Expanding the Field of Enquiry, in 2006. Four of the twelve univsities were selected in the Caribbean, and studies were facilitated by the UNESCO Office for the Caribbean and UNICA, the Caribbean Association of Universities and Research Institutions.

In this chapter, the summary findings of the four Caribbean case studies are republished. Four very different universities were selected, from the Dominican Republic, Haiti, Suriname, and the West Indies, and the universities were at very different levels of response. Summaries of the reports were developed by UNESCO, under the guidance of Justine Sass, and these are reprinted in this chapter. The full UNESCO report is available in print form, and all case studies are available on line at UNESCO's HIV and AIDS Clearinghouse, http://hivaidsclearinghouse.unesco.org . Professor David Plummer reviewed the methodology and Caribbean case studies and proposed an instrument for self analysis by Caribbean higher education institutions (see Chapter 22).

SURINAME – ANTON DE KOM UNIVERSITY OF SURINAME (ADEKUS)

Basic Facts	
Established:	1968
Status:	Autonomous
Location:	Paramaribo
Number of faculties:	3 faculties *(undergraduate only)* 5 Research institutes 4 Institutes
Total staff:	288
Total teachers:	256 *(of which 133 are part-time)*
Total students:	3,281
% students female:	66%
Student/ teacher ratio:	13:1

Anton de Kom University of Suriname (ADEKUS) is Suriname's only university. With the goal of becoming a centre of excellence in science and technology, the University is dedicated to high quality education, scientific research and public service.

There is no institutional policy or action plan related to HIV and AIDS and institutional leaders do not seem to be convinced that an institutional response is required. As one key informant explained, *'Of course we know that it [HIV/AIDS] is becoming a big problem in the society, but we do not experience the problem inside the university.'* This sentiment was echoed by the Dean, *'As long as we don't really feel the problem in the University, as long as we don't see a real impact, it is difficult to expect a response and to expect a deep reflection about the issue.'*

There is other evidence that suggests that students may be more vulnerable than is generally thought. As one Dean explained, *'Four years ago, when we asked our students if they knew someone living with HIV/AIDS, almost 100 per cent would say no. When we pose the same question now, 25 per cent of the students answer affirmatively. HIV/AIDS is getting closer to our students.'* Sex work and "sugar daddy" relationships to pay for school fees or to purchase material goods were also reported, although there was insufficient information to determine how prevalent these practices were.

HIV-related content can only be found in the curriculum of the Faculty of Medicine. This includes a seminar for third year students that presents information on the modes of transmission, and ways to prevent infection. The Head of the Public Health Department also noted during the seminar, *'We invite our students to talk freely and openly about HIV/AIDS.'*

The lack of integration of HIV into other aspects of the curriculum was reported by most faculty and administration officials to be due to overloaded curriculum and structural and institutional changes at the University. For example, the University President explained that Deans report that *'There is little space...to add additional topics and new areas of studies.'* In a separate interview, a Dean claimed, *'We really don't have space left for life skills training...There is no way that we can add new themes to the programme.'* Recent efforts to restructure the curriculum are believed to have led to a more technical approach to educational planning, creating fewer opportunities for broad-based educational programmes. As one Dean explained, *'Nowadays, we are more oriented towards the statement of educational objectives, in terms of knowledge and skills. We are less focused now on a more general preparation and education of our students for life in the society...we have started to focus more on measurable outcomes of education and less of general preparation of the students.'*

The Student Dean, however, stressed the responsibility of the University to offer opportunities for personal development and for a better preparation for life. There is a need, she explained, for *'...programmes that are holistic and that train students in a wide variety of skills that [they] need in life and in work.'* The Dean of the Social Science Faculty also saw the relevance of HIV and AIDS issues in the universities' programmes, although with a more limited application: *'I tend to say that it is not necessary to include the HIV/AIDS theme in all of the programmes, with the exception of sociology, where the AIDS theme could be part of the theme of Gender of Medical Sociology....If we add HIV/AIDS in all of our programmes, it would be purely to provide comprehensive training.'*

There was no evidence of other initiatives to develop or promote leadership in the field of HIV and AIDS. Non-formal educational activities related to HIV and AIDS were largely absent; no peer education programmes or support groups were reported and no periodic activities were planned for national or international days such as World AIDS Day. Students reported that activities were undertaken by campus student organisations during orientation for new students, although no further information was provided.

Some students and faculty members suggested during the review that students were informed and knowledgeable about HIV and AIDS. One student explained, *'The students at the university really know at lot about HIV and AIDS. They know how you can become infected, they know about condoms and how to use them, and they will not endanger themselves.'* Another student agreed but added that, *'Well, you can never have too much information. But maybe it not a lack of information that is the problem... although there is information on HIV/AIDS, the real problem is related to the acceptance of the reality of HIV/AIDS all around us...[and] stigmatisation–this is what we need to focus on.'*

Research related to HIV and AIDS is undertaken in the Faculty of Medicine, although some think that University should be more involved. A Member of Parliament and former President of the National AIDS Committee noted, *'The University can and should give an important contribution to research with regard to HIV/AIDS in Suriname. There are so many studies to be done: we really have a serious lack of reliable data on the development of the epidemic, the situation of specific groups, and the influence of contextual factors. The University has the experts who could conduct this research.'* Similar comments were made by the Presidents of the Prohealth and Lobi Foundations, NGOs active in conducting research on sexual and reproductive health.

No health services were available for staff or students although the President has mentioned the possibility of establishing condom distribution points on campus. ADEKUS is also preparing to establish a psychosocial centre providing social and emotional counselling and care for students, although no mention was made of specific counselling for HIV and AIDS.

Although public service is explicitly mentioned in the University mission, community outreach has been a matter of individual action. Some students are believed to be active in the activities of local NGOs, and one student is a Youth Ambassador of the Caribbean Community (CARICOM), involved in HIV and AIDS campaigns. However, there is no evidence of widespread commitment to community engagement, or of incentives offered by the University for outreach opportunities (e.g. course credits, certificates).

Most Deans seem to recognise that, in the long run, the University cannot stay isolated and will need to engage at the institutional and the community level on HIV and AIDS. As one Dean explained, *'The University will have to allow for a shift towards a more explicit presence...offering more support to society.'*

DOMINICAN REPUBLIC – PONTIFICIA UNIVERSIDAD CATÓLICA MADRE Y MAESTRA (PUCMM)

Basic Facts	
Established:	1962
Status:	Private, religious
Location:	Santo Domingo
Number of faculties:	4
Total staff:	N/A
Total teachers:	N/A
Total students:	7,927
% students female:	60%
Student/teacher ratio:	N/A

Pontificia Universidad Católica Madre y Maestra (PUCMM), part of the International Federation of Catholic Universities, is dedicated to teaching, investigation and community service. PUCMM promotes academic excellence, and the *'harmonious synthesis of reason, science, culture and life with the Christian faith.'*

The university does not have an institutional policy on HIV and AIDS, and not all university authorities are convinced that one is needed. Several Department Heads reported during the assessment that *'there did not seem to be a demand for the implementation of a policy on HIV/AIDS.'* At the same time, one Department Head noted that a policy addressing–at a minimum–universal precautions whenever the potential for exposure to blood or other bodily fluids exists *'would personally help a student or staff out if accidental contamination were to occur'*.

HIV and AIDS education is provided in the faculties of Medicine and Dentistry, typically consisting of biological-clinical-treatment aspects, with little focus on psychological aspects such as decision-making and problem-solving, stress management and coping, and communication and negotiation skills. However, the Health Sciences faculty reportedly was in the process in 2005 of evaluating the curriculum content related to STIs/HIV/AIDS to also provide skills on prevention and communication. Medical students interviewed showed a deep interest in the further integration of HIV and AIDS in their curriculum and all interviewed though it would be appropriate to include *'some class or classes about sexual matters in the first year of university.'*

University staff in general reported lacking training on HIV and AIDS. In 2003, the Centre for Integral Prevention, Formation and Investigation established a one-year postgraduate course for professors to enable them to integrate sexuality and issues into their courses; however, due to lack of funds, this programme was discontinued in 2004. The Centre has, instead, focused on training peer educators for the University's orientation programme.

Since 2003, PUCMM has established an orientation programme for first year students, addressing drug abuse, alcohol, HIV and AIDS, and physical and health aspects more generally. Initially a one day session, the programme will expand in August 2005 to be one week in duration and delivered by peer educators. The 2005 peer group (comprised of 20 medical students) was trained by the Students' Dean and the Centre for Integral Prevention, Training and Investigation on STIs/HIV/AIDS, alcohol consumption, drug abuse, psychological skills and nutrition and is responsible for monitoring, educating, and supervising newly-admitted students during orientation.

As a religious institution, abstinence is strongly encouraged, although other non-formal education activities addressing other aspects of prevention have been organised periodically by WHO, the Pan-American Health Organization (PAHO), COPRESIDA, and REDOVIH. These have included conferences and seminars on HIV-related themes and awareness-raising activities conducted in partnership with the Faculty of Health Sciences. Notably, students report that a large part of those participating are those within the Health Faculty itself, or *'those who already are generally well-informed about the epidemic'*. Further efforts need to be made to reach out to students from other faculties, such as Engineering, Telecommunications, and Architecture, who may have less access to information and skills-building activities.

Research on HIV and AIDS conducted within the university dates back to the mid-1980s, and includes legal and medical research, and KAP studies. Most research is undertaken by students completing degrees in Dentistry, Law, and Medicine; some are presented and/or published, although largely in local journals and conferences. To date the large majority of HIV-related theses focuses on medical aspects of the disease, and no studies have been undertaken on psychological aspects of HIV and AIDS or the social and cultural roots of the disease.

The Students' Health Centre is open to the entire university community, although professors reportedly only use the Centre for employment-related procedures (e.g. physical exams, the completion of a medical history form). The Centre does not have laboratory facilities, and as such, does not perform Voluntary Councelling and Testing (VCT). The staff has not received any training on HIV-related issues, and is largely used for general complaints such as headaches, stress, gastro-enteric complaints, and common respiratory ailments.

There is reportedly little demand at the Health Centre for HIV and AIDS information. A staff member could recall only two recent occasions in which students, both foreign, attended the Centre because they were concerned about having been infected with HIV. These students were referred to private health care professionals outside the institution, and no follow-up had been made by the Centre.

The University recently initiated an agreement with COPRESIDA to co-administer several peripheral public health clinics in Santiago. These clinics provide a range of HIV and AIDS services including information, counselling, testing, treatment, and care of people living with HIV. Initially including four clinics, coverage may be scaled up to the regional level in the future.

This agreement has the potential to expand the technical and financial resources available to PUCMM for HIV and AIDS-related work and to provide on-site training

for students and staff. PUCMM should capitalise on this opportunity to not only focus on serving the needs of *society* but also the needs of its *students and faculty* to the information, services, and skills necessary to reduce their vulnerability and risk to HIV.

HAITI – UNIVERSITY OF QUISQUEYA (UNIQ)

Basic Facts	
Established:	1988
Status:	Private
Location:	Port-au-Prince
Number of faculties:	6
Total staff: Total teachers:	N/A 173 (*of which 128 part-time*)
Total students:	1,600
% students female:	N/A
Student/teacher ratio:	N/A

The University of Quisqueya (UniQ) is Haiti's leading private university in terms of the number of students and the number of programmes offered. Committed to serving the needs of society, each faculty has a training programme that provides community service.

Political instability and insecurity in recent decades has reportedly affected enrolment rates, with greater numbers of students attending Dominican tertiary institutions. To promote a safer learning environment, UniQ is planning to move the campus to the northern outskirts of Port-au-Prince in 2006. There are no plans to establish on-campus student dormitories, meaning that students will continue to be required to commute.

There is no institutional policy or plan at UniQ related to HIV and AIDS. Key informants felt that any publicity concerning an HIV and AIDS policy would adversely affect the image of the University and have a negative impact on its enrolment. The Vice-President for Academic Affairs did, however, indicate that there was a tacit agreement that no staff or students living with HIV would be dismissed or asked to withdraw. There is evidence that fear of stigmatisation makes this a moot point as most persons prefer to resign or withdraw from studies as soon as they start having frequent bouts of illness.

There is no dedicated administrative or departmental structure for the coordination and implementation of the institution's response to HIV and AIDS, and related leadership appears to be the efforts of select individuals. This includes the Vice-President for Academic Affairs, and the Head of the Orientation Unit (a psychologist), who has been 'doubling' as a counsellor and mentor in sex education. Students have also been active, although there appears to be no mechanism to link the student- and staff-level initiatives.

UniQ reported being eager to spearhead the involvement of tertiary education institutions in the national response. In 2002, the university participated in the development of the Ministry of National Education, Youth and Sports' Strategic Plan for the Prevention and Fight against HIV and AIDS and produced a 12-page document entitled 'HIV/AIDS and the education community: UniQ gets involved'.[1] In this paper, UniQ committed to activities at three levels: HIV and AIDS education, research and community service.

Presently, medical students learn about HIV and AIDS at the advanced level of their course of study through courses on parasitology, virology, and infectious diseases, anatomopathology, and dermatology.

The first course on Sexuality, STIs, and HIV/AIDS was piloted in the 2004–05 academic year as a sex education course but within the framework of a peer education project. Students in select faculties (Education, Medical and Health Sciences, and Agronomy) followed the one-week course developed to prepare them to be HIV and AIDS peer educators. These participants—now part of a Network of Young People Committed to Combating AIDS (REJES)—were subsequently sent to conduct information sessions about HIV and AIDS in high schools. Reportedly successful, the administrators are currently considering introducing it as a compulsory foundation course.

UniQ has also developed, in collaboration with the Haitian Study Group on Kaposi's Sarcoma and Opportunistic Infections (GHESKIO), and Cornell and Vanderbilt Universities, a Masters in Public Health modular programme targeting health care professionals and social workers working in HIV and AIDS counselling and detection centres. The first course was in July 2005; evaluation of the programme is pending.

Medical students at UniQ have also established a club, ACTISTSIDA, which raises awareness among students about STIs, HIV, and AIDS. Activities are sporadic, and take place primarily during World AIDS Day. The impact of these efforts is not measured and there is no follow-up, making it difficult to ascertain knowledge or behaviour change among the student population.

There is no evidence of a body of knowledge being produced directly at UniQ on the various aspects of HIV and AIDS. The bulk of published Haitian research on HIV and AIDS comes from two main organisations, Partners in Health/Zanmi lasante and GHESKIO. Research findings were believed to be difficult to access at the University as book acquisition is reportedly a problem.

To reinforce national scholarly research on HIV and AIDS, UNESCO and UNAIDS are collaborating to create a joint UNESCO/UNAIDS professorial chair. It likely that this will be a rotating post, meaning the incumbent will visit a different university each year to conduct training and research.

There are no HIV and AIDS related services on campus as there are no health centres or sick bays. During the time of the assessment, there were no billboard displays or evidence of condom distributors nor were there emergency kits or Post-Exposure-Prophylaxis (PEP) available for incidents of exposure to staff and students (e.g. needle stick injuries, exposure to blood or other body fluids). Moreover, use of existing HIV and AIDS services off-campus, such as VCT, are reported by students to be low due to a) perceived lack of confidentiality; b) *stressful and frightening* counselling techniques; c) unavailability of counselling services; d) fear of stigma and ostracism; and d) the perception that HIV is a *'death sentence'*.

Efforts by UniQ to engage itself in the HIV and AIDS response are quite recent, and it is difficult at this stage to measure their effectiveness. The will seems to be there, although further steps are required to establish an institutional structure capable of delivering coordinated activities that are monitored for their overall impact on knowledge, attitudes, and behaviours among staff and students.

WEST INDIES – UNIVERSITY OF THE WEST INDIES (UWI)

The University of the West Indies (UWI) serves 15 countries in the Caribbean[2] on three campuses located in Jamaica, Trinidad and Tobago, and Barbados. All campuses are quasi-autonomous but integrated through centrally administered functions and operations at the Mona Campus in Jamaica.[3]

Basic Facts:	
Established:	1948
Status:	International tertiary institution
Location:	Jamaica (Mona Campus)
Number of faculties:	5
Total staff: **Total teachers:**	1,737 630
Total students: **% students female:**	10,781 68%
Student/ Teacher Ratio:	17.1:1

HIV and AIDS represent a major health tragedy in the Caribbean…UWI is positioned to play a central role in educating [partners and stakeholders]… and to fight HIV and AIDS. My vision is to expand and enhance our contributions in the effort to the community and we obviously need to have the same effort within the university…

-Vice-Chancellor, UWI

UWI developed its first policy on HIV and AIDS in 1995. Many stakeholders –largely from the academic community – participated in its development and the draft policy was reviewed and approved by WIGUT, one of UWI's staff unions, before its promulgation. Although the policy was not very comprehensive, it was perceived to be adequate at that time.

The policy was redrafted in 2004, again in collaboration with a range of stakeholders, to address a greater variety of issues. Research undertaken by Masters-level students in the Social Science department was believed to have fed into the current policy, which addresses: rights of affected persons; confidentiality; managing HIV and AIDS within the University with regards to treatment of affected persons, education and counselling, employee guidelines, medical/laboratory environments, and accidental exposure to HIV; staff and student responsibilities; gender-related issues; research; and the community. Stakeholders are reportedly committed to keeping the policy timely and relevant to current challenges.

The policy does not cover issues pertaining to the financial management of HIV and AIDS in the institution such as: employee benefits, inability of students to repay student loans or skills replacement and training costs. The policy does, however, make provision for staff and student welfare and for Anti Retroviral Therapy (ART) and access to PEP in the event of accidental exposure to blood products in laboratory settings and sexual assault. A separate policy on sexual harassment and assault also exists; but these policies exist in isolation from each other with no formal links between the two.

Even though an HIV and AIDS policy has been in existence for 10 years, the general feeling from many informants during the assessment was that the policy is not well-known among staff and students. No informant could recall if there had ever been a need to enforce the policy in cases in which an individual's rights were infringed.

Leadership at UWI has consistently demonstrated commitment to the regional HIV and AIDS response. The Chancellor, a distinguished medical professional, was previously a member of PAHO and currently carries special responsibility for HIV and AIDS in the region. He has indicated that he is more than willing to put his expertise at the institution's disposal. The previous Vice-Chancellor was also very supportive of HIV and AIDS initiatives, establishing the University's HIV and AIDS Response Programme (HARP) in 2001. The current

Vice-Chancellor is perceived to be central to HARP's successful functioning.

HARP is a multidisciplinary group dedicated to using the University's capacities to partner with government and NGOs to contribute to HIV and AIDS prevention and care, and to mitigate the impact of the epidemic. It aims specifically to:

• Accelerate action by UWI in response to the growing HIV and AIDS epidemic through research, education, training, and strategic engagement with the wider society;

• Develop and monitor institutional policies;

• Generate, attract, and manage resources to sustain the response to HIV and AIDS; and

• Serve as a clearinghouse for HIV and AIDS information, working in collaboration with and complementing national, regional and international agencies.

There is a notion within the institution that HARP is part of the Medical Faculty, perhaps because HARP's Coordinator is also the Head of the Department for Community Health. However, HARP's mandate is to look at the entire University's response. As a Senior Project Officer explained, HARP is placed in the Medical Faculty in terms of 'location but not vision.'

HARP began to gain momentum in 2002 when UWI collaborated in the Strengthening the Institutional Response to HIV/AIDS/STI in the Caribbean (SIRHASC) initiative. Funded by the European Commission, SIRHASC had five project outputs; UWI was one of the lead agencies for two outputs, namely 1) an increased pool of appropriately skilled personnel to contribute to effective policy development, planning and implementation of STI/HIV/AIDS programmes; and 2) more comprehensive and accurate information on the course, consequences, and costs of the epidemic through improved surveillance, monitoring and evaluation of national control programmes and through operational research.

UWI HARP has made strides in integrating HIV and AIDS into curricula. In 2002, HARP established a Curriculum Development Committee to identify opportunities across disciplines to integrate HIV and AIDS into existing courses and to establish stand-alone courses. The process was consultative and cooperative in nature and had impressive results: 23 of the 40 courses targeted for integration in the 2003-2004 academic year were successfully integrated with HIV content, and 17 new courses were developed. A total of 32 (15 existing, 17 new) of the courses were delivered, exposing nearly 1,000 students to this information.

HARP has also expanded the information resources available for teachers to use in their courses and provided training opportunities. It piloted, updated, and finalised an HIV and AIDS Teaching Resource Manual with multi-disciplinary teaching support material for lecturers which is now also available on CD-Rom. HARP further procured more than 60 new publications for the University libraries and distributed 170 HIV and AIDS videotapes to University academic departments. Under the SIRHASC initiative, UWI facilitated two two-day Trainer of Trainers (TOT) workshops in 2003, training a total of 60 academic staff and has provided regular training sessions on basic information on HIV and AIDS for non-academic staff members of one of the staff unions. The SIRHASC initiative also enabled UWI to recruit a Health Communication Specialist, and a Public Health and Health Promotion Specialist.

A peer education programme has also been established through HARP, with supervision provided by the Student Counselling Unit. While peer education generally forms part of the informal curriculum, peer educators have also been used by UWI in formal classes, where they have acted as assistant lecturers and discussants on a module on health and security.

HARP, the Campus Health Service, and the Campus Counselling have also engaged in periodic IEC activities on campus, generally distributing Ministry of Health materials. HARP itself has produced limited promotional materials in the past; many campus stakeholders have complained about a lack of funds to do so.

The University has made a significant contribution to the regional body of knowledge on HIV and AIDS across a range of disciplines. Current research includes: clinical trials; communication for social and behaviour change; gender and the position of women; health economics; community health and psychiatry; and education. The SIRHASC initiative funded a study on the psychosocial needs of women living with HIV, and two HIV and AIDS impact assessments (in Haiti and Suriname). The University does not, however, have a good monitoring system to gauge the various new and ongoing research initiatives and information-sharing across departments remains problematic.

HIV and AIDS services are notably comprehensive, and confidentiality is assured. The Health Centre has STI diagnosis and treatment, pre- and post-test counselling is provided to all individuals undergoing HIV testing and ongoing counselling is available in the Campus Counselling Unit to people who require further psychosocial care. Staff at the Centre are adequately prepared to diagnose and treat opportunistic infections and free ART is available onsite, along with adherence counselling. Four students were following treatment at the time of this assessment and were reportedly showing good adherence. PEP is available to staff and students in the event of sexual assault, needle stick injuries and to individuals working with patients and blood products in the University hospital and laboratories. Where necessary, referrals can be made to other external service providers.

The overall response of UWI and specifically the activities of HARP have made significant strides in mainstreaming HIV and AIDS into the life of the University. UWI has adopted a comprehensive approach, including policy development and implementation, integration of HIV and AIDS into curriculum, research, and numerous services for students and staff. It has the potential to become a 'best practice' for other institutions in the region and around the world.

Steps to formalise its status—with core staff in dedicated institutional positions—and a structure on the main campus (not in the medical school) would assist in conveying the independent and multidisciplinary nature of its initiatives. Core funding from the university budget would also defer dependency on donor funding and demonstrate it as a central part of the University.

NOTES

1. "Le VIH/SIDA et la communauté éducative: L'UniQ s'implique."
2. Anguilla, Antigua and Bermuda, Bahamas, Barbados, Belize, British Virgin Islands, Cayman Isalnds, Dominica, Grenada, Jamaica, Montserrat, St Kitts/Nevis, St Lucia, St Vincent & the Grenadines, and the Republic of Trinidad and Tobago.
3. This synopsis presents the findings from UWI's Mona Campus. Further details on campuses in Trinidad and Tobago and Barbados are available in the full case study: Crewe and Maritz 2005 (unpublished).

Section 2

Reflection on Critical Issues

9

The Challenge of Sexually Active School Children in the Caribbean in the era of HIV/AIDS

J. Peter Figueroa

Chief, Epidemiology and AIDS,
Ministry of Health, Jamaica

The Education Sector has a critical role in combating the HIV/AIDS epidemic in the Caribbean. In particular, the education sector has a special role in helping to prepare young people from becoming HIV infected when they become sexually active. This is a tremendous challenge especially given the sensitivity of the subject matter.

This chapter explores three questions: Are school children sexually active? What does the research on sex education and prevention tell us? How do we strengthen the response of the education sector to better prepare young people for when they become sexually active?

ARE SCHOOL CHILDREN SEXUALLY ACTIVE?

In the Caribbean sex begins at an early age so that many school children are sexually active. The percentage of girls sexually active under 15 years of age was 25% in Barbados, 15% in Guyana and 37% in St Vincent and the Grenadines. Among boys the percentage was 30% in Guyana and 63% in St Vincent & the Grenadines. A survey of school children aged 10–18 years in Saint Lucia found the median age of first sex to be 10 years for males and 14 years for females while in Belize the mean age of first sex was 16.7 years for males and 17.6 years for females. Several surveys in Jamaica have found the mean age of first sex to be 13.4 years for boys and 15.9 years for girls. Analysis of three population based national KAP surveys in Jamaica in 1996, 2000 and 2004 showed that the median age of first sex actually declined from 16.5 years for boys and 18.2 years for girls in 1996 to

15.7 years for boys and 17.2 years for girls in 2004. The evidence is overwhelming that throughout the Caribbean sex begins at an early age and many school children are sexually active before the legal age of consent which is 16-years in Jamaica and several other Caribbean countries.

Many of the children who are sexually active have multiple partners and do not use a condom during sex. One survey of sexually experienced 10–14 year olds in Jamaica in 1997 found that 80% of boys and 67% of girls had more than one lifetime sex partner and as many as 26% of boys and 15% of girls had six or more lifetime sex partners. The Jamaica Adolescent Study found that only 30% of boys and 65% of girls used a contraceptive method during their first intercourse. Among sexually active adolescents 15–19 years of age in 2001, 68% of males and 53% of females reported using a contraceptive method at last sex. Only 24% of sexually experienced teenagers in Saint Lucia used a contraceptive method.

Unfortunately, many children, especially girls, are forced to have sex against their will. In Saint Lucia a survey of school children found that as many as 63% of girls and 25% of boys reported being forced to engage in their first sexual intercourse. A school based survey of 10–15 year olds in Jamaica in 2005 found that one quarter of the girls stated that they had been forced to have sex on the first occasion (K. Fox et al., 2005). The Jamaica Adolescent Study found that in 1997, 11.8% of girls and 2.8% of boys were raped or forced to have sex at first intercourse. The main reasons given for having sex in this survey was 'to see what it was like' (63% of boys and 53% of girls), 'to show love' (18% of boys, 14% of girls) and 'convinced by boyfriend/girlfriend' (10% of boys, 16% of girls).

The consequences of early sexual activity include unplanned teenage pregnancy, induced abortion, sexually transmitted infections, infertility and HIV infection as well as disruption of education and dropping out of school. The consequences are much worse for girls than for boys and rates of HIV infection are on average three times higher among teenage girls than boys. In Jamaica, every year there are 300 to 400 births to girls under 15 years and approximately 1,000 births to girls 15–19 years. The number of terminations of pregnancy among teenagers is not known. We need to ask ourselves whether our education systems are adequately addressing the challenges and consequences of sexually active school children or whether this is a problem that is largely ignored.

TABLE 9.1:
PERCENTAGE OF ADOLESCENTS ANSWERING KNOWLEDGE ITEMS CORRECTLY, BY SURVEY DATE AND SEX

Item	September 1995 (n=945)		June 1996 (n=868)		June 1997 (n=719)	
	Girls	Boys	Girls	Boys	Girls	Boys
Time during menstrual cycle when pregnancy most likely occur	4.3	9.3	4.8	8.1	5.7	10.4
Pregnancy is possible at first intercourse	27.3	32.7	31.7	47.4	33.7	50.6
Condoms protect against STDs	52.5	77.7	60.2	81.2	57.4	78.0
Birth control pills protect against STDs	14.7	16.1	21.5	18.6	21.2	26.0
Sex with a virgin will cure an STD	16.4	28.8	27.8	32.7	27.0	44.2
Having sex while standing prevents pregnancy	14.9	30.3	23.4	41.4	27.0	46.1
Drinking Coke or Pepsi after sex prevents pregnancy	16.4	23.9	23.3	35.3	24.3	36.3

Source: *The Jamaica Adolescent Study J. Jackson et al 1998*

LIMITED KNOWLEDGE OF REPRODUCTIVE MATTERS

Although many children are sexually active their knowledge about reproductive matters is very low. The Jamaica Adolescent Study found that only one of seven knowledge questions (i.e. condoms protect against STDs) was answered correctly by at least half the students on all the survey dates. Even at the end of Grade 8, half of the boys and two-thirds of the girls did not know that pregnancy was possible at first intercourse.

While awareness of HIV/AIDS and how to prevent it is generally high throughout the Caribbean, myths and major misconceptions are relatively common. Many persons believe that you can catch HIV from a mosquito or from a person with HIV/AIDS who is preparing your food. Thus only 38% of persons 15–24 years in Jamaica in 2004 answered the UNGASS knowledge indicator correctly (i.e. percentage who correctly identified three ways of preventing sexual transmission of HIV and rejected major misconceptions).

Throughout the Caribbean, education systems have been responding to these challenges to varying degrees, but current programmes are not adequate to achieve the delay of sexual initiation and to support the practice of safe sex among those schoolchildren who are sexually active. Health and Family Life Education (HFLE) is taught in many schools throughout the Caribbean. However, surveys indicate that significant numbers of schoolchildren are not exposed to these courses. For instance, 57% of schoolchildren in Belize and 29% of females and 35% of males 15–24 years in Jamaica did not get any family life or sex education in school. Even for those schoolchildren who are exposed to HFLE the approach is mainly information sharing with limited values clarification, or addressing of attitudes and gender roles, or development of inter-personal skills as well as condom use and negotiation skills. It is well-established that purely knowledge-based programmes are unlikely to change sexual behaviour.

WHAT DOES RESEARCH ON SEX EDUCATION TELL US?

Recent reviews of the literature provide contrasting results with respect to the effectiveness of sex education programmes. An analysis of 26 randomised controlled trials (RCTs) among adolescents 11–18 years in developed countries by A. DiCenso et al. (2006) found that primary prevention strategies did not delay the initiation of sexual intercourse, improve contraceptive use or reduce pregnancies in adolescents. Most of the participants in over half of these studies were African-American or Hispanic, thus over-representing lower socio-economic groups. In all but five of the studies, participants in the control group received a conventional intervention rather than no intervention, which may have reduced the likelihood of the education programmes in the intervention groups showing an effect. On the other hand, data from five of the studies, four abstinence programmes and one school-based sex education programmeme, showed an increase in pregnancies in partners of male participants.

There is evidence that prevention programmes may need to begin at a much earlier age if they are to be effective. Eight trials of day care for socially deprived children under 5-years of age showed lower pregnancy rates among adolescents on long term follow up (B. Zoritch et al., 2000). The positive outcomes were attributed to the quality of staff training, favourable staff:pupil ratios, adequate materials and parental involvement.

One may hypothesise that the love and stability provided to these children promoted higher self-esteem and helped empower them to make better decisions as adolescents.

Observational studies have shown that adolescent pregnancy prevention programmes have had a positive effect on decreasing initiation of sexual intercourse, increasing birth control use and responsible sexual behaviour, and reducing pregnancy in females; and on decreasing initiation of intercourse and increasing responsible sexual behaviour in males (G.H. Guyatt et al., 2000). It may be that adolescents receiving the intervention in observational studies are more predisposed to the positive outcomes while those less receptive are more likely to be in the comparison group.

However, three recent reviews of the literature support the effectiveness of sexual risk-reduction interventions for adolescents. B.T. Johnson et al. (2003) reviewed 44 studies and 56 interventions and found that intensive behavioural interventions reduced sexual HIV risk, especially because they increased skill acquisition, sexual communications, and condom use and decreased the onset of sexual intercourse or the number of sexual partners. The magnitude of the effect for the two most critical risk-reduction outcomes, sexual frequency and condom use, was small with only five of the interventions yielding significant effect size for these measures. Providing condoms to participants improved condom use. Studies that spent more time per intervention session on active condom instruction and training achieved greater success. Behavioural interventions that pursue these strategies do not increase the frequency of sexual behaviour, the number of sexual partners, or the onset of sexual debut (B.T. Johnson et al. 2003).

L. Robin et al. (2004) reviewed 24 studies conducted in the 1990s with a quasi-experimental or experimental evaluation design. Their findings suggest four overall factors that may impact programme effectiveness: focus on specific skills for reducing sexual risk behaviours, programmeme duration and intensity, the content of the total programme and the training available for facilitators. Among frequently targeted behaviours, the least consistent impact was found for delayed initiation of sexual intercourse and the most consistent for condom use. Only one programme focusing primarily on delayed initiation of sexual intercourse reported positive effects without also reporting negative effects (Jemmott JB et al., 1998).

D. Kirby et al. (2005) reviewed 83 evaluations of sex and HIV education programmes in developing (18) and developed (65) countries. Most of these programmes encouraged abstinence but also discussed or promoted the use of condoms or contraception if young people chose to be sexually active. Fifty-nine per cent of the studies measured impact for a year or longer and 22% measured impact for two years or longer. Twenty-two (42%) of these programmes significantly delayed the initiation of sex for at least 6-months, 29 (55%) found no significant impact and one (in the USA) found the programmeme hastened the initiation of sex. Of the 34 studies measuring number of sexual partners, 12 (35%) found a reduction, while 21 (62%) found no significant impact. Of the 31 studies measuring frequency of sex, 9 (29%) reduced the frequency, 19 (61%) found no significant change in frequency and 3 (all in developed countries) found increased frequency of sex. Of the 54 studies measuring programmeme impact on condom use, 48%

showed increased condom use, none found decreased condom use. Fourteen of 28 studies that developed a composite measure of sexual activity and condom use, found significantly reduced risk-taking while none found increased sexual risk-taking.

Overall, 65% of the studies found a significant positive impact on one or more of these sexual behaviours or outcomes, while only 7% found a significant negative impact. The evidence was strong that many programmes had positive effects on relevant knowledge, awareness of risk, values and attitudes, self-efficacy and intentions. Analysis of the effective curriculum led to the identification of 17 common characteristics of the curricula and their implementation. These had clear goals of preventing HIV/STI and/or pregnancy, focused on specific behaviours, included multiple activities to change the targeted risk and protective factors, used instructionally sound teaching methods that actively involved participants and helped them to personalize the information (D. Kirby et al., 2005).

FACING REALITY

It is essential that we face up to the reality that many schoolchildren in the Caribbean are sexually active and that there is the need for a comprehensive sex and HIV/STI education programme in schools. The new Health and Family Life Education curricula provides a good starting point for this programmeme, but it needs to be implemented fully and become an examinable subject. Sex education must begin at an early age, with material appropriate to the age group. Sex education should be provided in a context of promoting family values, life skills and a healthy lifestyle. Young children need to be fostered to develop emotional intelligence, resiliency skills, good interpersonal relations and conflict management skills while addressing gender equity and stereotypic gender roles. A loving, supportive environment is essential for the normal development of children. This is a tremendous challenge given the widespread violence in society.

Schools should be considered as 'no sex' zones and abstinence encouraged. However, simply preaching about abstinence is not enough. Children must be free to talk about sex and human sexuality must be discussed. Recognition of diversity and tolerance among persons is important. Children need to learn how to say no to sex and myths concerning not having sex need to be combated. Education for abstinence must be more creative and fun.

At the same time, youngsters need to be prepared for when they become sexually active. They need to learn condom skills before they start having sex. There are 12 different steps to properly using a condom. Many adults have no understanding of proper condom use and hence are reluctant to use it. Condom demonstrations using a dildo are essential to learning proper condom use. Only a minority of schools recognise this and are already doing them. Condom demonstrations need to be a standard activity in the Health and Family Life sex Education curriculum. Condoms, male and female, must be readily available for these demonstrations.

Parents need to be actively involved in the schools' sex education and health and family life programmes. Students have articulated the need for parental involvement in these programmes and for better communication with their parents. The truth is that there is no coherent programme for educating persons about parenting and this is a serious deficiency.

Even with an established high quality sex education programme and an effective health and family life education curriculum we can expect some young persons to be sexually active and to remain so following counselling. These youngsters need ready access to contraceptives in order to avoid pregnancy, HIV and other STI. Youth friendly health services need to be readily available. In Brazil, the Ministry of Health is introducing condom machines into schools. A UNESCO Study in Brazil found that two-thirds of the parents surveyed support the Government offering teenagers free condoms and sex education. We need to consider discrete access to condoms at schools through a few selected teachers and peer educators who are trained to manage and monitor the process. This could help to reduce teenage pregnancy and HIV infection among youths. For instance, almost one-third of all ever pregnant women aged 15–24 years in Jamaica become pregnant while still in school. Only 16% of them returned to school after the birth of their child (Morris et al., 1995).

STRENGTHENING THE RESPONSE OF THE EDUCATION SECTOR

The response of the education sector to the HIV/AIDS epidemic needs to be strengthened. An overall policy and strategic plan are needed to guide the response of the education sector. For instance, Jamaica has a National Policy for HIV/AIDS Management in Schools which is commendable. However, this policy does not provide any guidance to schools on how to manage sexually active school children. The Jamaican Government does have an excellent policy with respect to the provision of contraceptives to minors, which guides health providers. However, educators generally do not see this policy as also applying to the education sector. An education policy should address these matters and make Health and Family Life Education mandatory.

Teacher training colleges must prepare teachers to address HIV/AIDS and to teach the new Health and Family Life Education curriculum. A whole institution approach is best as this involves all members of the school community and uses a variety of different strategies and activities.

Schools do not need to wait for their Ministries of Education in order to implement HIV and sex education. The principal can initiate a multi-faceted programme to meet the specific needs of their pupils. Involving all sectors of the school community in the development of the programmeme is essential, as well as getting the endorsement of the school board. A small committee of interested persons can be formed, training sessions held and resource persons identified.

In conclusion, there is no doubt that many of our young people are sexually active at an early age without the prerequisite knowledge or skills to abstain or practise safe sex. The consequences of early sexual activity such as teenage pregnancy, HIV and other STI infections and disruption of education are far too common in the Caribbean. The scientific evidence clearly indicates that abstinence only programmes are inadequate and that investing in comprehensive sex education, that includes support for abstinence, but also provides risk-reduction information and skills would be a more effective HIV prevention strategy for young people.

REFERENCES

Assessing the Efficacy of Abstinence-Only Programmes for HIV Prevention among Young People. www.amfar.org. (2): 2006.

Brazil vows to install condom machines in schools. wl_nm/brazil_condom_schools_dc accessed February 7, 2007.

DiCenso A, Guyatt G, William A et al. Interventions to reduce unintended pregnancies among adolescents: systematic review of randomised controlled trials. BMJ (324) 2002.

Fox K, Gordon-Strachan G. Jamaica Youth Risk and Resiliency Behaviour Survey 2005 School-based Survey on Risk and Resiliency Behaviours of 10-15 year olds.

Guyatt G, DiCenso A, Farewell V et al. Randomised trials versus observational studies in adolescent pregnancy prevention. J Clin Epidemiol (53) 2000:167-174.

Jackson J, Leitch J and Lee A. The Jamaica Adolescent Study. Women's Studies Project, Family Health International 1998.

Jemmott JB, Jemmott LS, Fong GT. Abstinence and safer sex: a randomized trial of HIV sexual risk-reduction interventions for young African-American adolescents *Journal of the American Medical Association (279)* 1998:1529–1536.

Johnson BT, Carey MP, Marsh KL et al. Interventions to Reduce Sexual Risk for the Human Immunodeficiency Virus in Adolescents, 1985-2000. Arch Pediatr Adolesc Med. (157) 2003: 381-388.

Kirby D, Laris BA and Rolleri L. Impact of Sex and HIV Education Programmes on Sexual Behaviours of Youth in Developing and Developed Countries. Family Health International Youth Series Working Paper No. 2 2005.

Morris L, Sedivy V, Friedman JS, McFarlane CP. *Contraceptive Prevalence Survey: Jamaica 1993. Volume IV. Sexual Behavior and Contraceptive Use Among Young Adults.* Kingston: National Family Planning Board. March 1995.

Robin L, Dittus P, Whitaker D, et al. Behavioural Interventions to Reduce Incidence of HIV, STD, and Pregnancy Among Adolescents: A Decade in Review. J Adoles Health (34) 2004: 3-26.

Zoritch B, Roberts I, Oakley A. Day care for pre-school children (2000) Day care for preschool children, *The Cochrane Library,* Chichester: John Wiley & sons Ltd

10

Is Learning Becoming Taboo for Caribbean boys?

DAVID PLUMMER

COMMONWEALTH/UNESCO REGIONAL PROFESSOR OF EDUCATION[1]
(HIV HEALTH PROMOTION), SCHOOL OF EDUCATION, UNIVERSITY OF
THE WEST INDIES, ST AUGUSTINE, TRINIDAD

This book promotes the role of education as a key ingredient of the institutional response to the HIV epidemic. It assumes a demand for education and a universality of supply. Yet in recent years, gender dynamics in education in the English-speaking Caribbean have undergone significant shifts. On the one hand, educational access, retention and attainment by girls have improved significantly and should be celebrated as key success stories. On the other hand, retention, completion and attainment by boys appear to be slipping. The question at the centre of these changes is whether the decline for boys is relative (boys only appear to be declining because girls are doing so much better) or real (fewer boys are reaching their potential than was the case in the past). To explore this question preliminary data from a larger qualitative project on Caribbean masculinities were examined. As a result of this work new perspectives have emerged that may help to explain boys' changing educational achievements.

The importance of achieving a gendered identity is impressed upon us from our earliest years. During childhood we are provided with the means of constructing that identity essentially by modelling behaviours that differentiate us from the 'opposite' sex. Importantly, these behaviours and practices are not fixed - the paths to achieving 'legitimate' manhood vary widely between cultures and within cultures over time. It is in this context that changing educational achievement appears to present us with an interesting challenge.

In the past, academic excellence was largely, if not entirely a male domain. However, with education increasingly becoming 'common ground', boys are left with fewer opportunities to establish their gendered identity through education; and academic achievement furnishes those needs less readily. In contrast, fundamental biological differences means that physicality has been preserved as a way of asserting masculine difference, and the 'outdoors' remains boys' territory. In the Caribbean, outdoors physicality seems to have gained pre-eminent importance for developing a boys' identity. While this 'retreat to physicality' may well benefit sporting achievements, there are also important negative consequences. Opportunities to prove one's gender identity through physical dominance are increasingly driven towards hard, physical, risk-taking, hyper-masculine, sometimes antisocial acts including bullying, harassment, crime and violence. Meanwhile, the classroom no longer holds as much value for boys in establishing their masculine identity and it is therefore less attractive to them (a 'flight from academic achievement?'). Indeed boys who do achieve in academic pursuits are at risk of being considered 'suspect' by their peers and of becoming the subject of gender taboos. This includes boys who show a preference for reading, who regularly reported receiving homophobic criticism, perhaps the deepest of all masculine taboos.

Although this chapter does not specifically explore consequences of findings for schools as vehicle for reducing new HIV infections, it is included to stimulate dialogue among readers on gender considerations that will need to be factored in to ensure effectiveness of HIV strategies through formal and non formal education.

INTRODUCTION

Recent decades have witnessed important shifts in educational outcomes in the Commonwealth Caribbean for both boys and girls. These shifts are cause for both celebration and for concern.

On the one hand, educational outcomes for girls have improved significantly: girls now constitute the majority of secondary school enrolments in the region (Reddock 2004: xv) and girls' school attendance and retention rates exceed those for boys for all age cohorts (Chevannes 1999:11).

These trends are in evidence at the tertiary level too*. The number of women graduating each year from the University of the West Indies now exceeds the number of men (Figueroa 2004: 141; Reddock 2004: xv). Not surprisingly, this has not always been the case. Between 1948 and 1972, males occupied a sizeable majority (over 60%) of places at the University (Figueroa 2004: 142–143). However, this situation has been changing for some years now so that by 1974 female enrolments at the Jamaican campus passed 50% for the first time and by 1982 they exceeded 50% for all campuses. This trend has continued even further: by late 1992, 70% of graduates from the Jamaican campus were female (Reddock 2004: xv).

Of course, these changes might simply reflect a shift in the types of course offered by the university. Indeed, Mark Figueroa notes that the gender balance in registrations is not uniform over all disciplines: for example, in Jamaica 54% of law enrolments are female;

in agriculture this figure drops to 33%; and in engineering 10%. (Figueroa 2004: 142–143). Nevertheless, it remains the case that subjects that were once dominated by men are no longer so.

While we should rightly celebrate the achievements of women, we should also examine what is happening with the men. In this regard, there is mounting evidence that the educational status of boys and of young men is not faring nearly as well: boys' enrolment, retention and completion rates are lower throughout the system. There is little doubt that boys' performance has declined relative to the growing successes of girls, but what remains unclear is whether the data reflects a real decline or a relative decline? That is to say: boys only seem to be slipping because girls are now doing much better or are boys less likely to reach their potential in real terms compared with how boys performed in the past?

In an attempt to understand the situation better, and to add meaning to the accumulating quantitative evidence, interview data from a larger project on Caribbean masculinities were examined. I would like to thank the Commonwealth for funding this work. This project involved interviewing young men in their late teens and early twenties about their experiences of gender while they were growing up, particularly in peer groups and at school.

To date interviews have been conducted in three Caribbean countries: Guyana, Trinidad and St Kitts. The findings being reported here are preliminary and further interviews are planned for the coming year along with more detailed analyses. Nevertheless, these findings along with cumulative evidence from other researchers is building a compelling case that academic achievement is indeed becoming taboo at least among certain cohorts of Caribbean boys.

POLICING MASCULINITY

The interview data confirms that achieving a gendered identity – being able to project yourself as successfully masculine – takes centre stage for most boys as they mature. There is a sense that boys both aspire to masculine status and that their behaviour is policed to ensure that it conforms to prevailing masculine standards. Central to this policing process is the peer group, which the data reveals to be a formidable force in boys lives. According to Barry Chevannes:

As the boy approaches pre-pubescent years…the peer group begins to exercise its magnetic pull. (Chevannes 1999: 29)

Indeed, the present research reveals that for many teenaged boys the authority of the peer group at least competes and frequently exceeds the authority of any of the adults who feature in the boys lives. In that respect the data corroborates the words of Barry Chevannes who says:

The peer group virtually replaces mother and father as the controlling agents or, if not entirely a substitute, a countervailing force. (Chevannes 1999: 30)

So while it is popular to blame parents, teachers and the media for boys' adverse outcomes, more often than not it is the peer group that exercises the most profound influence. And as we will see shortly, this influence has wide-ranging social ramifications from educational achievement through to crime.

Of course peer group influences are not necessarily bad – but they can be. In fact they can be very bad. Here are the words of Bailey and colleagues in Jamaica;

The worst and most individualistic and predatory aspects of the street became the norm for youngsters who found validation for their behaviour in their peers and in the larger environment. (Bailey, Branche, McGarrity & Stuart 1998: 82)

The present research found strong linkages between peer groups and gang-related activity – to such an extent that a core research question that emerged was at what point does a peer group become a gang?

In time, some of these groups become fundamental identity –bearing groups that not only impose themselves on the behaviour of the young men but separate them competitively and conflictually from other similar groups of young men (Bailey, Branche, McGarrity & Stuart 1998: 59)

It seems as if in the absence of sufficient restraint, for example where there is lack of supervision or a 'power vacuum' for whatever reason, the peer group readily occupies that space. Often this occurs on the streets, where the peer group really comes into its own.

But these peer groups have to get this behaviour from somewhere? Someone must be responsible? The answer to this question is both yes and no. Yes, it is the case that the rules of masculinity arc comprehensively coded into our cultures. Moreover, parents, teachers and adult 'role models', including women, contribute significantly to setting the standards that boys emulate. As Wesley Crichlow reports:

> [My mother] *instilled in me a very rigid hyper-male gender prison* (Crichlow 2004: 193)

And when Crichlow then 'acted out' the hard masculinities that were instilled, he notes:

> ... *these activities demonstrated "power" to parents, women, teachers and friends, who were proud to see that a young man was not a buller, a sissy or a coward.* (Crichlow 2004: 201)

I draw your attention to the term 'buller' in the above example. This term is used in Trinidad and Barbados to denote a homosexual. We will return to the significance of this term shortly.

As for the 'no' case concerning whether some external agent is responsible, the research found that young men are not simply cultural sponges; the peer groups themselves are able to actively fashion dominant masculinity. Here is Barry Chevannes again:

> *An adolescent boy's friends exact an affinity and a loyalty as sacred as the bond of kinship as strong as the sentiment of religion. They socialise one another, the older members of the group acting as the transmitters of what passes as knowledge, invent new values and meanings.* (Chevannes 1999: 30)

This phenomenon I have previously called 'rolling peer pressure' (Plummer 2005: 226). Rolling peer pressure identifies a mechanism that explains how the cultures of boys and young men can be semi-autonomous and in effect take on a 'life of their own'. Codes and standards are continually passed down the chain from older to younger boys often

at arms length from adults. As a result, peer groups have a culture generating role that is, on reflection, highly evident in most modern societies. It also means that neither parents, nor teachers nor the media can be held primarily responsible for social movements that emanate from youth culture, including the problems that accompany them.

ASPIRING TO BE BAD: THE RISE OF HARD MASCULINITY

For many boys the constant social 'policing' of masculinity literally becomes a straight-jacket. These young men find themselves caught in a vice, occupying a narrow space of authorised masculinity while simultaneously being cut off from vast fields of social life which are rendered taboo by the same masculine standards they are under pressure to conform to. The rhetoric of the young men who were interviewed and their descriptions of the powerful influence of peer groups provided revealing insights into the standards against which boys are judged and the penalties for failing to conform. At the forefront of these standards is hard, physical, narrow, polarised masculinity. As Bailey et al. note:

> *It appeared as if the younger teenaged boys had embraced, in the most uncompromising way, the [prevailing] male gender ideology.* (Bailey, Branche, McGarrity & Stuart 1998: 82)

The relentless policing of 'manliness,' relies on boys being closely scrutinised. This scrutiny is particularly intense from peers. As a result, boys learn to choose their styles carefully and to craft an image for projection to the outside world, which partly reflects their personality but also carefully attests to their allegiance to the prevailing standards of masculinity endorsed by their peers. Elaborate codes arise which govern acceptable clothing, the designer labels to be worn, the deployment of 'bling' (jewellery acceptable to men), authorised styles of speech, striking a 'cool' pose and so on. For many boys image was everything – it sustained their masculine reputation.

Of course, image is more than merely appearance, it also stems from what you do. In contemporary male culture, masculine status is enhanced greatly by displays of sexual prowess, physical toughness and social dominance. Having multiple sexual partners earned respect while being faithful meant loosing face as Bailey et al. found:

> For males, multiple partnerships could become a matter of status… (p 65). The term 'one burner' applied to a faithful male in some Jamaican communities was a phrase of derision. (Bailey, Branche, McGarrity & Stuart 1998: 66)

Moreover, there was considerable social pressure to 'take' more than one sexual partner and this practice was bolstered by homophobic stigma for men who 'failed to measure up'.

> Someone who did not have as many women as they did was sick", "suspected as a buller" or not "the average young black male". (Crichlow 2004: 206)

The implications this data has for HIV prevention are significant. It is at the level of gender roles that sexual risks become deeply embedded in our cultures and safety can be steadfastly resisted as a result – despite wide awareness of HIV and the commonsense ways of avoiding it.

But the valorisation of hard and risky masculinities goes even further – this phenomenon constitutes the very foundations of many of our most profound social problems. There is strong pressure to resist adult authority, to earn status by taking risks and to display your masculine credentials in hard, physical and sometimes antisocial ways.

> In an attempt to temporarily secure my masculinity or hyper-masculinity and hegemonic heterosexuality, I participated in events such as stealing…breaking bottles with slingshots or stones on the street, engaging in physical fights, and "hanging on the block" with boys until late at night. (Crichlow 2004: 200)

It is here that the links between the prevailing standards of masculinity and crime start to emerge. In effect, crime becomes the ultimate symbol of the forms of masculinity that a society promotes – it stems from boys emulating the ways 'real men' are supposed to act according to the culture they grew up in:

> The so-called inner-city don is a role model not only because of his ability to command and dispense largesse, but also because he is a living source of power, the power over life and death, the ultimate man. Among the youth, a common word for penis was rifle. (Chevannes 1999: 29)

MASCULINE TABOOS – ENFORCING 'NO-GO' ZONES

Almost as noticeable as the symbols of masculinity that are widely flaunted, are the human qualities that go 'missing in action'. An early casualty is the ability to cry, or to be more accurate the ability to cry is not lost (the tear ducts still function), however crying in public is conscientiously suppressed. Most of the rest of the boy's emotional repertoire soon falls under similar heavy restraints, particularly those that denote tenderness.

However, not all emotions are expunged, some are actively cultivated – for example aggression and anger – precisely because these have come to symbolise masculinity.

In the following quote, Brown and Chevannes describe how boys use aggressive acts as a substitute for other emotions:

> *Boys greet each other with clenched fists and backslaps, and often use other forms of aggression to express their feelings.* (Brown & Chevannes 1998: 30)

Of course, there are always two sides to binary phenomena: aggression is both an expression of masculinity and a simultaneous public disavowal of tenderness. Here is Wesley Crichlow's perspective:

> *Our fights usually indicated an "overt disdain for anything that might appear soft or wet – more a taboo on tenderness than a celebration of violence".* (Crichlow 2004: 200 quoting Morgan)

It becomes increasingly clear from the present research and from the cumulative findings of other Caribbean researchers that much of the 'macho' acting out that is seen among boys and young men simultaneously affirms one's allegiance to prevailing standards of masculinity while publicly attesting to what is being rejected: soft, feminising and castrating 'failed' masculinities.

> *Boys have a real macho image to live up to. If a boy acts in an effeminate way he will be targeted and teased by the other students.* (Respondent quoted by Parry 2004: 176)

> *The culture demanded physical responses from boys and made toughness the hallmark of the real male. Young boys knew that if they performed outside the*

> *expected, traditional roles they would be ridiculed and labelled 'sissy' by boys and girls.* (Bailey, Branche & Henry-Lee 2002: 8)

IS BOYS' EDUCATION A CASUALTY OF THE RISE IN HARD MASCULINITY?

The combination of masculine obligation and taboo narrows boys' potential down and cuts them off from large areas of social life, which can only disadvantage them. Embracing hard, risk-taking, often antisocial 'hyper-masculinities' puts the lives of young men in danger: sexually, on the road, in the gang, and potentially in conflict with authority. By disenfranchising boys from activities that have been rendered taboo by their own codes of masculinity, boys are denying themselves access to considerable social benefits. For example, if being safe is considered 'sissy', then driving small low-powered cars at a safe speed potentially comes at a cost to one's reputation – and many opt to place themselves (and others) at risk in order to affirm their masculine status instead. Likewise, if youth culture has come to equate education with their own feminisation or with deep homophobic taboos, then getting an education is no longer something that a 'real man' would want to do. Yet this is exactly what the present research has found and these findings have been corroborated by the accumulated evidence of other Caribbean researchers as the following quotations confirm.

First, in a quote from a Jamaican boy to Barry Chevannes:

> *"School is girl stuff!" This declaration by an eight-year old inner-city boy...reveals the association built up in the minds of many boys.* (Chevannes 1999: 26)

Second, in the words of Wesley Crichlow, we see both homophobic and misogynistic taboos undermining the educational aspirations of boys:

> *Many young men in Trinidad argue that academic subjects such as mathematics, physics and English are for bullers and women, while trades are for men.* (Crichlow 2004: 206)

Third, from Mark Figueroa, we see misogynistic prejudice underwriting contempt for education by boys:

> *There is evidence that boys actually actively assert their maleness by resisting school. This is particularly true with respect to certain subjects that are seen as "feminine". Male-child subculture therefore exerts considerable peer pressure on boys to be disruptive in school and to underrate certain subjects.* (Figueroa 2004: 152)

Fourth, we see these same taboos reinforcing an anti-academic ethos of contemporary Caribbean masculinity in the work of Odette Parry:

> *The homophobic fears expressed by staff and the resulting censure of attitudes and behaviours which were felt to be "effeminate", "girlish", "sissy like" and "nerdish" reinforce a masculine gender identity which rejects many aspects of schooling as all of the above.* (Parry 2004: 179)

DISCUSSION

The educational achievements of Caribbean women over the last couple of decades are an important success story that deserves both recognition and praise. Unfortunately, these successes are at risk of being overshadowed by changes in boys'

education, which by-and-large show that male educational achievement is declining. Some commentators assume that these two changes are linked – that the progress made by Caribbean girls is at the expense of Caribbean boys. The implications of such a proposition are profound and demand careful analysis.

In 1986 Errol Miller published his work 'The marginalisation of the black male: insights from the development of the teaching profession'. Miller's thesis – that Caribbean men were being marginalised by social forces largely beyond their control – struck a chord which still reverberates 20 years later, especially in popular culture. Likewise his thesis stimulated vigorous debate in academic circles and has been the subject of many academic critiques over the years. In addressing the issue of 'male marginalisation' Barry Chevannes drew the following conclusion:

> *Are males being marginalised? Certainly not if the main factor being considered is power.* (Chevannes 1999: 33)

Mark Figueroa took the argument further by arguing that changes in male educational outcomes are a paradoxical effect of traditional male privilege rather than of marginalisation. According to this theory, males traditionally enjoyed privileged access to public space which they dominated, whereas women were largely restricted to private domestic space. In the context of education, this male privileging of public space worked against academic endeavours whereas women being largely confined to the domestic sphere were inherently better placed to study.

While Figueroa's thesis reconfigures the debate from marginalisation to male privilege, it seems to perpetuate the cross linking of girls' achievements and boys' shortcomings as the following quote suggests:

Increasingly, as women "take over" so-called male academic subjects, the options for boys will be more and more limited. Ultimately, there will be little that boys can safely do without threatening their masculinity. (Figueroa 2004: 159)

Moreover, in the past, boys' education and men's academic pursuits were privileged male domains too and an explanation is still needed why boys might be vacating the area with apparent alacrity.

Data from the present research adds a further dimension to the analysis of Caribbean boys' educational achievements. The research supports previous findings that boys' affinity with public space and physicality is linked to the development of masculine identity. Moreover, in contemporary Caribbean settings, this identity seems to preferentially elevate hard, aggressive, dominant masculinity as the epitome of manhood – perhaps increasingly so in recent years. Certainly, gang culture and music laced with violent allusions have become more prominent in the Caribbean in the last couple of decades. But the present research adds additional data concerning the role of masculine taboos in creating a range of pressures that create social 'no-go zones' for young men – one of which increasingly seems to be education.

A surprising but important finding that has emerged is the role of homophobia in stigmatising boys who are academically inclined. This stands out as a consistent and deep seated phenomenon, not a minor diversionary issue. In the first instance, the role of homophobia seems difficult to account for, but it starts to make sense in the light of recent research that has found homophobic

abuse to be a mechanism primarily for policing manhood (by stigmatising boy's transgressions and 'failed' masculinities) and is only secondarily concerned with sexual practice (Plummer 2005). In this sense, as a repository for 'failed manhood' and as a mechanism for policing the standards of masculinity, homophobia is rightly seen as being a gender prejudice – one which impacts on the lives of all men. Gender in development programmes therefore need to take a much more active interest in it.

So where do these findings leave the 'male marginalisation' thesis? The conclusion from the present work is that if boys are being marginalised, then it seems likely that they are in fact actively marginalising themselves in order to escape the stigma of masculine taboos. The process of developing male identity involves adopting and displaying shared symbols of masculinity while simultaneously disavowing any hint of failed masculinity. Lately, education seems to have become increasingly associated with feminising and homophobic taboos. This may well have coincided with the progress made by girls in education, but there would seem to be no reason why this has to be the case: greater access by women to education does not explain why males should necessarily have lesser access, unless it becomes taboo. It is the misogynistic and homophobic taboos that alienate boys from large areas of social life that they would be much better off having access to. Central to this process is how peer groups police certain activities that do not accord with peer-endorsed norms of manhood and/ or they come into tension with prevailing taboos. These norms and their associated taboos are endorsed and manufactured by the peer group. While this occurs in the context of wider social expectations of masculinity, the groups themselves actively manipulate masculinities as our highly visible youth cultures constantly demonstrate. In Barry Chevannes's words:

In a way we are all responsible. We [Society] provide the building blocks, the young people design and construct their own edifice. (Chevannes 1999: 31)

CONCLUSION

The final point to consider is whether the data offer clues as to ways forward. In this regard, there are a number of possibilities (see table 10.1). First, while associations have been made by some commentators between girls' accomplishments and boys' difficulties, it is important to recognise that this does not have to be the case. If anything, the link between the two elements is supplied by masculine taboos which tend to make simultaneous achievement by males and females mutually exclusive (the taboos most prominent in the data are misogyny and homophobia). In the case of these taboos, the problem clearly lies with the prejudices indoctrinated into men and boys rather than with girls and women

being responsible (they are just as much a victim of these prejudices as the boys are, but in different ways). But for as long as they play a role in the development of young men's identity, then they will impact on educational outcomes. On the other hand, if those taboos can be alleviated, then boys will find it much easier to engage with the education system and in more constructive ways. At least this particular social domain will no longer be seen as belonging to one gender or the other, but as a site where both sexes can develop in fulfilling and meaningful ways. Girls' accomplishments in education need to be celebrated and sustained. In addition, we need to take a much more strategic approach to boys' education. The assumption of a link between girls' achievements and boys' difficulties needs to be exposed as unnecessary as it is harmful. Moreover, men need to realise that prevailing contemporary masculinities which are both narrow and hard are leaving young men in a difficult situation. It is masculinity that is at the root of many of boys' educational problems: hard, narrow, polarised masculinities must be resisted. Well-rounded, diverse male role models

TABLE 10.1
THE WAY FORWARD

- Celebrate girls' educational successes as important Caribbean accomplishments
- Take a more strategic approach to promoting boys' achievements
- De-link girls' successes from boys' difficulties
- Recognise that contemporary dominant masculinities are problematic
- Resist hard, narrow, polarised masculinity
- Counterbalance hard, physical, narrow masculinities with well-rounded male role models
- Embrace diverse masculinities and alternative male role models
- Re-associate masculinity with education and academic prowess
- Engage more fully with peer group dynamics
- Confront the taboos that cause boys to flee from educational pursuits and retreat to hard, physical masculinity
- Reject homophobic and misogynist prejudices
- Support research into masculinities, masculine taboos and peer group dynamics

need to be visible and accessible. Notions of masculinity need to be reconnected with educational achievement. The complex and powerful role of male peer groups needs to be carefully studied and sophisticated strategies developed to intervene in their anti-social potential. Taboos have to be confronted if progress is to be possible. Based on the evidence from the present research and the corroborating evidence from other Caribbean studies, this necessarily includes addressing misogyny and homophobia.

I would like to express my appreciation to the Commonwealth and the University of the West Indies for supporting this project.

REFERENCES

Bailey W (ed.) (1998) *Gender and the family in the Caribbean.* Mona, Jamaica: Institute of Social and Economic Research.

Bailey W, Branche C, McGarrity G, Stuart S (1998) *Family and the quality of gender relations in the Caribbean.* Mona, Jamaica: Institute of Social and Economic Research.

Bailey W, Branche C, Henry-Lee A (2002) *Gender, contest and conflict in the Caribbean.* Mona, Jamaica: SALISES.

Brown J, Chevannes B (1998) *Why man stay so – tie the Heifer and loose the bull: an examination of gender socialisation in the Caribbean.* Mona: University of the West Indies.

Chevannes B (1999) *What we sow and what we reap – problems in the cultivation of male identity in Jamaica.* Kingston, Jamaica: Grace, Kennedy Foundation.

Crichlow WEA (2004) History, (Re)Memory, Testimony and Biomythography: charting a Buller Man's Trinidadian Past. In: Reddock RE (ed.) Interrogating Caribbean masculinities. Mona, Jamaica: University of the West Indies Press (pp. 185-222).

Reddock RE (ed.) (2004) *Interrogating Caribbean masculinities.* Mona, Jamaica: University of the West Indies Press.

Miller E (1986) *The marginalisation of the black male: insights from the development of the teaching profession.* Kingston, Jamaica: Institute of Social and Economic Research.

Parry O (2000) *Male underachievement in high school education.* Mona, Jamaica: Canoe Press.

Plummer D (2005) Crimes against manhood: homophobia as the penalty for betraying hegemonic masculinity. In: Hawkes G & Scott J (eds.). *Perspectives in human sexuality.* Melbourne: Oxford University Press.

11

HEALTH AND FAMILY LIFE EDUCATION: ADDRESSING CHALLENGES TO EFFECTIVENESS IN CARIBBEAN SCHOOLING

MORELLA JOSEPH, *CARICOM*

ELAINE KING, *UNICEF, BARBADOS AND EASTERN CARIBBEAN*

CONNIE CONSTANTINE, LYDIA O'DONNELL, ANN STUEVE AND

CHERYL VINCE WHITMAN, *EDUCATION DEVELOPMENT CENTER, INC, USA*

The history, evolution, and current status of the Health and Family Life Education (HFLE) initiative is examined. Over the past several years, HFLE has sought to improve the long-term health and prospects of Caribbean children and youth by making a life skills-based[1] education programme an essential core of the overall school curriculum. This chapter traces the roots of HFLE and explores the set of factors – including the threats that Caribbean children face and the foresight of the region's education and health leaders – that led to the programme's creation. The process of developing a Regional HFLE Framework under CARICOM leadership is summarised. An update is given on the progress in developing a common curriculum guided by the HFLE Curriculum Framework. Finally, the authors describe the ongoing efforts to gauge HFLE's effectiveness in achieving its intended objectives. In conclusion, the authors reflect on key implications for institutionalising and sustaining the HFLE intervention. The HIV related topics of CARICOM's Regional HFLE Framework is given in Chapter 21.

INTRODUCTION: INVESTING IN THE WELL-BEING AND FUTURE OF CARIBBEAN CHILDREN

Caribbean children and youth are increasingly vulnerable to new threats to their development. On a daily basis, they face many challenges – sexual abuse, alcohol and drug abuse, sexually transmitted infections (STIs), HIV and AIDS, early pregnancy, crime and violence, obesity, dysfunctional families, and neglect – with which they are ill-equipped to cope. Emanating from fundamental and complex changes in socio-economic and cultural patterns of living, these challenges prevent children and youth from maximising their true potential for learning and personal development. They also negatively influence the health and life opportunities of children and youth.

Research has shown that parents, caregivers, and families can play a vital role in protecting children and youth and preventing risk-taking behaviours that arise from environmental stressors. Yet, families are just one of the many sources that shape young adults' acquisition of knowledge and development of healthy and positive attitudes, values, and beliefs. The media and peers, for example, can send powerful and conflicting messages that leave young people vulnerable and at risk. Further, many families are, for various reasons (e.g. poverty, illness or unemployment) unable to provide and sustain the supportive and nurturing environment that is so critical to personal development and healthy lifestyles.

Consequently, adolescents and youth respond in a mal-adaptive manner that poses a threat to their health and development and contributes to a deterioration of family and community life.

Almost 20 years ago, the Caribbean Community (CARICOM) Ministers of Health and Education, joined by other education personnel, recognised the adverse impact of escalating social problems on children and youth and consequent erosion of the quality of life for all of the region's citizens. These leaders identified the need to engage the education sector more deeply in empowering young people with the knowledge and skills to make informed choices about their health and well-being.

Whilst the challenges that children and youth face are manifested both within and outside the school system, Ministers perceived that high school enrolment rates (1993 regional average of 93% at primary level and 54% at secondary) render schools the ideal setting for an intervention designed to enhance the welfare of children and youth. Educators have the opportunity to equip students with accurate information that enables them to make healthy lifestyle choices. They can also help foster students' development of essential life skills and aid students in making the link between their day-to-day choices and their overall health and safety. Thus, the Ministers began to chart a course to build schools' capacity to help reshape students' attitudes, values, practices, and behaviours and to ensure that educational opportunities were available and accessible regardless of gender.

Beginning in 1988, the Ministers passed a variety of resolutions at meetings of the Council on Human and Social Development (COHSOD). These resolutions supported the development and implementation of a comprehensive HFLE approach by CARICOM, the University of the West Indies (UWI), and other partner agencies. A brief overview of highlights in the Ministers' and other leaders' early support for and evolving vision for HFLE follows:

- In 1994, the CARICOM Standing Committee of Ministers of Education passed a resolution supporting a comprehensive approach to school-based health education programme – which they agreed to call Health and Family Life Education (HFLE).

- In 1996 a comprehensive strategy for strengthening HFLE in CARICOM countries was developed and endorsed by CARICOM Ministers of Education and Health. The Ministers agreed to support the development of national policies to incorporate HFLE as part of the core curriculum for all pre-primary, primary, and secondary schools.

- In 1997, participants in the Eighteenth Meeting of the CARICOM Heads of Government agreed that the sustainability of an efficient and productive work force ultimately depends on the full realisation of the potential of children and young people. The Conference of Heads also agreed that children and young people should experience programmes such as the life skills-based HFLE that support their development towards the 'Ideal Caribbean Person.'

From 1998 to 2003, the effort to move health education in schools from a series of vertical, single subjects to a broader, more comprehensive life skills-based HFLE curriculum met with some challenges. Even as attempts to incorporate HFLE throughout the school system intensified, it became evident that the programme was very knowledge-based and focused on the dissemination of information. At the same time, students' informal feedback revealed that they lacked the ability to apply their new knowledge in relevant settings.

Being cognisant of some of these concerns, participants in the April 2003 special meeting of the Council for Human and Social Development (COSHOD) – which focused on education – reaffirmed the Ministers' commitment to the comprehensive implementation of HFLE in schools. COSHOD called for the development and implementation of a life skills-based curriculum guided by a Regional HFLE Curriculum Framework which could be adapted by CARICOM member states to meet their specific needs. And, in 2004, the CARICOM Ministers of Education endorsed the development of the HFLE Regional Curriculum Framework for children and youth ages 9–14.

In the pages that follow, we discuss the process used to develop the Regional HFLE Curriculum Framework.

The Regional HFLE Curriculum Framework was developed to guide countries in adapting and upgrading their national HFLE curricula to strengthen the skills-based component.

A Regional Health and Family Life Education (HFLE) Curriculum Framework, which outlines both the philosophy and standards for teaching, and the desired student knowledge, skills and behavioural outcomes for students, was completed in 2004. The HFLE Framework document provides a tool for curriculum planners, education officers, teacher educators and teachers to review, develop and strengthen in-country HFLE curriculum and, by extension, harmonise curricula across the region. A strengthened HFLE curriculum has the potential to address many health and social challenges in the region, including HIV/AIDS, violence and substance abuse. Hence CARICOM and UNICEF were particularly keen to have this regional HFLE Framework translated into national curricula and implemented in classrooms, to provide students with information and skills to address some of the challenges to their health and well-being.

FORMING THE HFLE ADVISORY COMMITTEE

Working in partnership, the CARICOM Secretariat and UNICEF established a small HFLE Curriculum Advisory Committee to advise and guide the development of the Regional HFLE Curriculum Framework. The Advisory Committee included independent HFLE professionals as well as representatives from the Organisation of Eastern Caribbean States (OECS), UWI, national governments, and CARICOM and UN agencies – UNICEF, PAHO, UNESCO. This group of expert advisors was charged with overseeing the development of a Framework that addressed the needs of Caribbean countries for curricula that promote pro-social behaviours and mitigate behaviours that can lead to adverse outcomes. Education Development Center, Inc. (EDC),[2]

DEVELOPING THE REGIONAL HFLE CURRICULUM FRAMEWORK

The Regional HFLE Curriculum Framework was developed to guide countries in adapting and upgrading their national HFLE curricula to strengthen the skills-based component

Health and Human Development Programs (HHD) was recruited as technical consultant to lead the Framework development process.

FOCUSING RESOURCES AND PRODUCING MATERIALS

Sufficient resources were not available to complete the Regional Framework for the full range of pre-primary through secondary school students. Therefore, in appreciation of the spurt in brain development around age 11 that affects emotional skills and increases the capacity for abstract thinking, the Advisory Committee decided to focus its initial development efforts on the most critical 9–14 age group.

Working in concert with the Committee, a core, four-member technical writing team – expanded at times to include other technical experts – devised four central themes for the Regional Framework – Eating and Fitness, Sexuality and Sexual Health (including HIV prevention), Self and Interpersonal Relationships (including gender relationships and protection from sexual harassment and violence), and Managing the Environment. Through a process of consultation and collaboration, team members then developed materials for each of the four themes in a modular format that included standards, desired student knowledge, skills and behavioural outcomes for each age group, sample lessons, and teaching resources. The sample lessons included life skills development, interactive teaching strategies, and forms of alternative student competency assessment that went beyond pencil and paper approaches. The lessons also outlined the philosophy and standards for teaching HFLE and provided examples of approaches that educators could use to engage students.

Throughout the development process,

the technical writing team used several approaches to ensure that the Framework was academically sound, rigorous, and relevant to the unique needs of CARICOM countries:

- The team infused all aspects of the Framework's format and content with evidence-based research.
- The team made a special effort to ensure that the content and information in each theme reflected and addressed cultural differences among Caribbean countries and in addition, due attention was paid to gender equality.
- The team engaged HFLE coordinators and teachers in the development of the Framework and to reflect the concerns of classroom teachers as well as students.
- The team utilised the expertise of the Advisory Committee. At several points in the process, the Committee reviewed drafts of the Framework and provided feedback.

NOTES

1. UNICEF defines life skills-based education as an interactive process of teaching and learning that enables learners to acquire knowledge and to develop attitudes and skills which support the adoption of healthy behaviours.

2. Education Development Center, Inc. (EDC) is a publicly funded organisation headquartered in Boston, Massachusetts which provides consultancy services in a number of areas including health promotion, education, technology, and human rights and works in several countries across the globe.

12

RESPONDING TO THE NEED FOR INSTRUCTIONAL MATERIALS: THE CASE FOR PARTNERSHIP

IAN RANDLE

CARIBBEAN PUBLISHERS' NETWORK

A case is made for partnership between government and private sector publishers in the production of appropriate and culturally relevant instructional materials for HIV and AIDS education. It is argued that the development, production and use of such materials is an essential component of the education response to HIV and AIDS in the Caribbean region.

CURRENT PRACTICES

Instructional materials should be given high priority in policy formulation both at the national and regional levels because of the tendency in the past to treat this component, not as a core element of overall policy, but as an add-on or even at times something that will take care of itself. This often results in the poor articulation of instructional materials and curriculum goals; selection and use of materials that are dubious in their cultural relevance; and the overall availability and price to users being left entirely to market forces.

Happily, some governments of the region have moved away from this 'default' policy approach to the role of instructional materials in delivering the core curriculum, most notably Barbados, Jamaica, St Lucia and Trinidad and Tobago. These governments now clearly recognise at both a policy and implementation level the importance of instructional materials as one of the crucial links in the process of delivering quality education. At the implementation level, this ranges from the establishment of in-house instructional materials development units whose mandate is to produce classroom materials that have either been state published or published in partnership with private sector entities (for example, in Jamaica), to textbook evaluation committees where materials are evaluated and selected with reference to clearly developed guidelines that are in the public domain and familiar to private sector publishers (for example, in Trinidad and Tobago). In all these initiatives, partnership with private sector publishers is increasingly becoming the norm and this has resulted in the accelerated development of the educational publishing sector in the Caribbean, something for which these government ministries must be given credit.

These observations are made not with the aim of praising or 'buttering up' our Ministers of Education but to emphasise the fact that in developing their national and regional responses to HIV and AIDS education, a workable and effective template already exists in respect of instructional materials. These observations also make the case for Ministry policy initiatives towards HIV and AIDS education to be treated as if they were part of the core curriculum. Some good work has already been done in the form of the regional Health and Family Life Education (HFLE) curriculum, which has been developed and tested with national inputs, and which provides the basis for the development of a wide range of instructional materials at the national and regional level. Commitment to, and support for, the development and production of such materials as a high priority issue is necessary, given that HFLE is currently not seen as a core subject area and because of the low level of professionalism among those who teach the subject. Having said this, we have to be realistic and acknowledge the fact that given the demands on all governments of the region to find the necessary resources to deliver the core curriculum, it is difficult to make the case for the development and production of HFLE materials to be funded within existing and even future budgetary allocations to Ministries of Education. Therefore, from the outset, funding for the development and production of such materials has to be conceived as extra-budgetary items and sourced through agencies that already exist, and through programmes already developed specifically to support HIV and AIDS education initiatives. Representatives of many of these agencies and programmes are represented at the CARICOM Special Meeting of COHSOD on Education and HIV/AIDS, and this forum is being challenged to highlight instructional materials development and production as a priority area for support funding.

THE ROLE OF THE CARIBBEAN PUBLISHING COMMUNITY

The following section discusses the role of Caribbean publishers as partners with governments, Ministries of Education, regional and international agencies in the creation and production of instructional materials for HIV and AIDS education. Recognising that Caribbean publishers had a crucial moral, social and commercial role to play in halting the spread of HIV and AIDS in the Caribbean, the regional network of publishers, CAPNET, with support from UNESCO, convened in May 2005, a landmark international conference in Montego Bay to discuss a publishing response to the HIV and AIDS epidemic. We were also concerned by the realisation that the publishing community (as distinct from the general media) in the Caribbean and indeed throughout the world, had not been engaged in the dialogue about the HIV and AIDS epidemic and specifically about what role, if any, they might play in the vital area of education.

There had already been some halting efforts in this direction. For example, *The Caribbean Aids Epidemic* jointly edited by Glenford Howe and Alan Cobly and published by the University of the West Indies Press was the first book by a Caribbean publisher to address the HIV and AIDS issue in the region. Then in 2005, Ian Randle Publishers collaborated with UNESCO's Office for the Caribbean to publish the seminal work *Education and HIV/AIDS in the Caribbean* (2005) by Michael J. Kelly and Brendan Bain, as well as the pioneering novel for teenagers entitled *The Silent Killer*, written by the Barbadian Barbara Chase. But these were isolated efforts rather than coordinated or clearly defined publishing strategies aimed at a long-term outcome. The Montego Bay conference therefore had the potential to be the catalyst in mobilising an industry response through sustained development of reading and other instructional materials for HIV and AIDS education. The first of its kind to be held anywhere in the world, it attracted sizeable delegations from Southern, East and West Africa who were not only keen to share their experiences of effective publishing interventions, as in the case of Uganda, but also eager to learn from Caribbean and other colleagues about curriculum and publishing initiatives that might be effectively adapted for use in their respective countries. Box 12.1 provides a summary of the end of conference conclusions.

In assessing the outcome of that conference from a Caribbean perspective, there is no question that Caribbean publishers not only left with a heightened awareness of what it meant to be doing business in an environment under threat from the HIV and AIDS epidemic, but also for the first time were presented with the challenges and opportunities provided by the implementation of the regional HFLE curriculum in their respective countries. On a practical publishing level, participation by Macmillan Publishers from the UK opened up the opportunity for publishing the first ever Caribbean textbook on HIV/AIDS, *Teaching about HIV and AIDS for the Caribbean*. But we were preempted at the

BOX 12.1
Summary of the conclusions from the CAPNET Montego Bay Conference, 2005

- We anticipate that more publishers from the Caribbean region and beyond will recognize both the importance and commercial viability of publishing for HIV and AIDS.
- There will be new collaborative efforts between publishers across the African, Caribbean and Pacific countries and the South in general, and as part of this process, HIV and AIDS publishing will be fast-tracked in countries where little or no publishing in this area currently exists.
- Through the capacity-building component, editors will be better equipped to work with teachers, authors and persons living with HIV and AIDS to produce more books on the subject and to do so in sensitive language and in a non-discriminatory way.
- There will be greater collaboration between commercial publishers and materials production units, in government agencies and NGOs particularly, both in publishing and distribution.
- Through discussions among publishers, greater focus will be brought to bear on the special education needs of rural communities and of women, and practical publishing ideas and proposals developed to address their needs.
- By becoming involved in publishing for HIV and AIDS education, publishers will, by example, become active agents in helping to reduce the stigma and discrimination associated with the disease.
- Institutions such as the University of the West Indies will recognize the need to initiate research on the effectiveness of published HIV and AIDS materials that will inform the publishing industry.
- Information providers, including Ministries of Education, health educators and librarians, will become aware of the range of materials available for immediate procurement and use or adaptation.
  Publishers will become sensitized to the epidemic, its social and economic implications and their corporate responsibility in the face of the global consequences.

international level: our Nigerian colleagues, acting immediately on contacts that were made at the Montego Bay conference, successfully adapted a South African textbook series which, with the personal intervention of the Nigerian President, is now being used in all schools throughout the country. I would also like to think that, although they were not participants at the Montego Bay conference, Oxford University Press were inspired by the deliberations there to produce a new series of readers specifically for the Caribbean market. The discussions at the conference and the practical outcomes outlined above reinforced the importance and validity of South–South cooperation at all levels, but especially in the area of instructional materials and the possibilities for adaptation from one region to another. In this regard, the Deputy Minister of Education of South Africa will be pleased to note that a series of books originally published for his country have been piloted in both Guyana and Jamaica under the auspices of UNESCO, with overall positive results both for use in their original editions as well as for adaptation. At the same time, evaluation of these pilot materials has confirmed the validity of infusing HIV and AIDS learning concepts through general readers into the curriculum – an outcome that has been welcomed by the Ministers of Education. In the case of Jamaica, the Jamaican Library Service (JLS) has gone a step further and purchased a number of these books for use in schools.

So there is a platform on which we can build, and given the urgency of the response required from the education sector, all the available options need to be considered, including the adaptation of existing materials, particularly from countries of the South. Publishers in the Caribbean have been slow to enter the field of publishing materials for HIV and AIDS because we are not aware of any country in the region in which there exists any systematic effort by governments to equip schools and their libraries with books and other instructional materials designed specifically for targeted age groups. The JLS purchase described above is the only one of which we are aware and while one might be able to point to the availability of international NGO-produced materials in some of our institutions, these tend to be generic and broad-based in their approach and hence are not necessarily in line with national strategies.

Short of developing whole new programmes, which both take time and the kinds of resources that few of our governments have at their disposal, we would like to commend for your urgent consideration a strategy that lends itself to immediate or short-term implementation without the attendant high project costs. That strategy calls for the infusion of HIV and AIDS teaching and learning concepts in new editions of textbooks across the curriculum and to make it mandatory for such concepts to be infused in all new textbooks presented for use in schools. Textbook Evaluation Committees, such as the one that works so effectively in Trinidad and Tobago, would have a powerful and crucial role to play in making this one of the key criteria in the evaluation process and by doing so would make publishers partners in the process of HIV and AIDS education.

The Caribbean publishing community is keen to follow up on these initiatives. At the same time we wish to declare to the governments of the region that Caribbean publishers and their international colleagues, especially those with a long history of publishing textbooks for the region, are fully behind you in your efforts to fashion appropriate instructional materials for HIV and AIDS education.

We urge an extension of the burgeoning partnership relationship between Ministries of Education and private sector Caribbean publishers that is working so effectively for the core curriculum, to encompass new initiatives for instructional materials for HIV and AIDS. This should be within a policy framework that allows for private sector initiated projects to be developed within national and even regional curricula, supported by government approval, adoption and purchase though bilateral and multinational funding programmes. Such initiatives may be supplementary to curriculum materials projects developed by Ministries of Education with private sector publishing participation. Outsourcing of the publishing and distribution functions by Ministries of Education is now seen as a legitimate and cost-effective policy option even as these Ministries maintain control of the content, quality of the production and even the price at which such materials are delivered to the consumer.

At the same time I make no apology in going to bat for the regional publishing industry. Caribbean-based educational publishers have shown that they not only have the capability to produce and deliver quality educational materials, but have been key partners and supporters of governments in the production of instructional materials to support the delivery of national curricula at the primary level, particularly in Jamaica and Trinidad and Tobago. Local and regional publishers are in a unique position to ensure that the materials they develop are sensitive to persons living with HIV and AIDS, to cultural nuances and practices and also to the overall aims of national curricula. We have come a long way but we have not yet come of age. Our limited resources, of necessity force us to focus almost entirely on the demands of the core curriculum subjects, allowing little room for investment in what might be regarded as marginal areas such as HFLE. The fact that we have no ongoing publishing programmes for HIV and AIDS education to bring to the table at this forum does not denote a lack of interest or commitment but is rather the stark reality of limited financial resources. In this scenario, there is a danger that, unless Ministries of Education adopt a proactive approach of partnering with local and regional publishers, the 'crisis' of HIV and AIDS education could benefit extra-regional publishers by default, given their wider access to resources and their ability to invest in 'new' areas of the curriculum.

To summarise, Caribbean publishers bring to the table:

- A commitment to the regional response to the HIV and AIDS epidemic born out of a sense of moral obligation, shared responsibility and commercial self-interest,
- Willingness to invest in and publish for national curricula against the prevailing norm and at great commercial risk,
- Proven track record created within relatively short period of time of producing high quality, pedagogically sound and culturally appropriate textbooks for both national and regional curricula,
- Solid and mutually respectful working relationship with curriculum bodies and Ministries of Education, and
- Membership of a regional network of publishing professionals committed to the concept of regionalism, continued professional development among its members and the industry generally.

A REGIONAL APPROACH

The limitations faced by local and national publishing companies outlined above also apply to national governments. As the CARICOM region opens up into an effective Common Market with free movement of people, curricula across all subject areas will, over time, have to be amended to reflect the new realities of increased cultural as well as economic integration. Although it is some way off, we are likely to see the gradual blurring of national differences in cultural and societal practices even though we might remain geographically and politically separate. In this context the imperative for a regional approach to HIV and AIDS education, and, by extension, the development and production of instructional materials, not only becomes a national imperative related to costs but a regional one given the ideal of a 'borderless' Caribbean region. A regional approach to the development and production of instructional materials would not only achieve economies of scale but would also spread the cost among governments and assist those who would not be in a position to develop nationally-based projects but for whom the need is equally great. A regional approach also minimises the problem of distribution, which remains the single most intractable problem facing the producers of educational materials in the region.

CARICOM MEETING ON EDUCATION AND HIV/AIDS

It might be remembered that some initiatives in the 1970s and 1980s by governments to develop regional publishing projects never got off the ground and, in the one of the few instances that one did, it failed to remain sustainable.

I urge you not to be dissuaded by these past failures. The fact is that we cannot afford to fail, because in the spread of the HIV epidemic we are bound to each other. Besides, the Caribbean is a different place than it was 25 to 30 years ago. The infrastructure and institutions for functional cooperation are much more highly developed and our leaders are much more open to the concept of production integration in the region as evidenced by serious discussions about Jamaican and Guyanese bauxite being supplied for an aluminium smelter in Trinidad. In book production, Jamaican publishers today develop, edit and design textbooks for the national curricula that are printed in Trinidad, which has the most sophisticated printing plants in the Caribbean.

I would like to propose not only the endorsement of the principle of a regional approach to the development of HIV and AIDS instructional materials, but that our Ministers go beyond that to agree on the development of one or more series of readers that would include life stories of persons living with HIV and AIDS, contributed by each CARICOM country and edited, designed and produced in partnership with regional publishers and printers. Such personal life stories will be important in highlighting as role models persons who have responded to their situation not with despondency and depression but with courage and leadership through advocacy and outreach. At the same time, one or more international partners should be invited to fund the development and production phases, but equally important, the free distribution across the Caribbean region. Obviously such distribution would not be feasible on a one-on-one basis, but the regional free distribution effort might then be supplemented by national efforts to effect wider country by country distribution. Caribbean publishers stand ready to participate meaningfully in such a regional initiative.

The Caribbean publishing community is grateful for the opportunity to address the issue of instructional materials specifically related to HIV and AIDS education.

REFERENCES

CAPNET. 2005. Report of the Fourth International Conference on Publishing in the Caribbean: Publishers Against Aids. Kingston: Caribbean Publishers Network.

Chase, B. 2005 *The Silent Killer*. Kingston: Ian Randle Publishers.

Howe, G. and Cobley, A. (eds.). 2000. The Caribbean Aids Epidemic. Kingston: University of the West Indies Press.

Kelly, M. and Bain, B. 2005. *Education and HIV/ AIDS in the Caribbean*. Kingston: Ian Randle Publishers in association with UNESCO and IIEP

UNESCO. 2006. Report of the Review of HIV/ AIDS African Materials/Readers. Kingston.

13

African HIV/AIDS Instructional Materials: Adopt, Adapt or Start Over?

Diane Browne

Instructional materials specialist

The Ministry of Education, Jamaica, and the UNESCO Office for the Caribbean commissioned a study in 2005 on the suitability of selected African HIV/AIDS instructional materials in the Jamaican school setting. The findings were presented at the conference of the Caribbean Publishers Network in May 2005 (see previous chapter). This chapter presents the final report of the researcher. The recommendations that certain books could be adopted as is have influenced procurement of HIV materials by ministries of education in Guyana, Jamaica, Belize and elsewhere. The author has subsequently been engaged by Macmillan Publishers in adaptation of an African teacher training textbook on HIV, published in 2006, and an African reader to be published in 2007.

BACKGROUND, OBJECTIVES AND DESIGN OF THE STUDY

Throughout the world, the young, the generation to drive the engine of development of a nation, is the group most at risk from HIV and AIDS. Consequently, with this or any other intervention which seeks to address attitude formation or change, the target audience should be students in school and those who will teach them, the teachers and student teachers. Moreover, in the case of HIV and AIDS, it is even more challenging as it is realised that 1) at risk behaviours may well start at the primary level, and 2) awareness of the dangers of the disease itself may be either unknown or cultural beliefs may challenge the acceptance of any knowledge which does exist.

In Jamaica, although work has been done towards awareness and sensitisation, both by the government and NGOs, there have been as yet no instructional materials put out by the Ministry of Education, Youth & Culture (MOEYC) which would facilitate the classroom teacher in delivering effective instruction in this area.

One of the ways of mounting an intervention which deals with sensitive social issues is to use stories (supplementary readers), as well as the more obvious textbooks, to attain the objective. In this study, the books provided for this purpose are African, with cultural situations and illustrations which depict the African experience. Although these books would seem suitable for use in a region facing a similar manifestation of HIV and AIDS, one cannot presume acceptance of the material.

Indeed, the message about HIV and AIDS is only as good as the messenger, in this case, not only the reading material, but also those who will use it with the students. Evaluation of the African material, therefore, must not only examine the books, the content and visual images and their relevance to this region, but also seek to establish the opinions of the tutors in teachers' colleges and teachers in schools concerning the use of the material. The purpose of this research therefore, is to evaluate or trial this reading material, which speaks to literacy and HIV and AIDS prevention/mitigation, prior to a pilot which would allow for greater exposure within the system. This evaluation would also take into consideration the need for developing indigenous material, if it is considered to be the best way to deliver the message.

OBJECTIVES OF THE STUDY

These were to:

(i) evaluate African books already produced for HIV and AIDS education,

(ii) target not only classroom teachers and students, but also teachers' colleges and student teachers,

(iii) discover from this process which of this reading material is appropriate for the various target groups (as are, or with modification), and

(iv) to establish whether there is a need for material to be produced which better responds to the needs of the Jamaican society.

The design of the evaluation indicated that the focus would be on (i) sensitisation to and use of the materials by the tutors/lecturers in teachers' colleges with their students, (ii) the sensitisation to and potential use of the materials by the student teachers when they become classroom teachers, and (iii) sensitisation to and use of the materials by classroom teachers with pupils at the primary level.

This evaluation process involved: selection of the materials to be evaluated, selection of institutions and the participants from these institutions, training of the participants at a workshop in the use of the evaluation instruments, sensitisation in the same workshop of stakeholders in the MOEYC and schools/colleges, evaluation process to take place in the field.

SELECTION OF MATERIALS

Materials were selected based on initial reports from MOEYC officers who had previously examined the books, and the experience of this consultant in writing supplementary reading material, textbooks, editing of same, and as publishing manager in educational publishing. The titles chosen for the evaluation are listed in the Annex.

The books to be used were all developed for African children, and titles were selected from the following commercially published courses:

1. Health Education Readers *Maskew Miller Longman (Pty) Ltd, South Africa* Sara Series *Maskew Miller Longman & UNICEF.*

2. Stars of Africa Series *Maskew Miller Longman (Pty) Ltd, South Africa.*

3. Junior African Writers Series (JAWS) *Heinemann Southern Africa.*

4. Young Africa Series and Project Literacy *Heinemann Southern Africa.*

These were the books made available to the consultant by the Ministry of Education, Youth and Culture at the beginning of the consultancy. Selection from the available books was based on theme, approach to the subject and packaging, towards presenting a variety of material which might best carry the message, and was in no way influenced by the products of any particular publishing house. This is important to state, as there may be publishing houses which feel their books should have been included. Moreover, all publishers may be informed by the findings. More importantly, however, is that we discover what appeals to teachers/tutors and students, and whether they feel they need material specific to our region, and what form it should take.

The texts used in the trial reflected a number of approaches: series/single books which have a textbook approach, series which consist of supplementary readers which focus on one character, or which present stand-alone story books, as well as informational books. Some books had teacher's guides; others, questions placed in the back of the text. Some books dealt directly with stories/material related to experiences with HIV and AIDS, while others could be considered sensitisation by way of dealing with life experiences, such as loss and bereavement, family ties, and so on.

Two books were deliberately omitted by the consultant from those selected for the study. These were *Sara and the Boy Soldier* and *Daughter of a Lioness*; the first, because it had negatively stereotyped images of persons in dreadlocks, which are not negative images in our culture; the second, which was about female circumcision, totally alien to our culture.

BOOK PROCUREMENT

All titles selected by the consultant were requested for the workshop, a set for each institution. Further procurement needs were to arise from the trial itself or from a further pilot if one was done. It was envisaged that for some titles, for example, books in a series, class sets would be required. These class sets should ideally be one book per student. Should this not be possible, then at the very

least, there should be one book between two students. However, for novels, fewer numbers might be needed as these may not require that all students have access to the same book at the same time. As suggested by the consultant, a set of books was made available for each institution for the trial.

SELECTION OF SCHOOLS AND TEACHERS COLLEGES

Fourteen institutions were selected, ten schools with primary departments, and four teachers' colleges which train teachers for primary. Some of these, in particular the teachers' colleges, had expressed interest in being included in this trial. Two of the colleges were literacy colleges, seen as especially relevant to be included as the findings could inform the use of supplementary readers in initiatives such as this.

Choice of these institutions reflected areas of high population density, which are identified as areas with a high incidence of HIV and AIDS. Consequently, five institutions were located in Kingston, the capital, and its environs; four in the environs of Montego Bay, the second city and a tourist area; four, including a literacy college, although in rural/urban or rural areas, may be considered catchment areas for Ocho Rios, another tourist area. The final institution, located in a somewhat isolated rural area, is the other literacy college.

The mention of tourist areas is not to indicate that HIV and AIDS and tourism have a causal relationship, but as Kelly and Bain (2003) suggest, tourist areas, with the interaction of people from many different countries, constitute an additional risk factor.

Further selection of schools within the specific areas mentioned above was affected by other variables. For example, some of these schools are demonstration schools, which under the Primary Education Support Project (PESP), an MOEYC/IDB project, are to demonstrate best practice in a symbiotic relationship with teachers' colleges. Moreover, these schools have chosen literacy, as an area for improvement under PESP. Demonstration schools are also perceived as a testing ground for any innovation to do with the Revised Primary Curriculum recently implemented in the schools. Other schools are connected to colleges, in that colleges use them for practice teaching, although they have not been stipulated as demonstration schools. In addition, some of the schools were pilot schools for the Revised Primary Curriculum on the Primary Education Improvement Project (PEIP 11).

The schools for this trialing of material, therefore, would all have one thing in common, an environment in which innovations have taken place or in which innovations are taking place. In this way, one would expect to bring to the process persons who would not only be accustomed to educational initiatives, but consequently, also more likely to have a greater awareness of the significance to all stakeholders of an evaluation process of this nature. One school in particular was included because it was known to have already had contact with HIV and AIDS cases, either parents of students or students themselves, which it had dealt with compassionately as a school community. All of these schools were willing to be involved in the evaluation of the books.

The selection of these schools, while initially suggested by the consultant from her experience/knowledge of the schools in the field, was also subject to MOEYC suggestions/agreement. The number of schools and colleges chosen reflected that

which could be accomplished in the time allowed for the evaluation towards obtaining meaningful results.

PARTICIPANTS

The participants were to be principals/vice-principals, guidance counsellors, librarians and tutors in appropriate subject areas from each college. From schools, it was suggested that we invite principals/vice-principals, guidance counsellors, librarians, and teachers from grades 4, 5 and 6. In the primary schools all class teachers are required to teach all subjects, and at grades 1–3, to be able to deliver subject matter in a full integration mode. In addition, stakeholders from the MOEYC were invited.

Principals, vice–principals, librarians, guidance counsellors and classroom teachers attended from the schools. Not every school sent all these persons but the overall spread reflected these categories. From the colleges, there were Heads of Departments, other tutors and guidance counsellors.

PARTICIPATORY EVALUATION INSTRUMENT DESIGN

A workshop was held to sensitise the teachers/tutors to the HIV and AIDS challenge and to show them how to use the instruments for the trailing as well as how to use the books.

Two instruments were developed: the main one consisted of questions about the books and their use. The other listed the books so that persons could indicate why they had not used any particular book, presenting two choices; they had not had time or had thought the book totally unsuitable.

The main instrument was developed from the consultant's experience in book development and publishing, and based on a number of instruments for the evaluation of textbooks/supplementary material/fiction. Consideration was also given to the particular situation of this trial, that is, the introduction of a sensitive social issue using material which originates in a different social and cultural environment

This main instrument, which started out with 40 or so items, was finally distilled to 25, as one is aware that too long an instrument can be counter productive (see Annex). Items covered the following categories/areas:

- subject area and grade/year in which used
- who used it, that is, class teacher, guidance counsellor, tutor, student teacher
- packaging and readability, that is, the physical aspects of the book which facilitate or militate against reading/using the text effectively
- format preferred, comic or novel
- suitability, attractiveness and effectiveness of the illustrations in the text
- reading level and language
- the effectiveness of the message
- suitability for use with the curriculum
- whether the books required guides
- for what grades were the books best suited
- cultural relevance of text and images
- whether we could use these materials in our region as is, or they needed to be adapted
- whether we needed to write our own material
- for which age groups books were needed.

In the workshops the participants were sensitised to the challenges presented by the HIV epidemic throughout the world and in the Caribbean. In addition, information was given on the experience of the school previously mentioned, which had parents of children and a child dying from HIV and AIDS.

The participants did a cursory examination of the books, and the items on the main instrument were discussed in detail. They were told that they could suggest changes to the instrument if they wished to do so, and that they could include additional information on the back of the instrument form if needs be. This was to allow them to develop ownership of the process. No one saw any need for changes. The importance of the message and messenger was pointed out. It was explained that the books filled both these roles, and if unsuitable, the message would not be received by those who needed it. In addition, the participants were sensitised to the fact that teachers/tutors were also messengers. If these messengers were not comfortable with the message, or the delivery of the message to students, here again the message would be compromised. The importance of knowledge of the target audience was also indicated.

Finally, the participants were placed in groups, persons from colleges along with those from schools, so as to get as rich and multifaceted an interaction as possible. Each group had to select one of the books from the set given them, and prepare a lesson plan based on its use. They also had to indicate in what area they would use it, and how they would make linkages between the book and some aspect of the curriculum, theme/topics in that particular area. Each group made a presentation of its work which was commented upon by the other participants, as well as the consultant in the role of facilitator. The idea was not only that the participants would actually use the books, by way of familiarising themselves with the books and the process, but also that they would have input from others, within their group and from other groups. In addition, they would all be able to take away with them a prototype for using the books.

The participants were given the task, upon returning to their institutions, of deciding along with their principal, at what levels books would be used, and to explain the process for use to those teachers/tutors who would be involved in the trial.

PARTICIPATION IN THE EVALUATION PROCESS

There was a total of 26 books to be used by the institutions, excluding modules/guides. As it happened, the two books indicated as inappropriate by the consultant, were inadvertently sent out to the schools, thus giving a total of 28 books. Although there were 14 institutions involved in the trial, 150 responses were received. The four colleges returned 49 responses; the ten schools, 101. The greatest number of responses from any college was 31; from schools, 22. The greatest number of different books, including modules/guides used by colleges was 28, by schools, 17. Therefore quite a range of material was used by the institutions, as shown in the graph.

The findings were based on the analysis of the instruments as well as interviews. These findings also raise questions which will inform our decisions in using textual material for the HIV/AIDS campaign in schools and colleges.

FINDINGS: SUITABILITY OF THE BOOKS AS MESSENGERS

Who Used the Books? The books were mainly used by classroom teachers or guidance counsellors in the schools, and by tutors, guidance counsellors and students in the colleges.

Packaging and Readability The responses indicate that users found the packaging to be good, facilitating reading, as one would expect with such attractive, colourful books. Where this was not so, it was because the text was in black and white. Only one response from the total in the study was concerned that the soft covers of the books would not hold up under constant use.

The Message and the Need for Guides The majority of persons indicated that the message was effectively transmitted. Where the books had guides, these guides were thought to be adequate. It was felt that many books did not need guides. We recall, however, that many books do have questions at the end.

Reading Level The reading level and language was considered suitable for the age group with which the books were used. One must remember in this case, that teachers/tutors did have a choice, and therefore would have used books suitable to the target group.

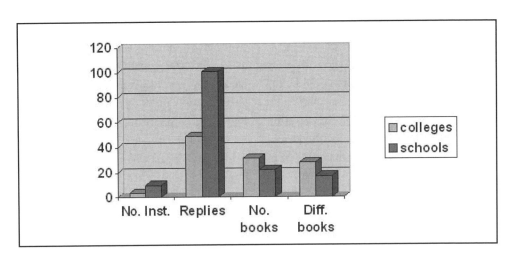

Where the same book was used for different age levels and still considered suitable, this might be an indication of the different reading levels amongst schools and within grades in any school.

One question asked was in relation to the Sara Series which had both novel and comic formats, and this was which format was preferred. There was a range of 20% to 83% across institutions indicating a preference for the comic. With such a range and an average of 44% preferring the comic, we might consider that as some persons said, both have their place. However, the reasons for preferring the comic are telling. Persons felt that the comic attracted the children, especially the boys. In addition, it was pointed out that this format could be used with all reading levels, and even those who had challenges in reading could enjoy it. Consequently, although this response may relate to format, it is included when considering reading levels.

Illustrations Persons very much liked the illustrations, except for some where they were in black and white, or where there was strong concern about cultural relevance.

Suitability for use with the Curriculum In general, persons thought the books could be fitted into the curriculum, including the aesthetics. More than one institution mentioned that their students acted out the stories/did role play, or planned to do so. (The institutions were allowed to keep the books.) So far, therefore, it would seem that the experience of using the African books in the institutions was a positive one. Indeed, for educators and publishers familiar with the books, this should not be surprising as the books are well crafted and produced.

Subjects in which used In schools, the books were used in the following subject areas: Language Arts, Reading, Social Studies, Science, Drama, Art & Craft, Religious Knowledge and Integrated sections of the curriculum. In colleges, the books were used in Social Studies, Educational Studies and Personal Development. The colleges considered that the books would be a good resource for the teaching of HIV and AIDS both in colleges and schools.

At What Level Used In the schools the books were used mainly at Upper Primary, that is, grades 4–6. Some were used at lower primary, at grades 2–3, and a few persons even felt that the books could be used from grade 1 through to grade 6. It must be noted, however, that those books used at lower levels tended to be those sensitising students to life experiences, such as love of family, friendship, loss and so on. In addition, although it does not pertain to the focus of this study, which is the use of the books at primary level, there were persons who felt that many of the books could be used at lower secondary.

The college tutors used the books with first and second years mainly. Some of the students in some colleges used the books themselves and some colleges even used the books in schools where they were doing practice teaching.

CULTURAL IMPLICATIONS: ADOPTION, ADAPTATION OR START-OVER? THE BOOKS AS MESSENGERS IN THE CARIBBEAN REGION

At this point the findings will speak to the main concern, that is, the cultural implications, which will address the matter of the possible need for material specific to the region. A number of persons felt that while the cultural experience through print was different from that of ours in the region, they could nonetheless manage these differences in their teaching. Consequently, it would appear that the books are effective messengers, which can find a place in both colleges and schools.

However, other persons felt that there were cultural challenges, either with the images, the vocabulary, in particular the African names, or more importantly, the cultural content. Those concerned about the cultural implications ranged from 10% to 54% of persons involved in the different institutions. This wide range, with an average of 38% is enough of an indication for us to consider how effective these books in their present stage would be for use in this region.

One would expect a similar number wished to develop our own books. Indeed the range of 9% to 50%, with an average of 30% would seem to bear this out. In fact, however, the same persons did not necessarily feel that we needed to develop books for this region. A number felt that we could use the books from Africa as well as develop our own. Nonetheless, with an average of 30% it is clear that we must consider the development of material specific to the region.

In addition, a specific area was identified by persons as needing book development. This was for lower primary, grades 1–3. Here again, there was a wide range amongst institutions, 6% to 50%, with an average of 28%. A few persons even suggested that we needed to develop books for Early Childhood, because they felt that sexual exposure occurred from this level. Some persons stated exactly what they felt was needed, that is, books which taught children about appropriate and inappropriate touching from adults, as well as what constituted abuse. The graph illustrates these findings.

THE TEACHER COLLEGE EXPERIENCE

It was indicated that the experience with the colleges would be discussed separately. There are number of reasons for this. Most importantly, it has been stated that the messenger, the teacher, is as important as the message. The colleges are the training ground for the future messengers. The tutors, as the teachers of student teachers, are in turn also messengers.

There were differences in opinions, both in colleges and schools, as the ranges of those finding cultural challenges in using the material, and so on, demonstrate. This is to be expected, because individual exposure, individual teaching styles, institutional culture, use of books at varying levels, and the

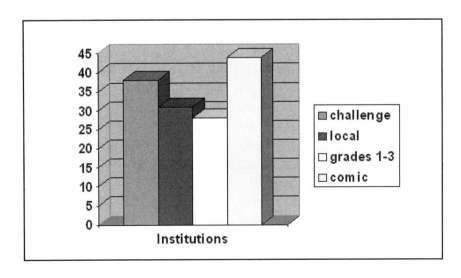

opportunity to choose from such a variety of books, must produce differences. However, although the findings in colleges overall are not that different from the schools, the differences amongst colleges stand out, and may be cause for concern. By way of example, these are detailed below.

One tutor said that he alone used the books as the other tutors said they were too busy. At another college tutors gave general responses on the questionnaire, leaving it to one tutor interviewed to fill in the gaps. On the other hand, the other two colleges, produced responses from tutors using the books with student teachers, student teachers using the books, as was suggested, and colleges using books with schools. Nineteen per cent of the number of responses in one case were from student teachers; 50% in the other. One of these colleges sent in 31 responses, the greatest number from any of the institutions.

Excuses given by those colleges where limited use of the books occurred, as mentioned previously, included tutors being busy in one college, and in the other, it was that practicum was taking place. The latter college did indicate that in the upcoming semester the books would be used when they were doing STDs. We know that the students and tutors in colleges feel that they are overburdened with work, that it may not be as easy to fit a book into subject areas as it is in schools. However, it is the differences in use between the colleges which raises questions.

In addition, there were two young adult novels among the books, ideal for the college population. The two colleges with limited responses, seemed to be unaware of these novels: one did recall their existence when I mentioned them in an interview. The other two colleges, the two with the far greater number of responses, had identified these novels and used them.

We are left to wonder if, apart from the matter of lack of time, there could be any sensitivity to the topic of HIV and AIDS, any denial or ignorance of its importance in some colleges, hence the seeming reluctance to using the books. This was denied when the question was posed in an interview, as indeed one would expect from a group which should be leading an initiative such as this. Perhaps only significant time in the field doing qualitative research, for which this consultancy did not allow, would give us the answer. However, we may have to consider whether there needs to be a further exposure to/a specific treatment in the use of material in the colleges.

ISSUES ARISING FROM THE FINDINGS

From this evaluation of books in the field, some matters arose for consideration, for those contemplating using the African books in the region, or even moreso for developing indigenous material.

Although the following anecdotes are not a part of the study in the field, they are nonetheless of note given the fact that one is led to wonder about the mindset of the tutor/teacher.

These examples are taken from interaction at one of the workshops, and speak to the comfort level with the topic as we consider the teacher/tutor as messenger. One teacher shared her distress and guilt at her reaction to a friend with HIV . The friend seemed by her actions, to wish to be literally embraced by this teacher, perhaps to establish that she was accepted by her. However, the teacher, with admitted knowledge that HIV and AIDS could not be transmitted by such contact, stated that she wished to avoid her friend and so visited her less. Another participant, married for over 30 years, stated that after so many years of marriage she could not bring herself to suggest to her husband that he use a condom. These concerns were discussed openly at the workshop, with positive reinforcement given by the MOEYC guidance counsellor in attendance. Nonetheless, there appeared to be no change in the emotional confusion on the part of the participants.

Although the above does not speak directly to using the books, it does indicate that there may be a need for greater sensitisation among the adult population expected to deliver the message. Having said that, we have to remember that attitudinal change takes much more time than the time devoted to sensitisation so far. Nonetheless, we must ensure that the message is delivered effectively in spite of lingering concerns by individuals.

Many books have teacher's guides, or if they do not, they have questions in the books themselves. Consequently, it is not surprising that many persons felt that they could manage the books without guides. Perhaps the questions in the books are adequate. Perhaps the teachers using them are very effective teachers. We recall that some even used role play to get the children more involved with the books, with very positive results.

It is of note, however, that some persons, when dealing with the books on life experiences, did not seem to see the relevance to the HIV and AIDS message. They did not see these books as precursors to the tolerance needed, the love and loss of life related to the HIV and AIDS experience. This may well speak to the need for guides.

A suggestion made by one college, interestingly enough, one of those which did not appear to participate as much as the others, was that even if we write our own books we should retain the African names. The reason given was that if we used our names (English names) we risked a child bearing the same name as a character who had HIV being teased mercilessly. The tutor interviewed stated that the other tutors felt very strongly about this and wished it to be noted. This would run counter to the concept of producing our own books because of the need for relevant material. However, it must be included here, as it again speaks to concerns, and any concern becomes important when considering how to approach the subject of HIV and AIDS. The idea of children being teased is not far-fetched. We must ask how does one get around that? How has it been dealt with in other countries?

We might be pleased that many of our participants were comfortable with using the African books. Perhaps we might conclude that this produces an immediate publishing solution. Perhaps using African books could serve as a good introduction to the topic, a distancing of oneself, a way of getting across the message, the imminent danger, without the target audience being overwhelmed. On the other hand, we have to consider that for us to understand, to internalise the danger posed, we will have to produce indigenous material, using our own setting and characters.

The two books mentioned previously, *Sara and the Boy Soldier* and *Daughter of a Lioness*, as being considered unsuitable by this consultant, were inadvertently included in the sets of books provided to the institutions. One school stated quite firmly that it did not include them in the trial. However, four other institutions, including a college, used them without any untoward comment, except for one of the schools which indicated cultural challenges with *Daughter of a Lioness*. Nonetheless, I stand by my original decision to exclude them.

One person, in relation to a particular book, felt that abstinence should have been stressed more. This class teacher also felt that the danger of sexual abuse should not only be focused on girls, but should relate to boys as well. It is of note that during the presentation of this paper at the CAPNET conference mentioned in the previous chapter, one tutor indicated that students had expressed their concerns about this very matter, abuse of boys not only by older men, but also by older women.

There is much that this research has unearthed. However, even as we discover that the findings will guide our decisions concerning our approach to the use of and development of material for HIV and AIDS, we must be mindful of the questions that arise, the questions that have not been answered.

CONCLUSIONS AND RECOMMENDATIONS

It has been indicated that at least one-third of the persons using the books found them to be culturally challenging, and wished us to produce our own material. Some felt that we could use ours along with the African material. Although we cannot generalise to the wider community from this trial, we should consider that we cannot afford the message on HIV and AIDS not reaching a third of the at-risk group in this region.

Developing and publishing our own books will take at least a year. There is, however, a sense of urgency in reaching the at-risk population. Consequently, we might consider using some of the books already published for Africa until we can produce

our own. This might, as indicated previously, provide an information bridge, a sensitisation for the time when we do publish for the region. In fact, some of the African books could remain in the system even after ours are produced, because they do speak to a universal concern, and many of the images are similar to those of our people.

One of the questions to be answered is whether we should adapt any of the books for use in this region. This is a matter to be discussed between publishers here and overseas, or publishers and the MOEYC, and will consist of copyright issues. There are books which most certainly can be adapted. The adaptation itself will take some time. I would recommend that it take the form of teachers/tutors/publishers/MOEYC in workshops discussing specific changes. Whereas a consultant or publisher could very easily suggest the changes, for books on this topic which will be in the system for some time and involve some investment, ownership by teachers/tutors is important.

Specific areas have been identified concerning the need for books, for example, grades 1–3. I feel that many of the life experience group produced for Africa can be used at this level, but the need has been stated and work should begin on indigenous material for this group as soon as possible.

At Early Childhood an HIV/AIDS curriculum is to be developed, so one presumes that books for this level will be addressed.

The comic format should be included, whether one is procuring books or developing them, for the reasons mentioned in the Findings: attraction for the students, especially for the boys, an at risk group, it appears, for so many things; and because this format is more easily used with challenged readers.

In the matter of teachers' guides, I think they are essential. This is a sensitive topic and teachers/tutors will need help, even if it is a section 'to the teacher' in the back of the book. It is especially important if the message is subtle rather than an overt one. One might also consider a training manual of sorts, a generic guide which might be used for the teachers of all age groups.

Should teachers/tutors be trained to use the books? This may well be something to be answered by those procuring the books or developing them. It may be a matter of economics. However, for a topic as important as this and as sensitive as this, one would hope that stakeholders would want to be sure that appropriate sensitisation and training take place. In addition, teachers/tutors will need to know how to introduce the topic seamlessly into other topics. One may even have to consider, as suggested by Sinclair (2004), a separate and set time in schools, for this and other life skills topics to enable the education of students for the twenty-first century.

At the Caribbean Publishers Conference on the subject of Publishing for HIV and AIDS (2005) there were varying opinions expressed by the participants concerning the strategies for teaching on HIV/AIDS; infusion, integration, the concern that areas like HIV and AIDS, if not subject to examinations would not be given the required importance, and so on. Although this is not part of this consultancy, it is mentioned because decisions about books may well be impacted by the strategies being employed in teaching. Important as these decisions are, they should not be allowed to delay unduly the need for sensitisation on HIV and AIDS in our educational institutions.

Although this study might lead to the conclusion that specific books be recommended for procurement, I do not think that it is in our best interest that this be done at this time, as there may be other books now available, equal to or better than those used in the trial. In an area which will impact the future of our children and the nation, what we need are the most appropriate books, the best messengers for both students and teachers/tutors.

Consequently, I would recommend that the decision-makers produce a blueprint, whether it be for books from Africa, African books to be adapted, or for the development of our own material, with a certain number of books assigned to each category, as follows:

- informational books,
- fiction – sensitisation to life experiences,
- fiction – stories focusing on the HIV and AIDS experience,
  (Also included in this could be series which identify with one or two characters, male and female - this would interest the students as they become involved with the life of the characters),
- books with a comic format, and
- young adult novels for the teachers' colleges.

We should bear in mind that some of the books used at the primary level can and should be used by the teachers' colleges, whether to give the student teacher exposure to the HIV and AIDS challenge, or for them to practice using books which they will then have to use in the schools.

Should there be a textbook series similar to that used in the trial, in effect a healthy living approach which does not focus on HIV and AIDS alone? This decision will be affected by the approach taken to the sensitisation process. If scarce resources are a consideration, we may well need to give this careful deliberation. We must be aware that an initial procurement/printing of books will not be enough for the challenge facing us. Sustainability of resources/books is essential. We may find that we already have textbooks which address the decision-making and values which lead to the healthy lifestyle of an individual, which include information on STDs and HIV and AIDS, and so decide not to duplicate that effort. Moreover, the concept of having special books to read about life experiences/skills related to HIV and AIDS, and the effects of HIV and AIDS itself, may not only be interesting for the target group, but may also bring to the topic the degree of importance needed.

REFERENCES

Kelly, Michael J, & Bain, Brendan, *Education and HIV/AIDS in the Caribbean*, Ian Randle Publishers/ UNESCO, 2003.

Sinclair, Margaret, *Learning to Live Together: Building Skills, Values and Attitudes for the Twenty-First Century*, International Bureau of Education, UNESCO, 2004.

ANNEX

**EVALUATION OF TEXTBOOKS/SUPPLEMENTARY READING MA24.
IN THE SARA SERIES, WHICH DO YOU PREFER FOR YOUR TARGET
AUDIENCE?**

Title of Book: _____

Series:_____

School/College: _____

College Tutor ( ):   Student Teacher ( ):   Classroom Teacher ( ):

Other: (please state): _____

Subject(s)/area(s) in which you used this book:

_____

Grade(s)/year(s) in which you used this book:

_____

Name: (optional) _____

This questionnaire is for the evaluation of books as suitable for use in Jamaican teachers' colleges and schools in educating our children and young people about HIV/AIDS.

If in answering any question, you wish to add other comments, you may do so on the back of the questionnaire. If you have any additional concerns or comments not covered by the questionnaire, you may also write them on the back of this instrument.

1.   Does the story carry the message? Yes ( )   No ( )

2.   Does the story engage the reader's interest and emotions, rather than preach?
Yes ( )   No ( )

3.   Are the concepts presented in a way which would facilitate
the reader's understanding? Yes ( )   No ( )

4.   If the setting of this book is not Caribbean, does the story nonetheless carry
across   cultural differences making it meaningful?   Yes ( )   No ( )

5.   Does the message conflict with any cultural norms, therefore making it less effective?
Yes ( )   No ( ) (If so, please explain on back of questionnaire).

6.   Is the story free of stereotypes and biases which would affect the message?
Yes ( )   No ( )

7.   Does the story present solutions which would allow for positive action on the part of the reader? Yes ( )   No ( )

8.   Are the illustrations attractive? Yes ( )   No ( )

9.   If the illustrations are not culturally relevant, do they nonetheless lend themselves to use in this region? Yes ( )   No ( )

10.   Do the illustrations assist in the understanding of the text? Yes ( )   No ( )

11.   Are there enough illustrations to hold the interest of the target group?
Yes ( )   No ( )

12.   Is the language appropriate to the reading level of the target group?
Yes ( )   No ( )

13.   Are there terms which would hinder understanding, thus making the book unacceptable to the target audience?   Yes ( )   No ( )

14.   Is the typesize appropriate for the target group? Yes ( )   No ( )

15.   Is the book appropriate in size and length for the target group? Yes ( )   No ( )

15.   Does the book lend itself to use with varying abilities/interests? Yes ( )   No ( )

16.   Does the book lend itself to use with topics/themes in the present curriculum?
Yes ( )   No ( )

17.   Does the book lend itself to the use of the aesthetics? Yes ( )   No ( )

18.   If the book has a teacher's guide, do you consider the teachers' guide adequate?
Yes ( )   No ( )

19.   Do you think the book needs a teacher's guide for it to be useful?
Yes ( )   No ( )

20.   Would you use the book in its present form with your students? Yes ( )   No ( )

21.   For what grade level (for schools) or year group (for colleges) is the book appropriate?

_____

22.   Do you think this book should only be used with certain modifications?
       Yes ( )   No ( )   (Please tick below as appropriate.)
       a) changes in cultural situations as depicted in the text   ( )
       b) changes to illustrations   ( )

23.   Having used this book, do you think we need to develop material of our own rather than use it? Yes ( )   No ( )

24.   In the Sara series, which do you prefer for your target audience?
       The comic format   ( )   The novel format   ( )
       (Please give reasons for your preference on the back of the questionnaire)

25.   Which grades do you think we need books for which have not been addressed in this selection of books?

TEXTBOOKS/SUPPLEMENTARY READING MATERIAL SELECTED FOR CLASSROOM EVALUATION

LIVING & LOOKING TEXTS AND TEACHERS' GUIDES

SARA SERIES: COMICS

Sara Saves Her Friend
Who is the Thief?
The Trap
Choices
The Empy Compound
The Special Gift
Skills for Life: Introduction, Modules, 1, 2, 3, 4

Sara Series: Novels
Who is the Thief?
The Trap
Choices
The Empty Compound
The Special Gift

Novels
The Insect
Take Care
Living a Better Life
Mbili's Story
Two Donkeys
Just Me and My Brother
Simon's Story
Friends for Life
Bucki Must Choose

Zainabu and Mumbi
Moraa's Fate
Blue Train to the Moon
Stronger than the Storm & Teacher's Guide
Positive People: Informataional Text

Informational Textbook
I am HIV-Positive

14

Ending the Silence of Teacher Education: The Case of the Jamaican Teachers' Colleges

Vileitha Davis-Morrison
Institute of Education, The University of the West Indies, Mona
Janice HoLung
Joint Board of Teacher Education, The University of the West Indies, Mona

This chapter traces the development of HFLE/HIV and AIDS education in teacher education institutions in Jamaica since the 1990s. It points to problems initially experienced, outlines the process of its growth, and describes the approach now being used in teachers' colleges to bring this critical area of skills and content into the formal college curriculum.

INTRODUCTION

The high prevalence of HIV in Jamaica and its impact on the sustainable development of the nation signal the urgency for all teacher training institutions to become directly involved in educational policy and practice that can stem the rise of HIV and AIDS. Of the many issues concerning HIV and AIDS which teachers colleges need to address are the vulnerability of young people to HIV which is manifested in the early age of infection; the increasing number of women affected by the disease; the rise in the number of children who have been orphaned by the disease and some who are living with and caring for infected relatives (Ministry of Health, Jamaica, 2005). Additionally, the discrimination associated with the disease is evident in schools where HIV-positive students have been denied entry or face expulsion.

Teacher education has a multiplier effect and, therefore, the inclusion of HIV and AIDS education in teacher training institutions has the potential to reach a large percentage of those infected and affected by the disease. By its impact on the entire education system, teacher education can be an agent of change, reducing both the rate of infection and the discrimination and stigmatisation associated with the disease.

However, before the teachers can initiate change, their own images – that is, their beliefs, dispositions and attitudes towards the disease, towards those infected and affected by the disease – need to be transformed. For such a transformation to take place, the preparation of the teachers will require the methods and techniques for the development of the whole person, that is; the building of self identity and esteem, the fostering of personal attitudes and values conducive to promoting healthy lifestyles and the development of life skills for positive healthy sustainable behaviour. These changes in teacher preparation approaches, together with implementation of policies, and changes in lifestyle are needed. Furthermore, to be effective, the approach would need to recognise the synchronisation of concepts, themes and skill development with other courses and areas in the college environment, as well as the involvement of the stakeholders in the process of change. The establishment of a democratic, safe, healthy and supportive environment, community participation, volunteerism and service learning would be integral to the approach. Such an approach goes well beyond the formal curriculum of the colleges.

Quality assurance, accreditation and the certification of teachers in Jamaica and other countries of the western Caribbean are the responsibility of the Joint Board of Teacher Education (JBTE). This 42 year old Board, established at the University of the West Indies' Mona campus, is a partnership in teacher education and is comprised of Ministries of Education, colleges training teachers, teachers' unions and associations, invited members of the public and the University of the West Indies. The Board provides ongoing professional development for teachers' college staff, participates in the preparation and moderation of examinations and provides support in curriculum development to ensure that college programmes are relevant and reflect current educational philosophies and pedagogies.

This chapter focuses on the need for the inclusion of Health and Family Life and HIV and AIDS education in college programmes, both as curricula and extra-curricula inclusions. It discusses the involvement of stakeholders from the 12 teacher training institutions in Jamaica in the initial phases of the programme towards the institutionalisation of HFLE and HIV and AIDS education, now being implemented in eight of these institutions. The process of institutionalising involved wide stakeholder participation, comprising approximately 1,700 students, 135 lecturers, and 90 administrative and ancillary staff members .

TOTAL SILENCE OR PARTIAL SILENCE?

There has been some recent discussion as to the response of teacher education in Jamaica to HIV and AIDS education. According to Clarke, (2005, 75), teacher education has been a neglected area in the education sector's response to HIV and AIDS. He states that it is particularly important that HIV and AIDS education is given appropriate priority in initial teacher education and that HIV and AIDS life skills should be integral components in the curriculum for the professional preparation of all new teachers.

The UNESCO strategy for HIV/AIDS Prevention Education (2004) noted the need for the reorientation of teacher education in dissemination, capacity building and modelling. According to the document, the integration of HIV and AIDS education in programmes, in addition to access to culturally and gender-sensitive instructional materials developed for use with teachers and students should have begun by 2005.

Clarke also contends that the Jamaican Ministry of Education Policy is silent on what is intended for teacher preparation for HIV and AIDS. In teacher education institutions, the development of new subject areas by the JBTE is undertaken in tandem with the Ministry of Education's school curricula. The

JBTE is advised by the MOEY when there is a need for teachers to be trained for the delivery of a subject and responds to provide the sector with the teachers it requires. Through the curriculum development arm of the JBTE, curricula are developed or revised in response to the need when they are articulated and addressed by the Ministry of Education.

When there is a need identified in particular areas, the Ministry of Education has been able to accomplish revisions and developments, often through project funding. In order to keep the synchronisation between the Ministry's developments and teacher education programmes in recent years, the JBTE has had to source its own funding. This is more often done through bidding for projects, which has indeed slowed down the process of review and development. Over the past decade, however, the JBTE has been involved in considerable curriculum reform and revision and has laid emphasis on student-centred, participatory, interactive teaching methodologies. Such developments were linked to the Ministry of Education and Youth and Culture's 'Reform of Secondary Education' (ROSE) project, 'Primary Education Improvement Project' (PEIP II) and the integration of environmental themes into Early Childhood subjects. However, there was no focus on HFLE or HIV/AIDS or on life skills methodology, despite the devastating impact of the disease on the nation, and despite the involvement of some teachers' college staff members and JBTE and other University staff in the development of the PAHO/CARICOM tertiary framework for Health and Family Life Education, which incorporated HIV and AIDS issues and concepts.

Although the Ministry of Education has recently embarked on a Revised Scope and Sequence Framework for infusion of Health and Family Education (HFLE) with greater emphasis on HIV and AIDS into all curricula from Grades 1–9 and has also developed an early childhood framework, it is still not clear on the place that HFLE will occupy in the school's curriculum. The nebulous position of HFLE in the schools, the need for synchronisation of school and college curriculum and the fact that the colleges have to be cognisant of the deployment of their graduates have influenced the informal place of HFLE in the college programmes (Brown 2003).

While there was no formal place for HFLE in college programmes, due to the continuing advocacy of some JBTE examiners and the commitment of certain college principals and staff, some colleges produced varying versions of Health and Family Life courses. These courses (non creditable, non examined) focused on providing skills and content relevant to the personal development of the individual and are compulsory for all students. Therefore, challenged as colleges have been to find a niche within the formal curriculum, they have used their own initiative to implement HFLE, and within it, to some extent, HIV and AIDS education. These initiatives are laudable but have occurred virtually on an individual basis and with differing levels of commitment. As a result, they have lacked consistency in both approach and implementation. An examination of the HFLE and Personal Development courses (and in some cases there was an absence of structured courses) revealed that although their concept of health was all encompassing, HIV and AIDS education was not explicit in several. However some college lecturers speak of the efforts that they have made to address HIV and AIDS issues in the HFLE course.

Ramsay (et al., 2005), and Davis-Morrison (2004) reported that there were other existing course offerings in the teachers' colleges that contained HIV and AIDS content and issues, some of which were explicit in some units and implicit in others. These varied across the teacher training institutions. Courses ranged from Healthy and Unhealthy Lifestyles in the Social Issues unit of the secondary and early childhood Social Studies programme, Contemporary Health and Family Life Education in Guidance and Counselling, Sports Medicine, Health and Wellness, Human Sexuality, Marriage and Family, and Human Development Courses. However the implicit nature of HIV and AIDS in some of these courses meant that such issues were not reflected in the objectives and were not necessarily taught by the lecturers.

Since 2003, there was an increase in activities concerning HIV and AIDS education within the Jamaican teachers college community. The University of the West Indies Advanced Training and Research in Fertility Management Unit (ATRFMU) worked actively under the leadership of Dr Phyllis MacPherson-Russell, a pioneer in this field, with one teachers' college to implement an HFLE/HIV and AIDS project over three years. This project encompassed the development of curricula for the early childhood and primary teachers as well as linkages and outreach activities with two nearby communities. (Report 2003–2005, 3). The students in this college were involved in awareness raising and professional development activities.

Despite these activities, one could agree with Clarke (2005) that HIV and AIDS education has not been given priority, in a systematic and structured manner in the formal college curriculum, and that the associated life skills have not been integral in the professional preparation of all teachers as late as 2005.

THE RESPONSE BEGINS: INSTITUTIONALISATION OF HFLE AND HIV/AIDS EDUCATION

The process of institutionalising HIV and AIDS education through HFLE in the teachers colleges may be divided into three phases.

Phase 1 In 2004, after extensive discussion between the JBTE and the UNESCO Office for the Caribbean, a meeting was held at the UNESCO office, drawing on stakeholders from the Ministry of Health, the Ministry of Education and principals of teachers' colleges. The meeting resulted in the formal commitment of the college principals to placing HFLE and HIV and AIDS education in teachers' college programmes in the time allotted for Personal Development sessions. Thus all students would be exposed to HIV and AIDS education and there would be greater autonomy and flexibility in customising the programme to meet the diverse and complex needs of the students, the school and community. The principals agreed on the need for a holistic approach to HIV and AIDS Education and decided to adopt a 'whole college approach', in which all stakeholders would be involved in the decision making and planning for HIV and AIDS education.

The 'whole college approach' would focus on both formal and informal curriculum development and, as well, on activities aimed at empowering administrators, teacher educators, students and other workers in the institution and members of the community to use the knowledge, skills, values and attitudes gained to embrace healthy lifestyles which would include HIV and AIDS prevention behaviours. Thus an HIV and AIDS education programme would be facilitated through interactive, collateral education that occurs through contacts between students and every group of college staff in formal and informal encounters. Learning would go beyond the walls of the college and allow for an interface with the community within which the institution is located.

Meanwhile, the project led by the ATRFMU at one pilot college, had begun actively preparing a draft syllabus and had also initiated community linkages, and had planned further actions.

During the academic year 2004-5, the JBTE collaborated with The University of the West Indies HIV/AIDS Response Programme (UWIHARP) in a Global Fund supported project encompassing all 12 teacher training institutions. The project took into account appropriate syntheses with the CARICOM Health and Family Life Education Curriculum Framework for the schools, PAHO/CARICOM framework for the Teachers Colleges, as well as community work being carried out by some of the colleges across the island. The broad objectives were to increase awareness of HIV and AIDS issues among the college stakeholders, to determine the needs of college lecturers and students in the implementation of HFLE/ HIV and AIDS Education and to produce a tertiary level training manual that would help to improve the delivery of HFLE /HIV and AIDS education in schools.

The methodology included focus group and key informant interviews, and needs assessment surveys involving students and lecturers from each of the colleges. Observations during participatory writing and sensitisation workshops were also used in data collection.

THE WHOLE COLLEGE APPROACH

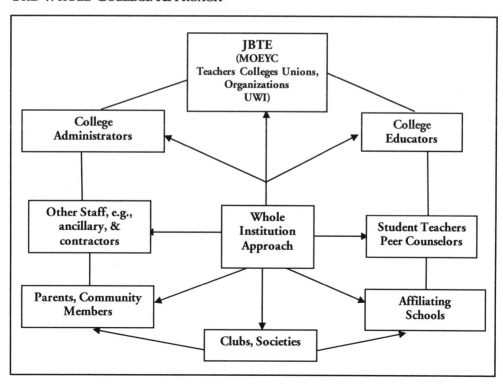

Phase Two. In 2005–2006 the JBTE continued this process under the HFLE/ HIV and AIDS Global Fund supported project in which four pilot colleges were involved. The implementation of the Whole College Approach, in which all sectors of the colleges were involved in action planning and the fruition of some of these planned activities, production of an HFLE/ HIV and AIDS education 30 hour/2 credit course, the continuation of the development of resource materials to facilitate teaching of the course and research publication and outreach programmes were major goals.

Data collection and analysis included surveys on students' knowledge and attitudes to HIV and AIDS education. The sample for the survey consisted of randomly selected students drawn from the pilot colleges. Observation and reporting on the implementation of the course was also done in four pilot colleges. Postgraduate work in educational studies in knowledge and attitudes of care givers in selected early childhood institutions was undertaken by a Masters Degree student, working in collaboration with the Project Implementation Unit.

The activities incorporated workshops to critically review and evaluate resource materials such as the Ministry of Education and Youth's HFLE Scope and Sequence curricula (Early Childhood, Primary Secondary), the Regional Framework for school and teacher education in HFLE and other available resource materials, in order to produce the four units of the 2-credit course on HFLE/HIV and AIDS for teachers colleges. Workshops were held to train tutors in interactive teaching, life skills methodology, and awareness-raising sessions for the college stakeholders and site visits were made for action planning and evaluation of the pilot course.

The project supported by the ATRFMU at one pilot college, had begun implementation of their own draft syllabus, and encouraged their third year students to incorporate HIV and AIDS issues into their practice teaching exercise, and deepened their community involvement by doing sensitisation work in neighbouring schools and health centres.

Phase Three Phase three, which began in September 2006, included four new colleges with activities comprising the continued evaluation of delivery of the 30 hours HFLE/ HIV and AIDS course, the development and implementation of scope and sequence for the infusion of HIV and AIDS concepts, themes and methodology into three courses across all levels and the development of a Health Promotion elective course. Peer educators from the colleges were identified and trained as peer counsellors. The policy for HIV and AIDS education and management in teacher education was developed and disseminated. Service learning, volunteerism and community participation in HFLE/ HIV and AIDS activities were highlighted as a result of the increased focus on the Whole College Approach to HIV and AIDS education.

FINDINGS AND ACHIEVEMENTS

The achievements over the past three years indicate that the institutionalisation of HFLE/HIV and AIDS education in the formal and informal curriculum in the teachers' colleges is now finally underway.

SURVEY FINDINGS

Some of the major findings from the key informant, focus group interviews and needs assessment surveys revealed that the Whole College Approach was accepted by the stakeholders as being the most desirable strategy for HFLE/HIV and AIDS education. One lecturer summarised that 'because this disease impacts on your entire life, it has to be something that is not just related to one area like a subject. Everyone needs to get involved.' However, the consensus was that not all persons would be suitable teachers to deliver HIV and AIDS education. An ideal HIV and AIDS educator needs to be 'equipped with the necessary knowledge, skills, values and attitudes; to be able to deal with their own fears, prejudices and misconceptions; to be comfortable with their own sexuality and to have real life experiences to relate to'. The important issue arising is the necessity for intensive training of whoever will be teaching HFLE/HIV and AIDS education.

All participants agreed that the approach used to address HIV and AIDS education prior to 2004 was inadequate. Some programmes had too limited focus on behaviour change and life skills development, which were considered necessary for the implementation of HIV and AIDS and sexuality education programmes in teacher training institutions. The lecturers also expressed the need for physical, human and financial resources in the implementation of any HFLE/HIV and AIDS course.

The surveys indicated that the students across several colleges have adequate knowledge of the disease such as how it is transmitted (except in the case of the unborn child) and how transmission can be prevented, as over 80% of these items were answered correctly. However, lower scores were evident in knowledge based questions on the developmental stages of the disease, prevalence in the Caribbean and on 'universal precautions'. There were high levels of empathy, tolerance and acceptance expressed towards teachers who are infected with HIV. Of importance is the finding that only a small percentage of students across the colleges believed that teachers are prepared (19%) and comfortable (21%) when teaching children about sex and sexual issues, and about HIV and AIDS issues (Holung 2006; Atkins 2006).

McClean (2006) in postgraduate research on the knowledge and attitudes of caregivers in selected Early Childhood institutions revealed the limited knowledge of caregivers on HIV and AIDS policies, universal precautions and, as well, the methodologies to teach HIV and AIDS issues to early childhood students.

TOOLS FOR AN HIV AND AIDS RESPONSE BY TEACHERS COLLEGES

Four main resources were developed to facilitate HIV and AIDS education in the teachers' colleges. These constitute (1) a profile of the HFLE/HIV andAIDS teacher educator, (2) an HFLE/ HIV and AIDS instructional booklet, (3) a 30 hour course (HFLE/HIV and AIDS), based on the life skills approach, and (4) a draft Workplace Policy for HIV and AIDS for colleges.

Profile of the HFLE/HIV and AIDS teacher educator

Aimed at helping teacher educators to reflect, to identify his/her strengths and weaknesses in the process of teaching and learning, and in making modifications to strive for the ideal. It was organised under the headings of knowledge and understanding, life skills and personal qualities which included values, attitudes and behaviour.

HFLE/ HIV and AIDS instructional booklet

Developed and disseminated to all 12 teacher training institutions. The booklet contained information on various instructional strategies useful for interactive approaches to teaching skills, especially focused on self examination and sexual health beliefs and practices, as well as sample lesson plans and exercises for both early childhood and primary student teachers.

NEW TEACHER COLLEGE COURSES

Major achievements were development and delivery of a 30-hour course (HFLE/ HIV and AIDS), based on the life skills approach, a complementary 90-hour Health Promotion course, which was synchronised with the Jamaican Ministry of Education's draft HFLE courses for students from pre-school to grade 9 and with the PAHO/ CARICOM HFLE framework for colleges; and the scope and sequence for infusion of HIV and AIDS concepts, and skills into three subject areas. The final draft of the 30-hour course was piloted to selected sets of students (approximately 250 students), evaluated and revised. The workshops to write, review and finalise the courses epitomised collaboration and inter-collegiate alliance.

The draft Workplace Policy was produced with wide stakeholder participation, and disseminated for further discussion, before final adoption and implementation. It takes into account existing policies, both National Jamaican policies, Ministry of Education's Policy for HIV and AIDS Management in schools, ILO/UNESCO Caribbean workplace policy for educational institutions and draws on policies of both the UWI and the University of Technology (UTECH) in Jamaica.

TRAINING OF STAFF AND STUDENTS

Lecturers were involved in interactive

participatory training sessions in the use of case studies, behaviour change communication, values clarification and role plays which provided them with the competency and skills to teach the pilot course. The training sessions utilised experts from a variety of organisations and the strategies included video presentations, activity sheets, case studies, games and simulation exercises. Thus, an important result was the training of a number of staff in both knowledge and methodology for HIV and AIDS education.

Students were exposed to a number of sensitisation and planning encounters, and a selected number were given intensive peer training for presentations, counselling and informal conversational activities. These peer counsellors were regarded as an integral part of the college dormitory life for fostering positive attitudes towards healthy sexual behaviours.

BEYOND THE FORMAL COLLEGE PROGRAMME

The institutionalisation of the whole school approach was realised to some extent. Sensitisation and awareness-raising workshops were held for selected groups of students, lecturers, administrative and ancillary staff members from eight colleges. These encompassed presentations by eminent persons as well as activities for both students, and staff members who were present.

College coordinators were nominated by their colleagues in eight colleges. The coordinators were responsible for assisting in coordinating planned events for the four colleges involved in the first phase. Action planning sessions were held, with students at the forefront of the suggested activities for the colleges. As a result of these sessions, and with the cooperation and support of the Project Implementation Unit, colleges implemented some of their suggestions within two months, examples being the preparation and presentation of an HIV and AIDS booth at a college Open Day fair, an exhibition of students' work at a college's Environmental Day celebrations, a two-day workshop at another college focusing on HFLE, and a dramatic presentation at an assembly.

RESPONSE OF THE STAKEHOLDERS

In a 2006 meeting, planned to introduce the newly appointed UWI Professor David Plummer, the college principals interfaced with a number of distinguished persons from the field of HIV and AIDS, and once again committed themselves to promoting HIV and AIDS education in the curriculum of the colleges, using the Personal Development course as the vehicle.

Workshop evaluations revealed that the majority of the participating lecturers felt that the training sessions were worthwhile, increasing their knowledge, developing skills and allowing them to clarify their own beliefs and attitudes towards the disease.

Lecturers were involved in the piloting of the 30-hour HFLE course. The methodology differed across the colleges. For two colleges, a team approach was adopted in which lecturers taught areas in the course which were related to their specialist area. During some sessions it was heartening to see the lecturers using the new approaches and using the materials utilised in the training sessions. During a three hour session observed at one college, an unusually wide variety of strategies including video presentation, questioning and reporting, group discussion and values clarification activity were utilised.

For one particular college, however, the method was still the didactic type, with the lecturer informing students about the new methodologies.

Despite the challenges experienced, the college coordinators all had positive responses to the programme. However, the experiences varied depending on the college context and, as well, on the expectations of the individuals. According to one coordinator, the process helped to improve her leadership and organisational skills. For another it helped her to confront several HIV and AIDS issues and changed her perspective that it was an 'overkill' issue (too much emphasis being placed on HIV and AIDS). Ancillary staff members expressed appreciation for the awareness raising sessions and in one instance, one member enlisted the help of the presenter to make arrangements at a nearby clinic for community members who were HIV-positive.

The students' response to the workshops on awareness raising, action planning, policy preparation and peer training was excellent. They participated very well in these workshops and training sessions, had interesting ideas and were able to implement some of the activities. They expressed great appreciation for the teaching of the pilot course, both with respect to the knowledge gained and to the strategies shown. They felt more knowledgeable about the subject and were also more comfortable with sexuality education. In one instance the students were very emotional, open and honest and the effectiveness of the session was a tribute to the esteem in which they hold the lecturer, who was their guidance counsellor.

The success of the awareness and action planning depended on the organisation and leadership skills of the coordinators and on the composition of their committees. At one college, the commitment and belief in the programme and collaboration among group members laid the foundation for planning and implementation of activities in a relatively short time. In contrast to the urban colleges, the rural college groups focused their ideas on the surrounding community. This brings to focus the difference in the relationship between colleges and communities in urban and rural areas and the implications for the community aspect of a Whole College Approach in urban colleges.

CHALLENGES IN IMPLEMENTATION OF HFLE/ HIV AND AIDS EDUCATION

There were several challenges impacting on the implementation of the recent work in the colleges. The lecturers noted the need for support in the delivery of HFLE/ HIV and AIDS content related matters, and also in teaching strategies and skill development. Areas such as information on sexually transmitted diseases, healthy diets and exercising for healthy living, first aid practices and environmental issues were those especially highlighted. Values clarification, conflict resolution, media watch activities and an emphasis on practicing critical thinking, self evaluation, self management were noted as aspects of skill teaching which were integral to HIV and AIDS education but which were not yet entrenched in pedagogy and needed further continuing support.

The need for effective communication and support from other members of staff for any initiative that they perceive to be outside of their area of subject matter specialisation was a grave issue. This led to difficulties faced by several coordinators in arranging events. At some colleges, therefore, events were loosely organised and it became difficult to assembly a core group of stakeholders for certain activities.

The lecturers cited time constraints,

curriculum overload and timetabling problems as challenges for collaborative planning. There was a great difficulty to organise, especially in respect of piloting of new courses and implementation of activities requiring a cooperative/team teaching approach. A major issue was the time frame involved in planning and the level of organisation that was essential. As one lecturer remarked, 'these had tired them out' and 'we had to plan well ahead of time'. It was also pointed out that the tutors were all presently teaching their maximum number of hours and many tutors felt inadequate or unwilling, to assist with clubs or societies or to engage in activities for a more holistic approach to an HFLE working programme.

There appeared to be the need for equipment and other resources to be used for teaching. Although the project was able to provide some colleges with multi-media projectors for the teaching of HFLE/HIV and AIDS focused and related courses, all voiced the wish for more equipment.

A major impediment to progressing in an HIV and AIDS education programme is the attrition of lecturers from the tertiary system, which affects the sustainability of the teaching practices and programmes in the colleges. Some of the lecturers trained in the delivery of HFLE/ HIV and AIDS education have already left the tertiary system and it will be necessary to support the training of substitutes as well as encourage peer training. The recent establishment of the M. Ed (Health Promotion) programme at the University of the West Indies, may, however, assist in this regard.

CONCLUSIONS AND RECOMMENDATIONS

The needed response has indeed begun. A variety of factors assisted its implementation. These included support and cooperation from all college staff, including the principals, coordinators, staff across the various sectors, the energetic and enthusiastic students, Global Fund financial support, assistance from the HIV and AIDS unit of the Ministry of Health, the Guidance and Counselling Unit of the Ministry of Education, and networking with other agencies and organisations.

The competition for time and space in the teachers' colleges must be addressed. Lecturers are finding it more difficult to participate fully in any intervention aimed at solving specific problems, which should take an integrated and holistic approach involving all stakeholders.

Continuous training in methodologies and strategies is required, which must include techniques for arriving at personal or collective solutions to problems. Such training should involve both counselling and teaching methodology and the lecturer would thus become empathetic but enabled to remain objective. The knowledge base of the HFLE/ HIV and AIDS lecturer must be extended and should include issues such as human rights, ethics and law reforms concerning HIV and AIDS.

The attrition of lecturers speaks to the necessity for the organisation of ongoing training, including peer training. The development of resource centres and access to internet facilities and improved library facilities, such as virtual library facilities at colleges, must be addressed.

The sustainability of the HFLE/HIV and AIDS education programmes at teacher education institutions will depend on the continuing support of stakeholders, the implementation of a health policy, the fostering of a health promoting environment within each college and the inclusion on the college calendar of special days such as World AIDS Day, Safer Sex Week and Environmental Days with activities to commemorate such events. Also, establishing an HFLE /HIV and AIDS course with an emphasis on service learning as a criterion for graduation, supporting of clubs and societies with HIV and AIDS college and community projects and assisting the lecturers with resources, will also help to foster sustainability. The incorporation of HFLE/HIV and AIDS education into the teaching practice exercise (the practicum), will be indicative of the extent to which the student teachers have consolidated the skills, attitudes, values and knowledge gained.

REFERENCES

Atkins, H.(2006) Knowledge, Attitudes about HIV/AIDS among College Students at Three Teachers' Colleges in Jamaica, Unpublished paper: Global Fund/ JBTE HFLE:HIV and AIDS Project.

Clarke, D. (2005) Response of the Education Sector in Jamaica to HIV and AIDS, UNESCO.

Brown, M. (2003) Health and Family Life Education in the Jamaican Teachers' Colleges, Presentation at the CARICOM HFLE meeting, Jamaica, 2003.

Davis-Morrison, V. (2004) the place of HIV/AIDS in the Teachers College Curriculum: Challenges and Possibilities: Presentation at the Seventh Biennial Conference of School of Education: Celebrating Achievements in Caribbean Education, Transformation, Diversity and Collaboration. April 15–17 2004.

Dexter, C; Meade, J.& Russel, P.(2006) Promoting Healthy Lifestyles in Western Jamaica, HFLE-HIV/AIDS Project Report 2003–2005, Advanced Training and Research in Fertility Management Unit UWI, Mona.

Holung, J.(2006) A Preliminary Survey of Teachers' College Students Knowledge and Attitudes towards Selected HIV Issues Unpublished paper: Global Fund/ JBTE HFLE:HIV and AIDS Project.

Ministry of Health Jamaica UNGASS Report. January 2003–December 2005, Declaration of commitment on HIV/AIDS.

Ministry of Health Jamaica (2005). National HIV/STI Prevention & Control Program, Facts and Figures. HIV/AIDS Epidemic Update January to June 2005.

Ministry of Education Youth and Culture (2001) National Policy for HIV/ AIDS Management in Schools Guidance and Counseling Unit Ministry of Education, Kingston Jamaica.

McClean, E. (2006) Knowledge, Attitudes of Care Givers in Selected Early Childhood Institutions. Unpublished M. Ed thesis UWI, Mona.

Pan American Health Organization Health Promoting Schools strengthening of the Regional Initiative Strategies and Lines of Action 2003–2012 (Original Spanish Health Promotion Series No.4) Washington, DC 2003.

Ramsay, H. J.Mullings, V Davis-Morrison, M Ruddock-Small. B. Bain (2005) Towards the Effective Delivery of HIV/AIDS Education in Health and Family Life Education in Teachers Colleges in Jamaica. Presented at the Third Annual Scientific & Business Conference "Towards a Strategic Framework for HIV and AIDS Research in the Caribbean: Emphasising Behaviour Change" Barbados May 5–8 2005.

Ramsay, H., Davis-Morrison, V., Mullings, J. (2005) Global Fund Intervention within the Teachers Colleges: Research Findings. Presentation to College lecturers, Knutsford Court Hotel. Feb. 2005.

UNESCO Education and HIV/AIDS Strategy 2004-2005 Enhancing the Response of the Caribbean education sector to HIV/AIDS.

15

The impact of HIV and AIDS on education in the Caribbean

Claire Risley, David J. Clarke,
Lesley Drake[1] and Donald Bundy[2]

1. Partnership for Child Development,
Imperial College, London
2. The World Bank, Washington DC

Recent research highlights the need for the assessment of the impact of HIV and AIDS on education in the Caribbean as integral to its mitigation. The analysis presented in this chapter is the first to attempt such an assessment. Although only preliminary evaluations of the effects upon the supply of education are made, it is clear that HIV and AIDS may have a significant impact on the education systems in the region. In addition to the quantifiable impact, the impacts of HIV and AIDS may be disproportionate in small states, which predominate in the region. There is a pressing need for the development of country-level multisectoral strategies, increased by the unusually high disparity between Caribbean states. A more in-depth impact assessment is clearly needed to inform this process.

IMPACT OF HIV AND AIDS

Where the HIV prevalence in a country exceeds 1%, the country is experiencing a 'generalised' epidemic, as the virus circulates by heterosexual sex in the general population. HIV infection can then threaten key areas such as the health and education sectors. Sixty-three per cent of Caribbean countries are experiencing such a generalised epidemic (data from UNAIDS 2006 and CARICOM 2004). Addressing the impact of HIV and AIDS on education can present a complex challenge for governments and it remains an area that is under-represented in national strategic responses (Kelly and Bain 2005).

The effects of the epidemic on social institutions, such as schools, are initially sporadic or hard to detect. However, as the epidemic progresses, the impact becomes more pronounced. For example, many sub-Saharan African countries are experiencing high levels of illness and death, orphaning and loss of key household and community members. In these contexts, the impact of HIV and AIDS on the functioning of the education system is considerable. In the Caribbean, some countries are at an earlier stage in the epidemic, where impact is at present negligible and increasing, while in others with higher HIV prevalence, impacts are already becoming substantial. Because small states may be more vulnerable to smaller shocks to the education system, the preponderance of small states in the Caribbean suggests it could suffer disproportionate impact.

THE INTERACTION BETWEEN HIV AND EDUCATION

The response to HIV and AIDS has often been considered to be the sole preserve of the health sector. Nowadays, the education sector is recognised to have a major role to play in efforts to control the disease. Schoolchildren are perceived as the 'window of hope' (World Bank, 2002) for the future because they have the lowest rate of infection of any age group and can be kept free of infection by the 'social vaccine' of a good education. On the other hand, the HIV epidemic is damaging the education systems, which can provide the 'social vaccine' and promote good health and nutrition of school age children. In countries with generalised epidemics, AIDS kills teachers, increases rates of teacher absenteeism, and increases the numbers of orphans and vulnerable children who are less likely to attend school and more likely to drop out. Girls are especially at risk from becoming infected and affected by HIV because of their socio-economic and physiological situation. Thus a paradox is apparent: education can prevent HIV infection, but HIV and AIDS damages, and has the potential to destroy, the system delivering this prevention. Understanding the likely consequences of HIV infection and AIDS on the education sector is a critical first step towards planning for and thereby mitigating their impact.

THE IMPACT OF HIV AND AIDS ON EDUCATION

The impact of HIV and AIDS is currently divided into three interrelated categories (Kelly 2000). These are the impact on:

- the demand for education;
- the supply of education; and
- the quality of education.

THE DEMAND FOR EDUCATION

A significant impact is evidenced in the increase of child vulnerability in terms of those orphaned and affected by HIV and AIDS. In the Caribbean region, the most recent estimate for orphans (UNAIDS, UNICEF and USAID, 2004) presents data for 2003 in ten Caribbean countries with an aggregate total of 1,035, 900 orphans due to AIDS, some 610,000 in Haiti alone. By 2010, the total is projected to increase to 1,087,000 in the ten countries. An increasing number of children are becoming infected by HIV, many of whom will have also experienced orphaning.

Additionally, the socio-economic impacts of HIV and AIDS include increases in household poverty that result in financial barriers to education (inability to pay fees, purchase uniforms, school materials and books, etc.) and opportunity costs when children may be called on to support household livelihoods; attitudinal impacts on participation in education, especially of those affected by HIV-related stigma and discrimination; and increased gender inequalities as girls are required to take on the responsibility for care of HIV-positive adults and affected siblings in the household.

THE SUPPLY OF EDUCATION

The impact can be separated into quantity and quality effects (Figure 15.1).

The most crucial effect on the supply of education is the decreased availability of experienced teachers. Two key questions are, therefore: how vulnerable teachers are to HIV infection and what steps need to be taken to support prevention at all stages of their career? The loss of teachers and other education sector personnel to other sectors of the economy is a phenomenon that is being encountered in generalised HIV epidemics as

FIGURE 15.1
QUANTITY AND QUALITY EFFECTS OF HIV AND AIDS ON EDUCATION SUPPLY

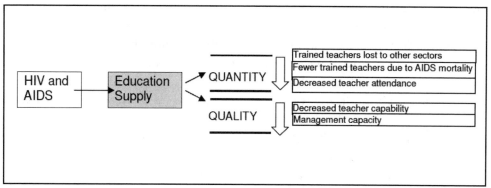

the impact on human resources progressively accumulates.

The impact on teacher productivity may manifest itself as, for example, a decreased and erratic school attendance and the loss of energy and motivation as AIDS progresses in severity in the infected individual (Kelly 2000). Other factors may include HIV-related illnesses in the family or community and attendance at funerals. Monitoring teacher attendance and productivity in the context of an HIV epidemic represents a distinct challenge for school management and for local education authorities. Access to antiretroviral therapy (ART), however, is a key issue and is critically important for maintaining the productivity of teachers living with HIV and AIDS.

THE QUALITY OF EDUCATION

The quality of education, in terms of learning outcomes and classroom processes, may be negatively affected by HIV and AIDS and it impacts on both demand and supply side factors.

- On the demand side, the psychosocial condition of children affected by HIV and AIDS in their households may reduce their ability to participate and to focus in class and learn, especially if they are grieving or being bullied because of HIV-related stigmatisation.

- On the supply side, the quality of education delivery will tend to be undermined by a combination of factors including the loss of trained and experienced teachers, the reduction in teacher productivity through illness and psychological stress and the loss of management capacity in the sector.

ASSESSING IMPACT

To date, no country in the Caribbean region appears to have undertaken any comprehensive impact assessment in the education sector and little is known, especially at the country level.

It has been advocated (Kelly and Bain 2005) that the education sector response in the region should rest on three pillars: 1) prevention of HIV transmission; 2) care and support for those who are infected or affected; and 3) management of the systemic and institutional impacts so as to mitigate negative effects. An HIV and AIDS impact assessment process is germane to the development of all three pillars in terms of sector policy, including workplace policy (ILO and UNESCO 2006), and strategic interventions aimed at capacity-building and programmatic response.

Assessing the impact of HIV and AIDS can be undertaken by using mathematical models that combine available information on HIV prevalence with education and financial statistics to project the likely impact. These analyses require good quality data, good communication with stakeholders, and are complemented by qualitative research in schools. The Ed-SIDA model of the impact of HIV was developed for the education sector (World Bank and Partnership for Child Development 2001, 2006; Grassly et al. 2003), which is a spreadsheet-format model incorporating UNAIDS HIV projections. Ministries of Education in 33 countries in sub-Saharan Africa are currently trained in using Ed-SIDA to manage and plan for HIV and AIDS in their education sector.

AN ASSESSMENT OF IMPACT ON THE SUPPLY OF EDUCATION IN THE CARIBBEAN REGION

Ed-SIDA was used to assess the impact of HIV and AIDS on Caribbean teacher supply. A country by country analysis was performed and the results were summed to provide regional projections. Presented here are: projections over the entire Caribbean region; those for the Organisation of Eastern Caribbean States (OECS); and Guyana and Trinidad and Tobago which illustrate the impact upon individual states. Results from other countries are available on request. The baseline analyses assume ART was provided to all teachers requiring it from 2005 to 2015.

The following data were input into the model.

- *Country-specific HIV prevalence* projections were based on antenatal clinic surveillance data and scaled to UNAIDS' (nine countries) or the Caribbean Epidemiology Centre's (22 countries) 2004 estimates.

- *Number of teachers* provided by UNESCO Institute of Statistics (UIS). Estimates were extrapolated from UN Population Division estimates of population size for those countries providing no teacher data.
- *Attrition and recruitment* data from Grenada (Junior Alexis, pers. comm.); rates were assumed to be equal across the region.
- *Financial* data were obtained from Fitzgerald and Gomez (2003) (anti-retroviral medicine cost); Lewin, 2002 (Teacher salary and training cost); country reports on social security at http://www.ssa.gov (funeral cost); and Jenelle Babb (Pers. comm.; Jamaica teacher training and salary cost)

Several assumptions were made. There are currently few data on HIV prevalence among teachers. However, Badcock-Walters et al. (2003) found that teacher mortality in South Africa was lower than that in pregnant women. It was consequently assumed that teachers have a prevalence and incidence of 80% of the country-specific projections. The efficacy of ART in preventing deaths and AIDS-related absences was assumed, conservatively, to be 50%.

RESULTS

Estimates of the number of HIV-positive teachers and AIDS deaths for the region are presented in Figure 15.2. The black line represents the median estimated prevalence scenario. The boundaries of the coloured sections represent the high- and low-prevalence scenarios. It is clear that under all these scenarios the number of both HIV-positive teachers and teacher AIDS deaths will increase. The projected number of teacher deaths shown would represent a significant impact on education supply in the region.

Figures 15.3, 15.4 and 15.5 present projections from OECS, Guyana and Trinidad and Tobago, respectively. The prevalence in Guyana and Trinidad and Tobago has reached generalised levels (2.4 per cent and 2.6 per cent, respectively in 2005 [UNAIDS 2006]), whereas in OECS there are still few people in the general population who are affected. It is assumed that all teachers in need are provided with ART from 2005 onwards; this results in a decline in the mortality rate, but is assumed to have no impact on the incidence of infection.

These projections indicate that both HIV positivity and AIDS deaths are likely to increase among teachers during the next few years. There will be more HIV-positive teachers primarily because if all teachers are given antiretroviral therapy, more HIV-positive teachers will remain alive. Despite this, deaths will continue to mount during this time as teachers who became infected during the initial peak in incidence at around 2000 die despite treatment. These charts indicate that countries with higher HIV

FIGURE 15.2
(A) HIV-POSITIVE TEACHERS AND (B) CUMULATIVE AIDS DEATHS AMONG TEACHERS IN THE CARIBBEAN

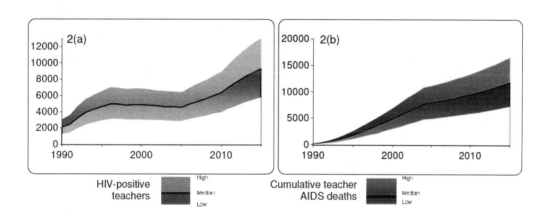

FIGURE 15.3
(A) HIV-POSITIVE TEACHERS AND (B) CUMULATIVE AIDS DEATHS AMONG TEACHERS IN THE OECS

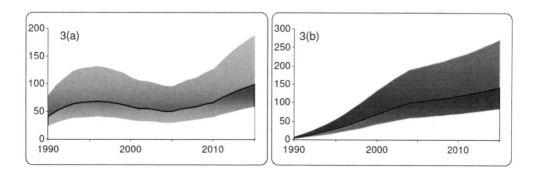

FIGURE 15.4
(A) HIV-POSITIVE TEACHERS AND (B) CUMULATIVE AIDS DEATHS AMONG TEACHERS IN GUYANA

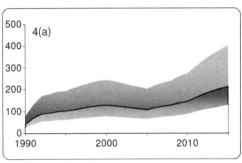
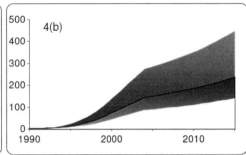

FIGURE 15.5
(A) HIV-POSITIVE TEACHERS AND (B) CUMULATIVE AIDS DEATHS AMONG TEACHERS IN TRINIDAD AND TOBAGO

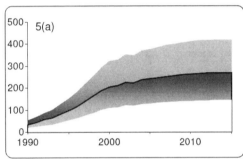
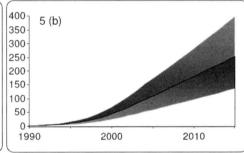

prevalence and larger populations would lose more teachers. However, smaller islands may be disproportionately affected by small shocks to the education system.

The special challenges of small states in educational development have been described (for example Bray 1991, 1992), and they include human resource difficulties in specialist areas resulting in the need for 'multifunctionalism'. However, the analysis and understandings need to be updated in the context of HIV and AIDS.

Even with the best data, the future of the epidemic is difficult to predict, especially at the country level. The results presented here are a preliminary analysis using limited data.

The loss of some 12,000 teachers in the Caribbean by 2015 represents a significant impact. Teacher turnover in Caribbean schools is fairly low compared to the UIS baseline of 3%, which results in a significant AIDS loss in terms of overall attrition. The smaller OECS countries are also among those with lower prevalence, resulting in lower numerical impacts, though the disproportionate effect on smaller states is a possibility already mentioned.

Given the results shown above, it is clear that HIV and AIDS will have a financial impact on the supply of education in the region. Figure. 15.6 shows estimates of the cost of HIV to the education sector.

Table 15.1
Estimates of number of teachers HIV-positive in 2015 and dead from AIDS by 2015

	HIV-positive teachers in 2015	Teacher AIDS deaths to 2015	AIDS deaths in 2015 as % of all attrition
Caribbean	9300	11800	13%
OECS	100	100	5%
Guyana	200	200	13%
Trinidad and Tobago	300	300	9%

Note: Data rounded to nearest 100, assuming a median-prevalence scenario and ART given to all teachers needing it (baseline attrition rate from Grenada)

It appears that, on current epidemiological trends, and without effective prevention measures, HIV and AIDS are likely to have significant consequences for the mortality of teachers. These consequences will be apparent over the next decade even if all affected teachers were provided with ART immediately. The major effects would be a need to recruit and train teachers to replace those who had died, at an estimated annual cost to the region of US$4–5M, and to provide ART to affected teachers, at an annual estimated cost of US$1.5M. The use of ART would prolong teacher's lives and reduce illness, resulting in an overall saving to the education sector of some $25M. Whatever is done now, these costs will be incurred by the education sector, and future budgets will have to accommodate these significant increases. Table 15.2, showing a comparison between the estimated annual costs in 2005 and 2015 indicates that, due to the increasing numbers of HIV-positive teachers and AIDS deaths, costs will continue to rise. A less conservative estimate of ART efficacy results in cost reductions between 2005 and 2015.

The model incorporates discounting for future costs, which accounts for the decrease in the cost of absenteeism in Trinidad and Tobago while HIV-positive teachers increase slightly.

This is a preliminary analysis, and does not include the human capital losses upon the death of a trained teacher. The cost-effectiveness of preventing teacher infection has also not been explored.

Table 15.2
Annual costs (1000 US$) associated with HIV and AIDS to the Caribbean education sector if ART were provided to all teachers needing it from 2005–15

	Caribbean		OECS		Guyana		Trinidad and Tobago	
	2005	2015	2005	2015	2005	2015	2005	2015
Absenteeism	$3062	$4468	$27	$45	$73	$100	$146	$118
Deaths	$7637	$5062	$67	$50	$200	$118	$186	$188
ART	$911	$1592	$10	$19	$22	$33	$48	$53

FIGURE 15.6
COST OF AIDS ABSENTEEISM AND DEATHS TO THE EDUCATION SECTOR FROM 2005–2015 THROUGHOUT THE CARIBBEAN REGION

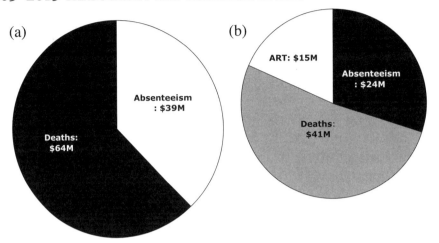

Note: (a) without ART, total cost $104M; (b) with ART provided to all teachers who require them, total cost $79M. $ are US dollars, 2000 equivalent. ART is assumed to cost $1000 per person per year.

CONCLUSION

It is clear that HIV and AIDS will have a significant impact on the supply of education in the Caribbean region. It is critical that a thorough analysis is made at the country level to allow disparities between countries to be accounted for. Multisectoral strategies need to be developed that support the three pillars of an effective response: 1) prevention of HIV transmission; 2) care and support for those who are infected or affected (including provision of ART); and 3) management of the systemic and institutional impacts so as to mitigate negative effects. To date, the education sector response to HIV and AIDS has concentrated, appropriately, on HIV prevention. While efforts in this area need to be strengthened, it is time to make a comprehensive impact assessment in order to mitigate the negative effects on education delivery in the future.

ACKNOWLEDGEMENTS

Thanks to Jenelle Babb and Junior Alexis for providing data and Manoj Gambhir for assisting with analyses.

SELECTED BIBLIOGRAPHY

Badcock-Walters, P. et al. 2003. Educator mortality in-service in KwaZulu Natal: A consolidated study of HIV/AIDS impact and trends. Paper presented at the Demographic and Socio-Economic Conference, Durban, South Africa.

Barnett, T and Whiteside, A. 2000. *Guidelines for studies of the social and economic impact of HIV/AIDS.* Geneva, Switzerland: UNAIDS.

Bray, M. 1992. *Educational planning in small countries.* Paris: UNESCO.

Bray, M. (ed.) 1991. *Ministries of education in small states: Case studies of organisation and management.* London: The Commonwealth Secretariat.

CAREC. 2004. Status and trends: analysis of the Caribbean HIV/AIDS epidemic 1982–2002. Caribbean Epidemiology Centre. Accessible at http://carec.org/pdf/status_trends.pdf

Commonwealth Secretariat. 1997. *A future for small states. Overcoming vulnerability.* London: Commonwealth Secretariat.

Fitzgerald, J. and Gomez, B. 2003. An open competition model for regional price negotiations yields lowest ARV prices in the Americas. In *International proceedings of the 8th World STI/AIDS Congress*. Bologna, Italy: Medimond.

Grassly, N.C., Desai, K., Pegurri, E., Sikazwe, A., Malambo, I., Siamatowe, C. and Bundy, D. 2003. The economic impact of HIV/AIDS on the education sector in Zambia. *AIDS* 17(7): 1039–1044.

ILO and UNESCO. 2006. An HIV/AIDS workplace policy for the education sector in the Caribbean. Port of Spain: ILO and UNESCO. Accessible at http://www.ilo.org/public/english/dialogue/sector/papers/education/carib-ed-policy.pdf

Kelly, M. 2000. Planning for Education in the Context of HIV/AIDS. Paris: IIEP-UNESCO.

Kelly, M. and Bain, B. 2005. *Education and HIV/AIDS in the Caribbean*. Kingston: Ian Randle Publishers.

Lewin, K.M., Keller, C. and Taylor, E. 2000, revised 2002. *Teacher education in Trinidad and Tobago: Costs, financing and future policy*. Multi-Site Teacher Education Research Project (MUSTER) Discussion Paper No. 9. Brighton, UK: Centre for International Education, University of Sussex.

Shaeffer, S. 1994. The impact of HIV on education systems. In Pridmore, P. and Chase, E. (eds) *AIDS as an educational issue*. DICE Occasional Papers No. 12. London: Institute of Education, University of London.

UNAIDS Inter Agency Task Team on Education. 2004. *HIV/AIDS and education: The role of education in the protection, care and support of orphans and vulnerable children in a world with HIV and AIDS*. Paris: IATT.

UNAIDS. 2004. Country fact sheets available at http://data.unaids.org/Publications/Fact-Sheets01

UNAIDS. 2006. *Report on the global AIDS epidemic* available at www.unaids.org/en/HIV_data

USAID, UNAIDS and UNICEF. 2004. *Children on the Brink 2004: A joint report of new orphan estimates and a framework for action*. New York.

World Bank and Partnership for Child Development. 2001. Modeling the Impact of HIV/AIDS on Education Systems: A training manual. The Ed-SIDA initiative. Washington DC: World Bank. First edition.

World Bank and Partnership for Child Development. 2006. Modeling the Impact of HIV/AIDS on Education Systems: A training manual. The Ed-SIDA initiative. Washington DC: World Bank. Second edition.

World Bank. 2002. Education and HIV/AIDS: A window of hope. Washington DC: World Bank.

16

THE PRICE OF PREJUDICE: THE CORROSIVE EFFECT OF HIV-RELATED STIGMA ON INDIVIDUALS AND SOCIETY

DAVID PLUMMER AND
ARDEN McLEAN

SCHOOL OF EDUCATION, THE UNIVERSITY OF THE WEST INDIES, ST AUGUSTINE CAMPUS, TRINIDAD AND TOBAGO

Stigma is an epidemic within an epidemic. It stalks people with HIV and those of us who are at risk. It cruelly denies care and compassion. It sentences people to isolation and poverty. It seems to justify callous insults and brutal treatment for our brothers and sisters when they are least able to defend themselves. And it shortens lives – significantly, considerably and, worst of all, needlessly. Stigma is a social evil that divides communities when unity is vital. It is the metaphorical opportunistic illness of AIDS – poised to strike whenever our defences are down. This paper seeks to expose six key ways that stigma takes its toll: It hides the epidemic. It wounds vulnerable people. It disrupts vital support networks. It impairs access to care. It licenses antisocial acts. It undermines political will.

INTRODUCTION

The Caribbean region with its heterogeneous face is made up of 30 territories and approximately 36 million inhabitants. HIV is not new to the region – it has been here from the very beginning when Haiti, in particular, was implicated in some of the earliest cases of AIDS. A quarter of a century later, the region now has the highest prevalence of HIV outside of sub-Saharan Africa and an overall prevalence of 1.6% (ranging widely from 0.1% in Cuba to 3.8% in nearby Haiti). There are currently at least 330,000 persons living with HIV/AIDS (PLWHA) in the region and these numbers are increasing in most jurisdictions (Caribbean Epidemiology Centre, 2004 and see www.unaids.org). The challenges posed by the epidemic are profound. A relentlessly expanding epidemic that seems to resist conventional interventions demands deeper analysis. This must include the role of stigma in aggravating and spreading the epidemic.

Advances in biomedical technologies over recent decades have been nothing short of remarkable. Yet the way that societies respond to disease still seems rooted in pre-modern approaches rather than being the fruits of evidence-based health care in modern open democracies. Nowhere is this more evident than for diseases that disproportionately affect marginalised populations or which are associated with taboo issues, such as sex and drugs. Why is the spectre of the 'grim reaper' so easily invoked by AIDS? Why does HIV conjure visions of isolation and quarantine, of leper colonies and the bubonic plague while other, more-infectious diseases do not? Part of the explanation seems to lie with the institutional frameworks, social traditions and cultural metaphors that underpin how we think about HIV (Brown, Macintyre & Trujillo 2003). For example, many of the laws that frame our public health responses are colonial relics – public health acts, prostitution laws, sodomy laws and so on. Moreover, our religious institutions (the backbone of our traditional health and welfare system) are experiencing profound difficulties in coming to terms with the epidemic too, largely because HIV is most commonly transmitted through sex.

The emergence of HIV as a pandemic with deep sexual and gendered dimensions poses unprecedented challenges to traditional social power relations. Central to these is how communities respond to and manage stigma – given the ancient metaphors and prejudices that HIV has unleashed. However, in order to manage the pandemic in a modern Caribbean context, it has never been more important than to meet HIV with fundamental social development and institutional reform. Indeed, HIV provides an unprecedented opportunity to mould kinder, more humane, sophisticated societies rather than resorting to the brutal methods and prejudices of our colonial past. To understand the task ahead, let us now turn to some of the ways that stigma exerts its adverse influence.

STIGMA HIDES THE EPIDEMIC

Stigma forces people into hiding. In doing so, it masks the epidemic and sets the scene for some seriously inadequate interventions (Kelly & Bain 2005). Stigma orchestrates a conspiracy of silence which renders HIV invisible even when it is surrounds us and is growing inexorably. Direct, personal engagement with a hidden epidemic is impossible. We are reduced instead to talking about HIV in the abstract atmosphere of meetings and policy documents – but not as it relates to real life and real death. The reality of a hidden epidemic eludes us, until it is simply too late.

'It's hard keeping my status a secret but I have to because there are some people who just wouldn't understand'. (Auguste 2006, 5).

A hidden epidemic entrenches denial. Denial is the classic symptom of a society that is failing to confront the epidemic in a genuine and significant manner. As long as our societies fail to engage with the epidemic in meaningful ways, then the epidemic will continue largely unrestrained. Risks will remain unchallenged. Prevention will be unable to gain traction.

Stigma creates social blind spots. Instead of living harmoniously with people with HIV in an open, healthy climate, everyday contact takes place without us even realising it. The only difference is disclosure. So should disclosure be forced? In a climate of stigma, forced disclosure would only distort our responses and aggravate the situation even further. If disclosure is forced in the presence of stigma, then people will suffer.

If stigma is addressed, then forced disclosure becomes irrelevant. Disclosure will be easy and the unnecessary suffering caused by stigma will wane.

Denial goes hand in hand with xenophobia – the wish to blame others (foreigners and marginalised groups) for our problems. In the Caribbean, the 'blame game' has played out in three key ways. First, in the travel and tourism sector, (which constitutes a major sector of the economy of many Caribbean states) foreign visitors are seen as having been primarily responsible for the epidemic. However, accepting this rationale leaves denial intact: local people can be portrayed as little more than helpless victims of hedonistic northern cultures and scant regard needs to be given to the indigenous local epidemic or to the participation of local people in risk activities that is necessary if the epidemic is to be sustained locally (which it is). Second, the mobility of Caribbean peoples among the various island states in the region is likewise implicated in xenophobic denial. In particular, the focus has been on people from countries with weaker economies who seek a better quality of life elsewhere. In this instance, the origin of the epidemic takes on an intraregional dynamic where blame is levelled at those from other, generally poorer, Caribbean nations. Third, social prejudices (such as homophobia) are at the root of HIV-related stigma. As a result, marginalised groups have shouldered much of the blame even though the Caribbean epidemic is largely heterosexual and affects ordinary people who did not take simple protective measures. In the final analysis, blaming 'others' is a sure sign that we are having trouble "owning" the epidemic ourselves. Unless we accept the epidemic as an internal problem – as our Caribbean problem – then meaningful action will evade us.

STIGMA WOUNDS PEOPLE

Stigma harms vulnerable people. By isolating people who are at-risk or infected, stigma intensifies their suffering way beyond the clinical impact of HIV. Moreover, stigma inevitably spreads to people nearby and exerts undue pressure on partners, family, friends and other social supports (Goffman 1963).

The school girl cried as she spoke. "Why are my friends treating me this way? What could I have done to stop my mother from dying of AIDS? I miss her so much. Now I have nobody who will talk to me". (DFID, u.d.p.1)

The vulnerability and suffering of people affected by HIV should be at the forefront of the AIDS agenda. One would have hoped that this point is self-evident, but stigma can obscure our vision of the epidemic. One explanation is that stigmatised conditions and vulnerable populations are more likely to be seen as deserving of their fate. It is then a short step to viewing 'them' as 'guilty' and therefore less worthy of state and community support. In short, stigma is an invariable basis for blaming victims and creating scapegoats (Heap & Simpson 2004).

'Families and their ill relatives are pointed at by others, talked about and shunned by the community of which they are part' (Hutchinson, 1998, 19)

If left unchallenged, stigma will continue to inflict grave injustices, and the scene will be set for dysfunctional interventions and rapidly spreading HIV. No one is guilty of having HIV and no one deserves it. Making people feel guilty will do nothing but further erode their self-esteem and intensify their vulnerability. We must collectively strive to preserve individual human dignity at all cost.

STIGMA DISRUPTS VITAL SUPPORT NETWORKS

Stigma breaks up families. As a result, an inordinate number of people with HIV die poor and alone. When family members are stigmatised their status changes – often dramatically. Rather than being embraced, people with HIV often report being disowned or estranged and made unwelcome in the family home. This is a telling outcome, because rejection is not the classic way that families cope with adversity. The difference in the case of HIV is due to stigma (Herek & Capitano 1997).

> *'I didn't tell my friend because I didn't know how she would treat me. I certainly couldn't tell my family–what would they think?' (Auguste' 2006, 5).*

People infected with and affected by HIV and those at risk can become socially isolated because of stigma. Social isolation has many detrimental effects, including depression, lack of care and support, poor access to food and services, and poverty (Ramsay, Williams, Brown & Bhardwaj 2004). In contrast, supportive networks sustain life. They are powerful promoters of health and well-being. Simply being able to get assistance with meals, transport to clinics, to have a shoulder to cry on and someone to laugh with are fundamental to health. The support of a family is as important as medical care. Cynthia, a 35-year-old Trinidadian living with AIDS, still allocates time to meet with other people with HIV to offer her support. She is able to do this because her family has been supportive of her. In her words:

> *'It is safe to take care of ill relatives just as if they have any other illness. You can hug, kiss them and love them just as you would if you had not known they were HIV positive.' (Staff Reporter Trinidad Guardian 1994, 10)*

Moreover, isolation does not overcome a desire for company, nor for intimacy – if anything loneliness intensifies those needs. However, in the face of sanctions, our deep human needs are increasingly fulfilled in furtive ways and in risky settings.

Paradoxically, the isolation induced by stigma can concentrate and amplify HIV risk. Moreover, greater openness and social integration can help to meet our basic need for company and support, while simultaneously reducing risk. The more connected people are to their supportive social networks, the less 'at risk' they become (see Levinson, Sadigursky & Erchak, 2004).

> *'HIV/AIDS patients need support and encouragement from their friends and family. It's not easy living with HIV/AIDS. Stigmatisation and discrimination make it difficult for those infected to openly speak'. (Dr Amery Browne, Technical Director of the National AIDS Coordinating Committee of Trinidad and Tobago in Woman Express, 2006, 16.)*

STIGMA IMPAIRS ACCESS TO LIFE-SAVING CARE

Access to quality medical services is a cornerstone of HIV care. Voluntary testing is often the first step to people taking some personal stake in the epidemic and to 'owning' their risks. Soliciting informed consent prior to testing is a key to making the epidemic real and meaningful. If people are unaware of having been tested and are not informed of the implications, it is hard to see how they might play a role in stopping HIV. Clearly, informed consent is in the interests of public health *as well as* individual rights.

Access to care substantially prolongs good quality life, especially when care includes anti-retroviral drugs (ARV). Significant benefits also flow to families and communities through sustained employment, reduced costs and infrequent medical visits – improved family well-being and social stability will follow.

There are many ways in which stigma interferes with access to care: for example, not feeling free to seek testing for fear of attracting undue attention and subsequent breaches of privacy (Jankie 2006). These issues are compounded in smaller communities such as those found on many Caribbean islands where people are often well acquainted with each other and with their community health workers, to whom they are often related. Additionally some people with HIV are unable to store medications at home for fear of discovery; and likewise, they fear taking them to school or work where there is the risk of being fired, expelled or bullied

Stigma also interferes with the delivery of quality care. It says volumes about our sincerity and our commitment to providing quality health care that stigmatised diseases often get the most neglected facilities. This neglect readily translates into eroded staff morale and contempt by administrators. Moreover, staff are drawn from the communities they serve, so prevailing prejudices can easily manifest as compromised care.

Paradoxically, some services in the Caribbean have been able to provide good facilities for people with HIV – only to trigger resentment. Here too stigma is playing its corrosive role. Resentment of good services reflects a belief that people with HIV are undeserving. However, for any other condition, improved facilities would be welcomed as part of the usual cycle of health service enhancements.

There is invariably resistance to making 'special' arrangements for HIV. It has been argued that all diseases need equal treatment and that HIV should not be the exception. On the surface, this claim seems reasonable except that HIV is spreading inexorably and has global repercussions. Extraordinary arrangements are justifiable on this ground alone. Further, no two diseases are alike, and it is fallacious to suggest that all diseases can be treated in the same way. Every health issue has its own special approach – in that sense HIV is no different. The principal factor affecting the delivery of HIV care is that it is deeply stigmatised. Indeed, many of the special arrangements that are necessary to cope with HIV have been implemented entirely because of stigma; otherwise more conventional arrangements would have sufficed.

Resentment of services for people with sexually transmissible diseases including HIV signifies a failure to accept the paramount importance of controlling HIV and that HIV can be found throughout society. It is long past the time when we could consider HIV services to be an optional extra: HIV services are core business at the frontline of a dangerous pandemic. It is stigma that makes HIV seem undeserving of core status alongside the other major health problems in the Caribbean.

STIGMA LICENSES ANTISOCIAL REACTIONS

Stigma is divisive. Segregating people into 'us' and 'them' creates destructive social splits at the very time when unity is essential. When division reigns, the only winner is HIV. Tugs of war about HIV prevention create dangerous mixed messages; and disputes about the services that people 'deserve' are further evidence of these divisions. If HIV spreads further and more people die prematurely, then the entire community suffers.

Stigma sows the seeds of hatred and instability. Turning a blind eye to HIV-related prejudice sets a precedent for accepting other forms of prejudice, discrimination and hate crimes. There are numerous reports from around the world where HIV-related stigma has resulted in cold-blooded attacks: murders of gay men; savage domestic violence; racist assaults; and infanticide, to name a few. In many cases, the victims may not even have HIV; such is the power of stigma. The presumption of risk or a malicious accusation is sometimes enough for people to lose their lives – not due to the effects of a virus, but at the hands of people who hate. This hate is driven by stigma.

But why do some people hate so deeply? Surely not because of the virus itself? We have known for years that HIV is difficult to transmit through casual contact. Caring for people with HIV should be simple, and not nearly as dangerous as working with drug-resistant tuberculosis, for example. Yet there is a sense that these facts are being resisted and the evidence looks suspicious. The inescapable conclusion is that stigma is at work here. Why? The most convincing clues come from health professionals themselves. We know of highly trained practitioners who refuse to treat people with HIV despite being acquainted with the facts and these same people would not refuse to treat tuberculosis. We are also aware of professionals who provide different classes of care depending how the infection was acquired: for example, caring for people with medically-acquired HIV because they are 'innocent', but refusing to treat others (who by implication are 'guilty'). Clearly, a fear of infection is not the real reason for refusing treatment. Stigma underpins this callous and unprofessional conduct.

"If I speak out publicly," said the leader of a gay rights group, "I will certainly be beaten or worse… and we don't put the office address on the web site, so that it is not burned down." (DFID, u.d.p.1)

But if stigma makes murderers out of ordinary people and licenses callous behaviour by practitioners, then society at large is the loser. Responding to callous and brutal treatment with indifference is a precedent that no community can afford. How can we be proud of a nation that tolerates such acts? How can we in the Caribbean, who have experienced slavery, brutality and genocide, celebrate emancipation while tolerating deep prejudices right within our borders? Surely there is unfinished business here! The symbolism of our inaction is just too important to ignore. There is more at stake than the inhumane treatment of people with HIV: we are creating a legacy for future generations. Can we be proud? Will they respect us?

STIGMA UNDERMINES POLITICAL WILL

Stigma influences public opinion. When this happens, political leaders are susceptible to yielding to the dictates of stigma to the long-term detriment of our social fabric and HIV control. Stigma often represents the views of a vocal, fairly extreme, segment of the population, and its influence on policy can be disproportionate. But even where stigma is widely held, the leadership choice is clear: to succumb to its dictates or to reject stigma for the greater good.

There are many significant parallels between HIV-related stigma and racism – including that both are completely unacceptable. Fortunately, nowadays our political leaders reject racism, although this has not always been the case. This profoundly important social change came about entirely because of national and grassroots leadership against racism. Likewise, our leaders need to take a principled stand to ensure that HIV-related stigma is unacceptable too. It is important to realise that stigma is neither inevitable nor is it a necessary ingredient for

HIV control – quite the opposite is true. The appropriate role of government is to act to restrain these antisocial tendencies and to protect the potential victims of stigma from discrimination. In doing so, important messages are sent about the standards a nation aspires to.

Despite our self-righteous statements and our claims to the moral high ground, guilt will be squarely on our shoulders if we do not explicitly name, challenge and reject stigma. While stigma invites us to believe impulsively that harsh responses will be needed to control HIV, in fact, human rights and HIV control go hand in hand. The alternative is that the epidemic becomes inaccessible because the very people needed to fight it will be forced underground. For this reason, there is a growing chorus from HIV/AIDS workers for comprehensive programmes to reduce stigma, to address marginalisation, to reform archaic colonial laws and to protect the vulnerable from prejudice and discrimination – including, the poor, sex workers, people who use drugs, and homosexually active men. The evidence is clear on this point: where sensible steps have been put in place to protect vulnerable populations against discrimination, HIV control has been effective. Where animosity, social divisions and conflict are rife, all sexually transmissible infections, including HIV, spread largely unrestrained.

Although the use of the media to change people's risky behaviour has met with mixed results, there is no doubt that the media exerts a powerful influence on public opinion (albeit not always in the direction one wants!). The media has an important role to play in creating a climate where HIV-related stigma is rejected. Appropriate roles for the media include showcasing good role models, denouncing stigma, fostering consensus

and establishing a constructive climate in which HIV can be defeated. A recent anti-stigma initiative developed by the Jamaican Ministry of Health is a case in point. This initiative showcases HIV-positive Jamaicans, who bravely came forward in support of the campaign. This case reminds us that leadership in HIV should not be thought of simply in terms of formal leaders – leadership shown by people at the grassroots and those of us with HIV is very powerful.

CONCLUSION: HIV REQUIRES LEADERSHIP; LEADERSHIP REQUIRES VISION

After decades of rising death rates and the relentless spread of HIV, it is easy to become fatalistic. Our nations need inspirational leadership to overcome the blurred vision that stigma induces. We need to envision a better world – a destination we all want to reach. Our collective vision has to see beyond the death toll and beyond the relentless spread of HIV. Our prejudices must be swept aside in order to see this epidemic with clarity. Sustained widespread protective behaviour change *is possible* and has been achieved in a number of settings around the world. In every case, an inclusive approach was taken with a heavy emphasis on social justice and inclusion and empowerment of those at risk and infected. Our vision has to anticipate the legacy that we will leave for future generations. Do we want countries crippled by hate and riddled with disease? No? Then stigma is the enemy. Do we want divided countries where our brothers and sisters are outcasts? Surely not! So our vision has to be of a compassionate, generous, loving response. The true heroes of the epidemic are those who reject stigma and who step up to help. The true heroes are people with HIV who endure so much unnecessary suffering on top of coping with a wicked infection. It is not 'them' who are 'guilty'; nor 'we' who are 'innocent'. If anyone should shoulder guilt, it is all of us for simply not caring enough. Our job is to 'own' the epidemic, to embrace those among us who are vulnerable and to offer our hand in support.

REFERENCES

Auguste, R.S. (2006, October 8). Living with HIV. *Woman Express*, p.4.

Auguste, R.S. (2006, October 29). Living with HIV/AIDS. *Woman Express*, p. 16.

Brown, L., Macintyre, K. and Trujillo, L. (2003). Interventions to reduce HIV/AIDS stigma – What have we learned? *AIDS Education and Prevention* 15(1):49–69.

Caribbean Epidemiology Centre. (2004). *Status and trends: Analysis of the Caribbean HIV/AIDS epidemic 1982-2002*. Port of Spain, Trinidad: CAREC.

DFID (UK Department for International Development). (undated). *Tackling HIV/AIDS stigma and discrimination in the Caribbean*. Retrieved September 20, 2006,

From http://www.dfid.gov.uk/case studies/files/south-america/carib.hiv.asp

Fraser, T. (2006, May 17). Fighting HIV/AIDS via the media. *Trinidad Guardian*, p.33.

Goffman, E. (1963). *Stigma: Notes on the management of spoiled identity*. Repr., New York: Simon and Schuster, 1986.

Heap, B. and Simpson, T. (2004). When you have AIDS people laugh at you – a process drama approach to stigma with pupils in Zambia. *Caribbean Quarterly* 50(1):83–98.

Herek, G.M. and Capitano, J. (1997). AIDS stigma and contact with persons with AIDS: Effect of direct and vicarious contact. *Journal of Applied Social Psychology* 271:1–36.

Hutchinson, L. (1998, June 8). People living with AIDS still shunned, report says. *Newsday*, p.19.

Jankie, A. (2006, June 5). Stigma makes patients shun AIDS clinic. Daily Express, p.16.

Kelly, Michael J. and Bain, B. 2005. *Education and HIV/AIDS in the Caribbean*. Kingston: Ian Randle Publishers.

Levinson, R.A., Sadigursky, C. and Erchak, G.M. (2004). The impact of cultural context on Brazilian adolescents' sexual practices. *Adolescence* 39(154): 203–27.

Ramsay, H., Williams, S., Brown, J. and Bhardwaj, S. (2004). Young children, a neglected group in the HIV epidemic: Perspectives from Jamaica. *Caribbean Quarterly* 50(1): 39–53.

Staff Reporter. (1994, December 12). AIDS-Caribbean families must be supported. *Trinidad Guardian*, p.10.

17

External funds relevant to the education sector response to school health and HIV/AIDS in the Caribbean region

Donald Bundy, Tara O'Connell, Alexandria Valerio and Mary Mulusa

World Bank

This chapter provides a preliminary estimate for the Caribbean region of the external funds that are currently available to support the education sector response to school health and HIV/AIDS. The analysis was undertaken on behalf of CARICOM as part of the preparations for the June 2006 Special Meeting of the Council for Human and Social Development (COHSOD) on Education and HIV/AIDS. The analyses are intended to help identify funding opportunities and to assist enhanced donor harmonisation in the region.

DATA COLLECTION AND ANALYSIS

Development partners in the Caribbean region were requested to provide information on their current support for:

- the national HIV/AIDS response, including support for the education sector response;
- the education sector generally, including support for components that might be relevant to the HIV/AIDS response, such as teacher training, curriculum development and education materials; and
- the education sector response to HIV/AIDS specifically.

Tables 17.1–3 show the data for the region as a whole as well as for specific countries, and show the level of support in the form of bilateral and multilateral financial commitments.

There are clearly important omissions and the estimate should be viewed as conservative. For example Table 17.4, which details projects and funding in the Caribbean region (see Appendix), does not include support from the Caribbean Development Bank. The information is not exhaustive and is based on responses received up to 26 May 2006. Note that all figures refer to US dollars.

TOTAL COMBINED EXTERNAL RESOURCES FOR HIV/AIDS AND FOR EDUCATION

Currently available information from development partners indicates that $849.2 million has been committed to the larger Caribbean region, comprising the CARICOM countries and the Dominican Republic. As shown in Table 17.1, the total for CARICOM countries alone is $624.6

million without the Dominican Republic, for which the figure is $224.6 million. Note that, in all tables, analysis is confined to CARICOM countries (exclusive of the Dominican Republic), unless otherwise specified.

Table 17.2 shows that three agencies contributed 92 per cent of the total: the Inter-American Development Bank (IDB), the World Bank Group (WB) and the President's Emergency Plan for HIV/AIDS Relief (PEPFAR). Other important contributors are the Global Fund for HIV/AIDS, Malaria and Tubercolosis (TB), the European Union (EU) and the Canadian International Development Agency (CIDA).

CURRENT ALLOCATION OF RESOURCES TO THE EDUCATION SECTOR RESPONSE TO HIV/AIDS

Table 17.3 shows that, of the total funding available, approximately 25.4 per cent is for HIV/AIDS and 74.2 per cent is for education. Neither of these figures could be clearly identified as being used to support the education sector response to HIV/AIDS. Only $2.7 million, 0.4 per cent of the total resources, was allocated specifically to the education sector response to HIV/AIDS.

TABLE 17.1
ANALYSIS OF FUNDS RELEVANT TO THE EDUCATION SECTOR BY RECIPIENT

	Total	% of grand total
Antigua and Barbuda	$0	0
The Bahamas	$18,000,000	2.9
Barbados	$100,500,000	16.1
Belize	$0	0
Dominica	$0	0
Grenada	$14,000,000	2.2
Guyana	$72,987,165	11.7
Haiti	$93,873,987	15.0
Jamaica	$109,465,340	17.5
Montserrat	$0	0
St Kitts and Nevis	$9,045,000	1.4
Saint Lucia	$18,400,000	2.9
St Vincent & the Grenadines	$12,200,000	2.0
Suriname	$17,833,432	2.9
Trinidad and Tobago	$141,000,000	22.6
Subtotal	$607,304,924	
Caribbean region shared funding	$17,265,500	2.8
Grand total	$624,570,424	100

Note: *$0 may be indicative of no data received rather than a lack of funds available.*

TABLE 17.2
ANALYSIS OF FUNDS RELEVANT TO THE EDUCATION SECTOR BY DONOR

	Total	% of grand total
CIDA	$5,263,100	0.8
EU	$3,246,519	0.5
Global Fund	$42,884,839	6.9
IDB	$338,895,000	54.3
PEPFAR	$72,235,966	11.6
WB	$162,045,000	25.9
Grand total	$624,570,424	100

POTENTIAL ALLOCATION OF RESOURCES TO THE EDUCATION SECTOR RESPONSE TO HIV/AIDS

There are two potential sources of external resources to support the sectoral response to HIV/AIDS: from multisectoral HIV/AIDS funds to the education sector; and from education sector funds to a specific sectoral subcomponent. Both sources are available in the Caribbean region but are underutilised.

- Current HIV/AIDS sector external support to the region is $158.5 million. Estimates of multisectoral programme support from other regions suggest that, on average, 5 per cent, $8 million is available to the education sector for the sectoral response to HIV/AIDS.

- Current education sector external support to the region is $463 million, of which 11 per cent is targeted specifically to the primary level and 26 per cent to the secondary level. Analyses from other AIDS-affected regions* indicate that some 5 per cent of education external resources are typically allocated to the sectoral response, which implies that approximately $23 million is available to the education sector in the Caribbean for the sectoral response to HIV/AIDS.

TABLE 17.3
ANALYSIS OF FUNDS RELEVANT TO EDUCATION BY SECTOR

	Health or HIV/AIDS	Education	%	Education & HIV/AIDS	Total	% of grand total
Primary education	–	$50,278,500	10.9	$0	$50,278,511	8.1
Secondary education	–	$119,200,000	25.7	$2,049,600	$121,249,626	19.4
Tertiary education	–	$0	0.0	$0	$0	0.0
Unspecified level / Youth	$158,588,337	$293,773,987	63.4	$680,000	$453,042,387	72.5
Grand total	$158,588,337	$463,252,487	100	$2,729,600	$624,570,424	100
% of grand total	25.4	74.2		0.4	100	

Note: *$0 may be indicative of no data received rather than a lack of funds available.*

IMPLICATIONS FOR FUNDING THE EDUCATION SECTOR RESPONSE TO HIV/AIDS

Current external funding for the education sector response to HIV/AIDS in the Caribbean region is estimated at $2.7 million. On the basis of funding experiences in other AIDS-affected regions, currently available external resources should be able to provide an additional $8 million from HIV/AIDS resources and an additional $23 million from education resources. This implies that only $2.7 million is currently being utilised to develop a sectoral response to HIV/AIDS out of a potential $31 million available.

INCREASING ACCESS TO CURRENTLY AVAILABLE RESOURCES

Analysis from other AIDS-affected regions indicates two key factors in securing support for an effective education sector response to HIV/AIDS.

- Ministries of Education should recognise that their strong leadership is the critical first step in mobilising resources for the education sector response to HIV/AIDS. In particular, accessing specialist technical assistance for programme preparation is a key element in developing an effective response.
- National AIDS authorities should recognise that among non-health sectors, education can make a particularly strong contribution to the mainstreaming of HIV/AIDS, and should give priority to the role of the education sector to HIV/AIDS prevention, provide resources for programme preparation and facilitate disbursement.

APPENDIX

FUNDS RELEVANT TO EDUCATION SECTOR RESPONSE TO HIV/AIDS IN THE CARIBBEAN REGION

The purpose of Table 17.4 (see following pages) is to map bilateral and multilateral funds available to the education sector of the Caribbean that are either specifically allocated for HIV/AIDS or might be used in support of HIV/AIDS work (e.g. teacher training, community involvement, curriculum development, or securing education materials) at the regional and country levels. The results of the study might allow us to better assess present allocation of funds as well as identify future needs and opportunities. They should also indicate gaps and strengths in funding for HIV/AIDS in education and assist in efforts at enhanced donor harmonisation in the region.

This study in not exhaustive and is based on responses received to a general request for information. The table does not include the Caribbean Development Bank.

Data from the following donors are included:
- CIDA – Canadian International Development Agency
- EU – European Union
- Global Fund – Global Fund to Fight AIDS, Tuberculosis and Malaria
- IDB – Inter-American Development Bank
- JICA – Japanese International Cooperation Agency
- PEPFAR – President's Emergency Plan for HIV/AIDS Relief
- WB –World Bank

TABLE 17.4
PROJECTS AND FUNDING RELEVANT TO THE EDUCATION SECTOR RESPONSE TO
HIV/AIDS BY REGION AND COUNTRY

Relevant projects	Funding
Caribbean region	
CIDA – Fighting AIDS Through Training and Education – with the Caribbean Family Planning Affiliation, Ltd, to be implemented in Anguilla, Antigua, Belize, Dominica, Grenada, Guyana, Jamaica, Montserrat, St Kitts and Nevis, St Vincent, and St Lucia. Goal to improve the sexual and reproductive health status of Caribbean youth by decreasing the incidence of HIV/AIDS and teenage pregnancy. Includes three strategies: a regional public education programme, regional training programme for service providers, and the strengthening and expansion of the Youth Advocacy Movement and peer helper groups that are part of family planning associations in the Caribbean into hard-to-reach communities	$1,484,600
Global Fund – Multicountry Americas (CARICOM). Primary focus on empowering people living with HIV/AIDS, particularly in the area of treatment and care. Efforts at scaling up existing capacity-building and advocacy programmes and establishing new programmes. Emphasis on advocacy around stigma and discrimination	$6,100,900
IDB – Caribbean Education Sector HIV/AIDS Response Capacity-Building Programme (Project No. ATN/JF-8627-RS). Will fund diagnostic analyses, preparatory studies, high-level meetings and capacity-building seminars to design a comprehensive strategy and a concrete programme that will enable the education sector to play a critical role in the prevention and mitigation of HIV/AIDS in the countries of the Caribbean region	**IDB, CARICOM/ PANCAP, UNESCO** – $680,000. IDB to contribute $565,000; CARICOM/ PANCAP Secretariats to contribute $35,000 in kind; UNESCO to contribute $30,000 in kind and the countries participating in pilot interventions to contribute a total of $50,000 in kind

Relevant projects	Funding
WB – Multicountry HIV/AIDS Prevention and Control Project. Includes components for preventive programmes that focus on behaviour change and strengthening national capacity for a response to HIV/AIDS	$9,000,000
Antigua and Barbuda	
None reported	
The Bahamas	
IDB – Support Programme for Transforming Education and Training – Phase I (Project No. BH-L1003). Includes components focusing on targeted programmes to facilitate inclusion of children of vulnerable groups into the preschool system. Efforts to strengthen Ministry of Education (MoE) capacity to inform intervention strategies across sector ministries. Emphasis on teacher training and capacity-building	$18,000,000
Barbados	
IDB – Education Sector Enhancement Program (EDUTECH) (Project No. BA-0009). Will help the Ministry of Education, Youth Affairs and Culture (MEC) implement reforms in curriculum, teaching practices, and assessment mechanisms. Finances formal training, workshops, classroom training, and the development of learning materials for teachers	$85,000,000
WB – HIV/AIDS Prevention and Control Adaptable Programme Lending. Includes components for prevention and control ($5,700,000) including HIV/AIDS Coordination Units being developed in each of the eight ministries, and management and institution strengthening ($3,500,000)	US$15,500,000
Belize	
None reported	
Dominica	
None reported	
Dominican Republic	
Global Fund – National Response to HIV/AIDS, Tuberculosis and Malaria. While primarily aimed at tuberculosis, also includes components aimed at HIV/AIDS. Includes the training of health personnel through, in part, designing and producing teaching materials. Much focus placed on vulnerable and at-risk groups, and promoting sustainability of work by ensuring civil society better responds to the needs of vulnerable groups and enhancing community-based help and volunteer groups	$14,698,774

Relevant projects	Funding
IDB – DR0112 Education Media (Secondary Education). Includes components for teacher training, curriculum development, development of a tutorial-based training system for teachers, and pilot programmes aimed at reducing violence and substance abuse in youth	$59,000,000
IDB – DR0125 Equity Enhancement Basic Education Programme. Efforts to increase quality in basic education. Emphasis on enhanced teacher training and teacher methodology	$80,000,000
WB – Early Childhood Education Project. Includes components for increasing early childhood development education quality including strengthening teacher capacity and teacher training ($20,320,000), and institutional strengthening in the education sector ($7,440,000)	$42,000,000
WB – HIV/AIDS Prevention and Control Project. Component aimed at mitigating suffering of and providing support to OVC. Support offered directly to the education sector	$25,000,000, with approximately US$3,900,000 allocated to the education sector
Grenada	
WB – Second OECS Education Development Project. Includes components for increasing equitable access through, in part, expansion and rehabilitation of secondary schools ; improving quality of teaching and learning ; strengthening governance and management ($1,570,000); and project management	$8,000,000 (IBRD/IDA blend)
WB – HIV/AIDS Prevention and Control Project. Includes components for promotion and behaviour change ($1,350,000), prevention and control ($1,890,000), and access to treatment and care ($1,040,000)	$6,000,000 (IBRD/IDA blend)
Guyana	
CIDA – Guyana Basic Education Teacher Training Project (GBET). Goal to improve the quality of basic education in Guyana by strengthening the country's basic education teacher training system. Was designed to address the prevalence of unqualified and untrained teachers, seen as one of the key factors contributing to low student achievement levels	$3,778,500 (1998 – 2003, with extension)
Global Fund – Strengthening Local Capacity to Respond to HIV/ AIDS through alliances. Includes, among other things, efforts to enhance education programmes and to reduce stigma and discrimination. Activities to achieve this include recruitment and training of individuals and the development, production, and dissemination of educational materials. Also effort to implement an integrated multisectoral response to HIV/AIDS	$8,881,686

Relevant projects	Funding
IDB – Education Sector Response to HIV/AIDS in the Caribbean Project. Funded by the IDB and with CARICOM as contracting management firm. Seeks to develop and support the implementation of effective intervention models for use by the education sector to reach in- and out-of-school youths. Two strategies will be employed: (1) community-based youth drop in centres providing HIV/AIDS education services to both school attendees after school hours as well as out of school youth, providing counselling and risk prevention skills, and (2) MOE contracting with NGOs to deliver HIV/AIDS services in school in a coordinated, cost-effective and systematic manner. The Education Development Centre INC. contracted to execute the programme	$565,000
PEPFAR – Guyana Country Project. Efforts for prevention aimed at reinforcing safer sexual behaviour and reducing stigma and discrimination. Behaviour modification messages aimed at in- and out-of-school youth. Community-based programmes to partner with the education system, among others, to enforce efforts at delaying the onset of sexual intercourse. Incorporating messages of abstinence and reproductive health into HFLE series being developed by MoE as well as into current Life Skills curriculum. Programme works with education partners and the MoE at local and national levels to support education of OVC, partially through school books and education materials. Also an emphasis on infrastructure development and capacity-building	$19,761,979 (planned FY05)
WB – HIV/AIDS Prevention and Control Project. Five-year project in the school system. Begun in 2005. Includes components to strengthen institutional capacity ($2,600,000) including within the non-health ministries, and scale up response by line ministries ($3,490,000) including the MoE. $54,292 disbursed for 2006 for sensitization, coordination and implementation of HIV/AIDS education for all MoE staff, PTAs and students. All head teachers will be trained	$10,000,000
Haiti	
IDB – Basic Education (Project No. HA0038). Includes efforts to build capacity at the MoE and throughout the system through teacher training, production and distribution of teaching materials, and school-based improvements	$19,400,000
IDB – Vocational Training (Project No. HA-0017). Focuses primarily on capacity-building and training aimed at skills for the informal sector. Includes emphasis on training and building links between civil society and the Government	$22,000,000
PEPFAR – Haiti Programme. Includes, among other things, efforts around prevention and care including education support for OVC, and the cross-sectoral strengthening of management and staff	$52,473,987 (planned FY05)

Relevant projects	Funding
Jamaica	
EU – Addressing HIV In Jamaica: A Holistic Response. Project aims to provide stigma and discrimination-free HIV prevention, care and support, information, and education to the most disadvantaged in Jamaica, including children and young persons from economically and socially marginalized communities. Will benefit seropositive and negative members of such groups by providing both targeted prevention information and holistic care and support. Efforts at stigma and discrimination-free testing, counselling, skills-training initiatives, community strengthening, performing arts, and other public education on HIV-related issues (including gender and sexual orientation), anti-stigma campaigns, rights-based advocacy on policies affecting target groups, and nutritional, material, and clinical support. Project implemented by Christian Aid	$953,389
EU – Sexual and reproductive Health (SRH). Aims to improve the knowledge of and provide tools for behaviour change in order to fully exercise one's sexual and reproductive rights. Emphasis on vulnerable groups including adolescents. Efforts to build institutional capacity to deliver high quality services to vulnerable groups. Implemented by UNFPA with the assistance of NGOs and Government agencies	$2,293,130
Global Fund – Scaling Up HIV/AIDS Treatment, Prevention, and Policy Efforts. Efforts include the promotion of safer sex practices particularly amongst high-risk groups including youth, behaviour change leading to reduced transmission, and reduction of stigma and discrimination.	$23,318,821
IDB – PESP Basic and Primary Education Programme III. Efforts to improve the delivery of quality primary education and strengthen school management capacity at the regional and local levels. Emphasis on teacher training including through the development of training materials and institutional strengthening	$29,000,000
JICA – Support the Ministry of Education and Youth HIV/AIDS Education Prevention Program. Carried out with support from partner agencies including UNESCO, UNICEF, various NGOs, the National AIDS Committee Education sub-Committee. Achieved through placement and dispatch of junior/senior volunteers to Headquarters of the MOEY and six volunteers to the six Regional Offices, and assistance in capacity-building for Education Officers, PTA Presidents, Board Chairpersons, principals, and Guidance Counsellors, aimed at benefiting teachers and students	Provides only human resource support
WB – Reform of Secondary Education Project II. Includes components for School Improvement Plans ($5,800,000), Reform Support ($3,600,000), Expanded Access ($7,800,000), and Monitoring, Evaluation & Assessment ($2,300,000)	$38,900,000
WB – HIV/AIDS Prevention and Control Project. Includes a component for prevention programmes aimed at behaviour change ($7,820,000)	$15,000,000

Relevant projects	Funding
Montserrat	
None reported	
St Kitts and Nevis	
WB – OECS Education Development Program. Includes components for improving quality of teaching and learning, learning resource centres, school-based improvement and extracurricular activities, and establishing a project management unit	$5,000,000
WB – HIV/AIDS Prevention and Control Project. Includes components for advocacy and behaviour change ($510,000), and prevention in high-risk groups including out-of-school youth ($1,130,000)	$4,045,000
St Lucia	
WB – OECS Education Development Programme. Includes components for expansion and upgrading of schools ($3,040,000), and improvement of quality of teaching and learning ($2,880,000)	$12,000,000 (IBRD/IDA blend)
WB – HIV/AIDS Prevention Project. Includes components for a line ministry response ($900,000) and strengthening institutional capacity ($2,660,000)	$6,400,000 (IBRD/IDA blend)
St Vincent and the Grenadines	
WB – OECS Education Development Project. Includes components for rehabilitation of secondary schools ($530,000), improving the quality of education ($2,700,000), curriculum development ($300,000), literacy enrichment and support including materials ($1,400,000), improvement of student services support ($700,000), and project management ($500,000)	$6,200,000 (IBRD/IDA blend)
WB – HIV/AIDS Prevention Project. Includes components for scaling up of line ministry response ($1,600,000) and strengthening institutional capacity ($2,550,000)	$6,000,000 (IBRD/IDA blend)
Suriname	
Global Fund – Suriname Country Project. Aims, among other things, to integrate comprehensive HIV/AIDS and tuberculosis counselling and referral services with primary health care (PHC) services, to scale up and upgrade a voluntary counselling and testing system, and to improve psychosocial care and support activities for PLWHA and their families. Activities include the upgrading of health education, the promotion of non-discriminatory attitudes in the work place, and the documentation and combating of stigma and discrimination. There is also emphasis placed on the process of behaviour change towards a healthy and safe sexual lifestyle	$4,583,432
IDB – Support the National Strategic Plan for HIV/AIDS (Project No. SU-T1007). Efforts at behaviour change around reduction of transmission, and stigma and discrimination	$750,000
IDB – Basic Education Improvement Project (Project No. SU0023). Aims to improve quality of primary education through school inputs and institutional strengthening	$12,500,000

Relevant projects	Funding
Trinidad and Tobago	
EU – Provide support to curriculum of courses either infused with HIV/AIDS or new modules developed; training of trainers among UWI staff to provide sensitization and education to others; two lecturers funded the Department of Economics, Health Economics Unit – they have also conducted Impact assessment of HIV studies in a number of Caribbean countries; provides internships for a number of students to focus on HIV/AIDS; UNESCO Chair at UWI St Augustine; Abstinence Clubs in secondary schools supported by both MoE and MoH; MoE (supported by UNESCO) strategic planning session facilitated by ECD	(data not available)
IDB – Secondary Education Modernization Programme (Project No. SEMP, TT-0023). Aims to reform and expand the secondary subsector through, among other things, institutional strengthening of the MoE, curriculum development, teaching and learning strategies, professional development, and the construction of new schools	$105,000,000
IDB – PIPELINE: Support for a Seamless Education System (Project No. TT-L1005). Focuses on early childhood education and development. Includes professional development of early childhood providers and a review of existing curriculum to ensure effective linkage to primary education	$16,000,000
WB – HIV/AIDS Prevention and Control Project. Includes components for prevention efforts ($8,055,000) focusing on promotion of behaviour change, in part, through heightened education efforts, project management, coordination and evaluation ($2,020,000) including a network of HIV/AIDS focal points in the ministries	$20,000,000

18

Building Sector Leadership: A Caribbean model, The Advocacy and Leadership Campaign

Connie Constantine, Cheryl
Vince Whitman and
Mora Oommen

Education Development Center, Inc.

In January 2005, seeking to amplify and apply this concept to the Caribbean region, the UNESCO Office for the Caribbean and Education Development Center, Inc. (EDC) developed and launched an advocacy and leadership campaign. The campaign entitled Leading the Way in the Education Sector: Advocating for a Comprehensive Approach to HIV and AIDS in the Caribbean *was designed to advance the education sector response to HIV and AIDS in the Caribbean.*

The overall goal of the campaign was to develop and support a cadre of leaders throughout the Caribbean region to become knowledgeable about the impact of HIV and AIDS and committed to influencing members of the education sector to create a more comprehensive approach to addressing HIV and AIDS issues. The campaign sought to bring information, skills, and resources to senior-level staff in the ministries of education to: (1) advance policies and programmes related to HIV and AIDS; (2) promote the greater inclusion of persons living with HIV and AIDS (PLWHA); and (3) advocate for a comprehensive approach to health promotion and the mitigation of the impact of the HIV and AIDS epidemic in the education sector.

BACKGROUND

'Advocacy at all levels is needed to mobilize all sectors of government in the struggle against HIV and AIDS and to trigger support and complementary actions by non governmental organizations, civil societies and the private sector.' (UNAIDS Inter-Agency Task Team on Education Strategy Framework).

Three landmark developments in the field of education and HIV and AIDS, and the fact that the Caribbean region has the second highest prevalence of HIV and AIDS in the world second only to Sub-Saharan Africa, provided the impetus for initiating this campaign. These developments included: (1) the publication of a groundbreaking, prevention-focused Health and Family Life Education (HFLE) curriculum framework; (2) the publication of a seminal book that charted a bold new course to combat the spread of HIV and AIDS; and (3) the efforts of a global task force that united to mount a comprehensive response to the epidemic.

First, CARICOM, UNICEF, the United Nations' agencies, and EDC's Health and Human Development Programs (HHD) division worked collaboratively to facilitate efforts to advance accomplishments in Health and Family Life Education (HFLE) and HIV and AIDS. In the fall of 2005, the *Caribbean Regional Curriculum Framework for Health and Family Life Education for Ages 9-14* was developed with four major themes: 1) Sexuality and Sexual Health including HIV and AIDS; 2) Self and Interpersonal Relationships; 3) Eating and Fitness; and 4) Managing the Environment. While the completion of the *Framework* was an important step towards addressing HIV and AIDS in the education sector, there was, however, a need to build leadership and capacity to scale up HFLE programmes.

Second, in October 2004, Professors Michael Kelly and Brendan Bain completed and published a seminal book, *Education and HIV/ AIDS in the Caribbean*. In this book, Kelly and Bain described the threat to the education system in the region, detailed the powerful role that educators can play in addressing HIV and AIDS, and identified ways in which the education sector needs to strengthen its response to HIV and AIDS. Kelly and Bain noted that for the first two decades of the epidemic, the response to HIV was largely concentrated in the health sector. At best, the education sector in most places around the world concentrated on disseminating information. The approach has rarely looked at what the whole system must do. Following the publication of this important resource, the need remained to disseminate its findings to a larger audience.

Third, at the global level, UNESCO convened the UNAIDS Inter-Agency Task Team (IATT) on Education to 'accelerate and improve the education sector response to HIV and AIDS.' By its very composition, the IATT on Education models a comprehensive, cross-sector approach to the epidemic – its members include the UNAIDS co-sponsoring agencies, bilateral agencies and private donors, and a wide range of civil society organisations. The IATT on Education has made great strides in building the knowledge base of effective strategies and disseminating information. The organisation sponsors international symposia and events, and its working groups have produced a rich array of online and print resources to guide a more comprehensive education sector response (http://www.portal.unesco.org). Yet, in nations around the world and in the Caribbean, few ministries of education have implemented the broad approach that the IATT on Education espouses.

The Caribbean region needed to coalesce around the need for a broad, systemic approach to HIV and AIDS that involved all sectors of society. In particular, the education system needed to rally around the development of a comprehensive approach to HIV that focuses on promoting and protecting the health of students and staff and mitigating the impact of HIV on the education system itself.

THE NEED TO ENGAGE EDUCATION STAKEHOLDERS IN HIV AND AIDS PREVENTION

Ministries of Education frequently ask, 'Why does the education sector need to play a more active role in addressing the issue of HIV and AIDS?' It is an important question, and the response is the crux of the campaign. Health and education are interdependent. Poor health can profoundly affect academic performance, achievement, and the quality of teaching. Ministries of Education form the natural hub of systemic change to promote health practices that foster the health and safety of students and teachers, ensure the creation of a productive workforce, and advance economic development.

The engagement of Ministries of Education in addressing HIV and AIDS in the Caribbean will positively affect the region's future, as well as its present status. First, increasing the number of years of schooling that students complete will result in citizens with long-term better health and well-being – this is especially true for girls. Second, increasing health education and support for teachers and staff will combat absenteeism, improve morale, and enhance the quality of learning. Protecting teachers and staff is essential for maintaining a quality education system.

The advocacy and leadership campaign purports to strengthen this 'hub of systemic change' to mount an effective, comprehensive response to the HIV and AIDS crisis in the Caribbean. The best way to tackle HIV and AIDS is with systemic management, as well as a public health approach in the education setting. Beyond its most basic function, a comprehensive approach to HIV means moving well-beyond a health promotion curriculum component alone to having the education sector use all means at its disposal to promote and protect the health of students and staff and to mitigate the impact of HIV and AIDS on the system itself. A comprehensive approach includes four key elements:

1. Overarching policy recognising that the education system is a workplace for thousands of government staff. Adapting and customising such policies as those

the International Labour Organization (ILO) has developed to meet the needs of the education sector is one such way. Education sector policy would also cover curriculum, the school environment, and services.

2. Curriculum and education based on effective strategies of behaviour change, skill development, and participatory learning set in the context of health promotion for responsible lifestyles as addressed by HFLE and the development of the ideal Caribbean person.

3. A healthy psycho-social school and physical school environment. Such environments are free of fear, stigma, and homophobia, promote gender equity, are free of sexual harassment and sexual assault, and have codes of conduct and facilities to ensure girls' attendance.

4. Services provided by trained guidance counsellors and mechanisms to coordinate with Voluntary Counselling and Testing and mental health and nutrition services in the community. These services make knowledge about and access to testing and care easy for education sector staff and students who may be sexually active.

CAMPAIGN DEVELOPMENT PROCESS

On February 1, 2005, EDC/HHD received the endorsement of the UNESCO Office of the Caribbean and the Director General of UNESCO for the campaign launch to take place in Trinidad and Tobago on February 16, 2005.

As a first step in each of the pilot countries (St Lucia, Trinidad and Tobago, and Belize) participating in the campaign, EDC conducted extensive research to identify 'leaders' from a variety of sectors. Project staff also considered the recommendations of UNESCO and ministry of education staff of each country when compiling a list of individuals to contact. After identifying a team of ten to twelve respected leaders in each pilot country to guide the development of campaign messages, strategies, and materials, EDC/HHD conducted a series of interviews with the teams. Individuals interviewed were key players across sectors from ministries of health and education, teachers' unions, youth groups, non-governmental organisations (NGOs), media, parent teacher associations, faith community, chamber of commerce, higher education, social services, business and industry, National AIDS Coordinating Committee, and PLWHA support groups.

Next, EDC/HHD developed an advocacy toolkit for the campaign leaders and senior-level staff of the ministries of education and launched a Website (www.caribbean leaders.org) with downloadable copies of the toolkit (other features include profiles of the campaign leaders and descriptions of campaign activities in each country). Available in print and on a CD, as well as on the Website, the toolkit includes a rich variety of resources:

- A series of country-specific fact sheets,
- A workbook on advocating for a comprehensive approach to HIV and AIDS in the education sector,
- A poster that depicts the comprehensive approach,
- A PowerPoint presentation that incorporates key campaign messages, and
- A simple guide about persuasion, influence, and social marketing that guides influencers about what to say, and how to say it, with strategies to customise messages.

In addition to working with the three pilot sites, EDC/HHD collected and reviewed similar materials internationally, and staff conducted an extensive literature search to pull together current data to inform the materials development process. In doing so, staff drew on their experience and expertise gained through projects globally, which address HIV and AIDS along the continuum from prevention to intervention and care, especially in the education sector in Southeast Asia, Africa, and the Caribbean. EDC/HHD's membership in several international partnerships – UNAIDS IATT on Education, the FRESH partnership (Focused Resources on Effective School Health), and INTERCAMHS (International Alliance for Child and Adolescent Mental Health in Schools) – has given staff the opportunity to learn about many existing HIV and AIDS materials and programmes.

IMPLEMENTATION OF THE CAMPAIGN

EDC/HHD used a multi-tiered approach to implementation that engaged stakeholders on two levels – the teams of local leader/advocates and senior-level staff of ministries of education – in the campaign. Prior to the launch of the campaign in each country, EDC/HHD conducted a leadership orientation for eight to ten leaders/advocates that EDC/HHD and UNESCO staff identified during the preliminary site visits and interviews. The purpose of the orientation sessions was to introduce the cadre of leaders/advocates to one another and to prepare them to advocate for a comprehensive approach to addressing HIV and AIDS in the education sector. During the session, the teams of leaders/advocates reviewed the campaign materials, discussed the elements of a comprehensive approach to HIV and AIDS in the education sector, and participated in professional development exercises on developing targeted messages and delivery systems for the audiences they wanted to reach.

The next step of this campaign was to conduct a one-day retreat with the senior-level staff of the ministry of education. The purpose of the retreats was to prepare senior management teams of ministries of education to advocate for and to implement a comprehensive approach to respond to the HIV and AIDS epidemic in the education sector. More than 175 senior staff, ministers of education, and permanent secretaries – from the ministries of education in Trinidad and Tobago, St Lucia, and Belize participated in the retreats. At each of the retreats, ministry participants worked in small groups to create plans for implementing a comprehensive approach to HIV and AIDS. The leaders/advocates played a key role in the retreats, giving presentations, interacting with the ministry staff, and facilitating group activities and discussion.

EVALUATION

Evaluation results from leader/advocate orientation sessions. Twenty-five participants in the three leadership orientations (7 in Trinidad and Tobago, 10 in St Lucia, and 8 in Belize) completed post-event surveys to assess the impact of the orientations. The survey used a scale of 1 to 5 (with 5 being the highest) to measure participants' level of satisfaction with the event. Analysis of the quantitative data revealed high levels of satisfaction with the quality of the orientation (average rating of 4.02), the quality of campaign materials (average rating of 4.4), and participants' understanding of the information presented regarding a comprehensive approach to HIV/AIDS (average rating of 4.16).

An analysis of qualitative responses to the survey revealed that participants could envision opportunities to use the campaign materials in schools, education councils and teachers' unions, conferences/meetings, training initiatives, one-to-one contact with key individuals, and national HIV and AIDS prevention efforts. One participant contacted EDC/HHD staff two months after the orientation to report, 'I use the toolkit as often as I can [to] meet with people where they are at. I've used it for training purposes, meeting with secretary in the Division of Education as well as churches and all my staff members.'

Survey respondents also said that they appreciated the opportunity to engage in peer networking, to participate in professional development on HIV and AIDS issues, and to learn more about advocacy strategies. One participant noted, 'I have a much better understanding of a comprehensive approach and this programme would certainly assist me immensely in my day-to-day activities . . . it presents me with the opportunity to further influence the needed changes in the education sector.' The seeds of a cross-sector approach were evident in the comments of another participant, who stated, 'Because I would be working with the entire Chamber of Commerce, I foresee the workload necessary to coordinate and implement the campaign . . . we will most likely execute the campaign via a roster of businesses.'

Evaluation results from ministry of education retreats. Seventy-five participants in the three ministry of education retreats completed evaluation forms (14 from Trinidad and Tobago, 33 from St Lucia, and 28 from Belize). Analysis of the quantitative survey data revealed that 87% of the survey respondents thought this retreat would have a profound impact on their work. Ninety-three per cent of the survey respondents were willing to make a personal level of commitment to support this initiative, and 89% were personally motivated to use a comprehensive approach to address HIV issues in their departments or units.

Campaign materials were effective in delivering key messages. An analysis of the qualitative responses to the survey revealed that many of the respondents believed they learned something new or gained insights from the retreats. Respondents expressed surprise about, 'the amount of persons infected with the disease in the country,' 'the rate of new infections among youth,' 'the age sex is being initiated—shows that we are at risk at an earlier age,' 'the damaging effects of labelling and stigmatization,' and 'the seriousness of our situation with respect to the continuing rate of infection.'

The majority of survey respondents said that to face challenges in implementing the campaign, they needed more resources, needed to engage stakeholders, and needed effective approaches to surmount people's prejudices. Respondents expressed concerns about, 'lack of support from teachers and their union leadership,' 'getting HIV-positive persons to become part of the action flow,' 'having individuals to accept and embrace the plan,' 'attitudes, political will, and lack of legislation,' and 'concerns of dealing with HIV infected persons in the work place.'

Survey respondents (including 75 per cent of all St Lucia respondents) also reported that testimonials from PLWHA at the retreat had a significant impact on them, as did presentations by local leaders. One respondent said, 'I realised that HIV positive persons can live a wholesome life, full of confidence and behaving as normal.' In terms of future actions to combat stigma and discrimination – a significant barrier – participants commented that they would like to involve PLWHA 'to be advocates for greater tolerance and caring – as spokespersons in our schools.' Another participant noted that, 'We would like to see more PLWHA be informed to participate in more workshops like these.'

KEY LEARNING AND RECOMMENDATIONS

Based on lessons learned from the implementation of the campaign, and to sustain the momentum created by this initiative, EDC/HHD recommends the following:

1. Replicate this campaign with ministries of education throughout the Caribbean region to assist senior-level decision-makers in all Caribbean countries to understand and address the impact of HIV and AIDS on schools, teachers, and society.

2. Institutionalise the messages in this campaign within the education sector by moving towards the development of HIV and AIDS policy, curriculum, services, and safe environments. Such actions will help countries reach the overarching Millennium Development Goal of reducing the incidence of HIV infection in young adults ages 15–24 in the Caribbean region.

3. Promote the engagement of HIV and AIDS leader/ advocates from within each country. During the development of this programme at the ministry of education retreats, almost all of the speakers at each retreat came from within the host country. Having already prepared and presented on the topic, each presenter can serve as an excellent resource to assist with disseminating the message to another audience or country. It is hoped

that the identified leaders will create a web of influential advocates who will commit to communicating the messages throughout the country and the region. It will be critical to promote the website, along with other ways of communication and exchange, as well as to support ongoing learning among the leaders. Such interaction and ongoing mentoring will enhance their confidence and skills, provide the needed energy and support for each other, and spark new ideas for advocacy and leadership activities to carry out.

4. Promote the participation of youth. Each country included the participation of a youth group. As these groups become more familiar with the message of a comprehensive approach, they can participate in various settings, such as schools, PTA meetings, and teacher professional development sessions.

5. Promote the greater involvement of PLWHA. At each of the retreats, a person living with HIV participated and presented. They spoke candidly and from the heart about their experience. Their participation was critical and seems to have had a profound impact on participants, possibly beginning a process of attitude change. However, in two of the three countries, the current social environment does not allow for PLWHA to speak publicly about their status. Perhaps this advocacy campaign in the education sector can contribute to changing that social norm as well.

6. Continue to strengthen the liaison between the National AIDS Coordinating Committee (NACC) and the ministry of education. At the start of the campaign, conversations revealed that NACC officials were very interested in increasing the organisation's collaboration with the ministry. During the development of the campaign, and the planning of the one-day ministry retreat, the NACC played an important role.

7. Enhance and support the capacity development of the HIV and AIDS managers in the ministries of education. In each of the countries in which EDC/HHD worked, the HIV and AIDS managers provided critical assistance by serving as point persons within the ministry. They took the lead in helping identify and invite participants for the retreat, and they participated in developing the one-day ministry retreat. It will be important to continue to support their professional development and to strengthen ways they can learn from and support each other.

REFLECTIONS

Education and HIV/ AIDS in the Caribbean presents a compelling argument for education sectors in the Caribbean region and around the world to rally around the development of a comprehensive approach to HIV. Initiatives that focus on promoting and protecting the health of students and staff have the power to mitigate the impact of HIV not just on the education system itself, but on the society as a whole. In the words of a participant in one of the ministry of education retreats, 'The problem of AIDS is everyone's business. Therefore a collaborative approach using difference agencies is needed.'

EDC/HHD and UNESCO believe strongly that the advocacy and leadership campaign will assist in developing a supportive environment for the efforts of the UNAIDS co-sponsors, including UNICEF, the World Health Organization (WHO)/Pan American

Health Organization (PAHO), ILO, the United Nations Development Programme (UNDP), and UNESCO. By gaining commitment from the leader/advocates, multiple audiences in various settings will hear the message of a comprehensive approach. Currently, the ministries of education are reviewing their draft plans and incorporating them into overall ministry efforts. In the coming years, EDC/HHD will continue to monitor the implementation of the campaign and to disseminate findings on the model's efficacy in affecting systemic changes related to HIV and AIDS policies and programmes.

SECTION 3

TOWARD POLICY AND CONCERTED ACTION

19

THE CARIBBEAN COMMUNITY DECLARATION ON EDUCATION, HIV AND AIDS

THE CARIBBEAN COMMUNITY

A special meeting of the Council for Human and Social Development (COHSOD) of the Caribbean Community was convened in Port of Spain, Trinidad & Tobago, June 9–10, 2006, with a focus on Education and HIV and AIDS. Senator Hazel Manning, Minister of Education, Trinidad & Tobago, chaired the special meeting, and her opening address set the agenda. At the conclusion, Ministers of Education made their first-ever declaration on the Education Sector's Response to HIV and AIDS. Several of the papers in this book were presented to Ministers. The Declaration is a benchmark document, and provides momentum for policy and concerted action.

OPENING ADDRESS: SPECIAL MEETING OF COHSOD

SENATOR HAZEL MANNING, MINISTER OF EDUCATION, TRINIDAD & TOBAGO

Colleague Ministers and Members of the Council of the Caribbean Community for Human and Social Development: The Nassau Declaration of 2001 was significant in that CARICOM Heads factored in, perhaps for the first time, the health of Caribbean people in relation to the potential of HIV/AIDS to deplete our human resource base and put the creation of wealth in our Region at risk.

In 2002 a commitment was made in Havana, Cuba to make *education* integral to the fight against HIV/AIDS. It was recognised that without the full involvement of the education sector, this disease would not and could not be overcome.

Today, I welcome all my CARICOM colleagues in education to this all important Special Meeting of the Council for Human and Social Development on Education and HIV/AIDS. This meeting is important because it brings together the education sector in the region to work on solutions to a common problem – one that threatens not only our quality of life but also our very existence.

As we join forces, reaching beyond our normal operational levels we search for a common thrust that will unite the education sector in the region and across disciplines, for the HIV/AIDS problem respects no boundaries. And so I welcome educational administrators and practitioners from early childhood care and development, through primary, secondary and tertiary levels as well as the adult education sector.

Over the past four years, the education sector in the region has received much technical and financial support from regional and international bodies to support various initiatives regarding HIV/AIDS. I welcome the representatives of many of these agencies who are with us today. The response of the education sector to HIV/AIDS must include commitment and support of many partners within our individual countries and across geographical and national borders. I welcome all our partners especially the Media who have a vital role to play in the fight against HIV/AIDS.

The education sector in the region is grappling with various programme initiatives to address the HIV/AIDS pandemic. However, we recognise that these responses have been inadequate to stop the unrelenting spread of HIV/AIDS in our region. The education sector in almost all our countries has developed programmes to address HIV/AIDS through (i) curriculum development, (ii) teacher training, (iii) materials development, (iv) guidance and counselling and even (v) aggressive awareness building campaigns.

Yet the epidemic remains a significant problem for us all. This tells us that we are dealing with a complex problem. One that is moving at a rapid pace and ravaging our people as recent data reveal that:-

1. The Caribbean has the second highest regional HIV prevalence rate in the world.
2. AIDS has become the leading cause of death among males and females ages 15–44 in the region.
3. If the current trend continues, close to one million people in the Caribbean will die of AIDS by the end of 2009
4. By 2009 there will be 243,000 new HIV infections and 334,600 new cases of AIDS in the Caribbean – a total of 577 persons infected with either HIV or AIDS - 3 per cent of whom will be children.

Here in Trinidad and Tobago there is an estimated adult HIV prevalence of 2.6 per cent. An estimated 27,000 persons were living with HIV at the end of 2005. We also know that 73% of infections occur among people between 15 and 49 years of age. AIDS remains a leading cause of death among young adults male and female. This is in keeping with regional and international trends.

With increased commitment by the Government and people of Trinidad and Tobago, and guided by a National Strategic Plan, we have made several strategic advances:-

• We now have a fully functional National AIDS Coordinating Committee in the Office of the Prime Minister.

• Cabinet has approved full-time Sector Coordinators for HIV in 8 key Government Ministries and Departments.

• We are seeing increased collaboration across all sectors in the fight against HIV, from:-

  o Trade Unions to NGOs
  o To the Private Sector
  o To Faith Based Organizations
  o To International Agencies
  o To support groups for persons living with HIV.

• We have been able to reduce mortality due to AIDS by 60% from peak levels.

• We have been able to reduce new cases of AIDS by 48% from peak levels, and

• We have seen a modest reduction in new HIV infections per year by 16% from 2003 to 2005.

Within the Ministry of Education, we have made a commitment to work relentlessly in a number of ways:-

1. We have developed a Strategic Plan for dealing with HIV/AIDS in the Ministry of Education.
2. Our Student Support Services Division

has a significant partnership with the National AIDS Coordinating Committee

3. We use Music, Drama and the Arts in the curriculum to build awareness in our schools and take the message to the wider community as demonstrated in the performances this morning.

4. We have an ongoing programme of teacher sensitisation and education as well as parent awareness on HIV/AIDS.

5. We have expanded our Student Support Services Division by 169% last year. Their work is already revealing the impact of all the social ills on the lives of students and highlighting the need for research.

The 2002 research study 'Children on the Brink' surveyed 41 countries around the world – 10 being Caribbean countries. Let me just single out one aspect of the research for our consideration. The study showed that by 2010, 313,000 children or 41% of the total number of children who lose parents in these 10 Caribbean countries will be orphaned because of AIDS. Our challenges are therefore varied and urgent.

Therefore I wish to highlight five challenges and raise a few questions:-

Our first challenge is to define a research agenda. Our seriousness about combating HIV/AIDS must be shown through our research agenda.

- Have we, individually or collectively, prioritised gaps in knowledge relating to the impact of, and response to, HIV and AIDS within the education sector?
- Do we know how many adults in the education sector have HIV/AIDS?
- Do we know whether they are receiving treatment?
- Have we reviewed the effectiveness of some of our prevention programmes to ensure quality, coverage, gender-sensitivity and comprehensiveness?
- Do we have an AIDS profile of our school system?
- Do we know how many of our children are living with AIDS? – or how many of our teachers are living with AIDS? Or how many children have parents living with AIDS? or dying from AIDS?
- Do we know the number of AIDS orphans in our schools? Or how cases of child abuse, street children and incarcerated youth intersect with being an AIDS orphan?
- Do we know how many of our students drop out because they are AIDS orphans? Or are likely to drop out or die from the disease? Or how many teachers are we likely to lose because of HIV/AIDS?
- Do we know how much of our investment in education is lost when we lose teachers and students to this disease? We need answers to questions such as these and we need them fast.

THE SECOND CHALLENGE IS TO DEVELOP AND MAINTAIN AN EFFECTIVE HIV AND AIDS MANAGEMENT STRUCTURE

Experience has shown that committees and part-time personnel are not effective enough to deal with the rapid and complex developments of the HIV/AIDS pandemic. If the education sector is to manage its response to HIV/AIDS while not losing sight of its core responsibilities, we need full time personnel and a budget committed to appropriately directing, monitoring and evaluating the education sector response. In Trinidad and Tobago, we have recognised this and so in the new school year, we will have a full-time coordinator for HIV/AIDS in our Ministry of Education.

THE THIRD CHALLENGE IS TO DEVELOP AN EDUCATION SECTOR POLICY ON HIV AND AIDS

Some territories like Jamaica and Haiti are already advanced in this area while others like Trinidad and Tobago, Guyana and the Bahamas are in the process of developing theirs.

The International Labour Organisation has completed an *'HIV/AIDS Workplace Policy for the Education Sector in the Caribbean'*, which is a useful resource for individual territories as we address their own policy issues and legislation especially where stigma and discrimination are concerned. In Trinidad and Tobago the Education Act prohibits all forms of discrimination against students and teachers. However in small societies we must use education to change attitudes so that stigma is reduced and eventually removed.

THE FOURTH CHALLENGE IS TO IMPLEMENT THE HEALTH AND FAMILY LIFE EDUCATION CURRICULUM

Thirteen Caribbean countries have an HFLE policy, but most use the HFLE Curriculum. For a long time aspects of health and family life education have formed part of the general school curriculum in the region. But by the late 1990s with the help of CARICOM there was a shift to a skill based HFLE Curriculum built around problem solving, critical thinking and decision making skills. The challenges however have been the training of teachers, the integration of this approach to HFLE into school curricula and the overall methodologies for the delivery of its concepts and modules. As Ministers of Education, with a mandate from CARICOM to create an ideal Caribbean citizen, we need to move with urgency to ensure that present and future generations benefit from a properly integrated and institutionalised Health and Family Life Education Curriculum in our school systems.

THE FIFTH CHALLENGE IS TO DEVELOP AN IMMEDIATE EDUCATION SECTOR RESPONSE TO THOSE CHILDREN INFECTED AND AFFECTED BY HIV AND AIDS

A comprehensive, co-ordinated approach that is research driven is needed to support our psycho social programmes for students affected by or infected with HIV/AIDS. The Education Sector needs to rapidly encourage persons and train Guidance Counsellors and Social Workers, as there is a significant lack of trained personnel in the region working in these much needed areas.

The Question is:- How do we do address these challenges?

We cannot do it in isolation. The collaboration effort cannot be over-emphasised. There is need for more effective organisation of partnerships locally, regionally and internationally. We need clarity as to who funds what so that we are better able to match response to need and make better use of the many opportunities for financial and technical assistance that exist.

The development of a comprehensive database of organisations that support education and HIV/AIDS is urgently needed, so too is networking across the region and the sharing of best practices. Therefore, I urge you to give your support to the recently formed *Network of Coordinators in HIV and AIDS in the Education Sector*, chaired by Belize, with Trinidad and Tobago as the Deputy Chair.

Colleagues, there is a lot of work before us. The challenges are many. The CSME heightens our awareness of a common labour force. Ours is the task to prepare future citizens for a life that is productive. We must, with haste, find common solutions to a disease that can destroy our capacity for economic growth.

Caribbean brothers and sisters, the education sector must make a difference over the next five years. We must be inclusive and relentless in our resolve. We must find ways during the course of this meeting to bring all sectors on board in a:-

- Sustained
- Comprehensive
- Research driven
- Evidence-based drive that puts this epidemic behind us.

Ladies and Gentlemen, we welcome you all on this historic weekend when our beloved Soca Warriors play their first World Cup match in Germany. We have made arrangements for you to share this wonderful moment with Trinidad and Tobago – the smallest Nation in the 2006 World Cup.

Let the symbolism of this moment be our beacon of hope in the fight against HIV/AIDS.

THE PORT-OF-SPAIN DECLARATION ON THE EDUCATION SECTOR'S RESPONSE TO HIV AND AIDS

MINISTERS OF EDUCATION OF THE CARIBBEAN COMMUNITY_

1. We, the Ministers of Education of the Caribbean Community, *along with* representatives of National AIDS Authorities, and other representatives of governments, organizations and agencies participating in the Special Meeting of the Council for Human and Social Development (COHSOD) on Education and HIV and AIDS in Port-of-Spain, Trinidad and Tobago 9–10 June 2006;

2. **Recall** that the Nassau Declaration asserts that the Health of the Region is the Wealth of the Region;

3. **Note with alarm** that we are facing an unprecedented human catastrophe and that a quarter century into the pandemic, HIV and AIDS continues to inflict immense suffering on the countries and communities of the Caribbean, that a total of 300,000 persons live with HIV in the region, including 30,000 who became infected in 2005, that the disease is the major cause of death in persons between 15–35; and that the prevalence rate in women 15–24 years is at least twice as high as men of similar age group;

4. **Recognise** that the extensive national, sub-regional and regional consultations under the joint collaboration of the Pan Caribbean Partnership Against HIV and AIDS (PANCAP) and UNAIDS were undertaken and resulted in recommendations and a roadmap for Universal Access to HIV and AIDS prevention, care, treatment and support (2006–2010);

5. **Also recognise** the political Declaration on Universal Access resulting from the High Level meeting of the United Nations General Assembly on HIV and AIDS, 2 June, 2006 as a basis for action;

6. **Affirm** that Education is a critical sector in the multi-sectoral response to HIV and emphasise our commitment *to achieving the targets set for Education for All and the relevant targets in the Millennium Development Goals;*

7. **Recognise** that comprehensive assessments of the impact of HIV on

the education sector at country and regional levels are urgently required to inform the development of appropriate response strategies, *and specifically those that focus on prevention;*

8. **Commit** to the development and implementation of national and regional sectoral policies on HIV and AIDS and Education and the integration of such policies into national and CARICOM/ *PANCAP* strategies;

9. **Commit** to the adoption of education workplace policies guided by the ILO Code of Practice on HIV and AIDS and the World of Work and the ILO/ UNESCO HIV and AIDS Workplace Policy for the Education Sector in the Caribbean;

10. **Pledge** to provide leadership for planning and implementation of national and regional sectoral responses and to facilitate accelerated access to resources from funds allocated for both education sector development and HIV and AIDS response;

11. **Commit to** the elimination of HIV-related stigma and discrimination in educational systems through leadership, policy, legislation, regulations and research, and in this regard, support the Champions for Change programme initiated by PANCAP;

12. **Affirm** the rights of people affected by and infected with HIV and promote their meaningful involvement in the education sector at all levels, including policy design and implementation;

13. **Request** the CARICOM Secretariat in collaboration with relevant stakeholders to develop a mechanism for accelerating implementation of GIPA principles in the regional response;

14. **Endorse** the development of professional and scholarly approaches to effective school health with urgent emphasis on HIV through training and research in selected regional institutions

15. **Commit** to professionalising the fields of HFLE, school health and sex education with attention to HIV and AIDS, to ensure timely, universal coverage and the development of career paths in those fields;

16. **Commit** to extending and deepening the coverage and professional development of educators to implement HFLE and HIV and AIDS education programmes;

17. **Endorse** the establishment and support development of the Caribbean Network of HIV Coordinators in the education sector as a CARICOM-led regional resource;

18. **Request** the Network of HIV Coordinators to develop a model for partnership between Ministries of Education and national organisations of PLWHA, consistent with the GIPA principles;

19. **Request the PANCAP** to develop a regional strategic framework for the education sector response in the overall regional response to HIV and AIDS;

20. **Request the CARICOM Secretariat** to establish a network and consultative mechanism among development partners to increase efficiency and effectiveness of their contribution to the regional and national strategic plans for HIV and AIDS and education, and to collaborate in the development of policies and the sharing of information and knowledge;

21. **Agree** to the inclusion of the education sector in the priorities identified in

the review of the Caribbean Regional Strategic Framework for HIV and AIDS to be undertaken by PANCAP in 2006, recognizing that the education sector response to HIV and AIDS also provides an opportunity to address other significant health and life style issues, with special emphasis on prevention;

22. **Agree to engage with CAPNET** to develop national and regional publishing projects to ensure provision of quality and culturally sensitive instructional materials to support universal coverage of HIV and AIDS education and to infuse HIV and AIDS principles into new instructional materials;

23. **Recognise** the importance of mainstreaming gender in all materials and methodologies used to address education with regard to HIV and AIDS

24. **Recommend that Ministers of Education** continue to advocate for appropriate attention to HIV and AIDS issues and keep the HIV and AIDS high on the agendas of COHSOD and national parliaments;

25. **Also call on all stakeholders** to advocate for, and contribute to the mobilization of resources in support of the national and regional programmes that would advance the role of education in the accelerated approach to HIV and AIDS;

26. **Request the Chair of COHSOD** to ensure that the issues related to Education and HIV and AIDS are brought to the attention of Heads of Government for their endorsement and support;

27. **Recommend** that targets established in the Regional and National Strategic plans for Education and HIV and AIDS be aligned with those established by the national, sub-regional and regional consultations for HIV and AIDS prevention, care, treatment and support and the UNGASS targets for 2006–2010;

28. **Ensure** access to educational opportunities at all levels for children in vulnerable settings and conditions with emphasis on those affected or infected by HIV and AIDS;

29. **Request** of the Caribbean Examinations Council that all appropriate syllabuses and assessment procedures for the three levels of secondary examination be urgently reviewed to ensure that knowledge and skills that will contribute to the education sector response to HIV and AIDS are included.

20

AN HIV/AIDS WORKPLACE POLICY FOR THE EDUCATION SECTOR IN THE CARIBBEAN

INTERNATIONAL LABOUR ORGANIZATION AND THE UNITED NATIONS EDUCATION, SCIENTIFIC AND CULTURAL ORGANIZATION

Education institutions and services play a vital role in teaching employees and students about HIV and AIDS, shaping attitudes to HIV, AIDS and people living with HIV, and building skills for reducing risk of HIV, promoting care and opposing stigmatization. Infection rates are increasing in the Caribbean region - prevalence rates are the second highest among regions worldwide. The education sector must take account of the fact that people who are HIV-positive can remain capable of normal work for many years. It is therefore critical for education services and institutions as workplaces to adopt and implement a policy, or, where such a policy already exists in the education sector or as a national workplace policy, to adapt it for use in education workplaces based on the principles and concepts of the present text. Either approach would enhance the education sector response in ways that protect the rights of all employees or students, prevent further HIV infection, and create a caring, safe and supportive learning environment. The ILO UNESCO Policy reproduced in this chapter is a model for Caribbean countries. Printed copies of the policy are available from the Caribbean regional offices of ILO and UNESCO, located in Port of Spain and Kingston respectively.

1. INTRODUCTION

This policy is based on the *ILO code of practice on HIV/AIDS and the world of work* (hereafter, 'the ILO code of practice'), adopted by an international tripartite meeting convened by the ILO in 2001, and includes key concepts and principles of the ILO code of practice. Development of the policy has resulted from collaboration between ILO and UNESCO.

The policy was carefully reviewed and modified by representatives of Ministries of Education and Labour, teacher trade unions, private employers and National AIDS Councils/Commissions from five Caribbean countries[1] during a tripartite workshop held in Kingston, Jamaica, 28–30 September 2005.

2. PURPOSE

The purpose of this policy is to provide a framework for addressing HIV and AIDS as a workplace issue in education sector institutions and services through social dialogue processes, in complement of other national workplace or overall education sector policies where they exist. It covers the following key areas of action:

- prevention of HIV,
- elimination of stigma and discrimination on the basis of real or perceived HIV status,
- care, treatment and support of staff and students who are infected and/or affected by HIV and AIDS,

- management and mitigation of the impact of HIV/AIDS in education institutions, and
- safe, healthy and non-violent work and study environments.

3. GLOSSARY OF TERMS

Administrator: Principal, Vice Principal, Dean or other officer who plays a managerial role at the education institution or services.

AIDS: the Acquired Immune Deficiency Syndrome, is a range of medical conditions that occurs when a person's immune system is seriously weakened by infection with the Human Immunodeficiency Virus (HIV). HIV injures cells in the immune system. This impairs the body's ability to fight the disease. People living with AIDS are susceptible to a wide range of unusual and potential life-threatening diseases and infections.

Antiretrovirals: drugs used to kill or inhibit the multiplication of retroviruses such as HIV.

Board: the governing authority of an education institution, public or private.

Community: local institutions outside the education institution which provide leadership or support on social, economic and political issues relevant to citizens, such as private employers or business, non-governmental social welfare organizations, health care providers, FBOs, cultural institutions, etc.

Decent work: an ILO concept covering the minimum desired content of jobs and occupations, which includes respect for fundamental principles and rights at work and international labour standards, employment and income opportunities for workers, social protection and social security, and social dialogue and tripartism at work.

Discrimination: any distinction, exclusion or preference made on the basis of HIV status or perceived HIV status. Discrimination consists of actions or omissions that are derived from stigma and directed towards those individuals who are stigmatized. Discrimination is action, which has the effect of nullifying or impairing equality of opportunity or treatment in employment or occupation, in accordance with the definition and principles of the ILO Discrimination (Employment and Occupation) Convention, 1958 (no. 111), and is understood to include for reasons of sexual orientation.

Education institution: the establishment or setting where the learning, whether formal or non-formal, takes place. For purposes of this policy, education institutions include pre-primary, primary and secondary schools, post-secondary vocational/technical training, further and higher education institutions, and places of adult and non-formal education.

Education service(s): other components of a nation's education and training system, public or private, other than an education institution.

Employee: an administrator, teacher or non-teaching support staff employed in an education institution or services.

Employees' representatives: in accordance with the ILO Workers' Representatives Convention, 1971 (No. 135), persons recognized as such by national law or practice whether they are: (a) trade union representatives, namely, representatives designated or elected by trade unions or by members of such unions; or (b) elected representatives, namely, representatives who are freely elected by the workers of the undertaking in accordance with provisions of national laws or regulations or of collective agreements and whose functions do not include activities which are recognized as the exclusive prerogative of trade unions in the country concerned.[2] For purposes of this policy, "undertaking" is understood to mean "education institution".

HIV: the Human Immunodeficiency Virus, a virus that infects cells of the human immune system, and destroys or impairs their function.

Legal age: the age at which an individual is considered a major and legally responsible for decisions according as defined by a country's legislation.

Non-teaching staff: a person engaged in support functions other than management or teaching in an education institution or service.

Parent: the biological and adoptive parents or custodians, or legal guardians of children.

Peer educator or counsellor: the trained employee or student who develops or implements a developmental counselling programme to meet the social, psychosocial and educational or training needs of employees or students in relation to HIV and AIDS.

Physician: a medical doctor licensed in accordance with the regulations of the State or other competent health licensing authority.

Post-exposure prophylaxis (PEP): measures to be instituted after possible accidental exposure to HIV infection.

Reasonable accommodation: any modification or adjustment to a job or to the workplace that is reasonable, practicable and will enable a person living with HIV or AIDS to have access to or participate or advance in employment.[3]

Screening: measures to assess HIV status, whether direct (HIV testing) or indirect (assessment of risk-taking behaviour), asking questions about health or about medication used in this policy in the context of exclusion from employment or education.

Sex and gender: there are both biological and social differences between males and females. The term 'sex' refers to biologically determined differences, while the term 'gender' refers to differences in social roles and relations between males and females. Gender roles are learned through socialization and vary widely within and between cultures. Gender roles are affected by age, class, race, ethnicity and religion, and by the geographical, economic and political environment.[4]

Sharps: objects such as a needle or other instruments used in health care that are able to penetrate the skin and potentially cause infection.

STI: sexually transmitted infections, which include, among others, syphilis, chancroid, chlamydia, gonorrhoea. They include conditions commonly known as sexually transmitted diseases (STDs).[5]

Social dialogue: any form of information sharing, consultation or negotiation (with or without formal agreements concluded) between educational authorities, public and private, and employees or their representatives (i.e., workers' representatives as defined below). In the context of this policy social dialogue is applied to students and other stakeholders.

Social protection: social protection corresponds to a set of tools, instruments, policies which aim at ensuring that men and women enjoy safe and decent working conditions. Social protection therefore covers income security, health and safety at work and the environment, conditions of work and family issues, pensions and retirement.

Stigma: a dynamic process of devaluation that significantly discredits an individual in the viewpoints of others.

Student: a person attending formal or non-formal classes or pursuing studies at a school, training institution, college, university, or any other education institution.

Teacher: a person engaged part-time or full-time in education of students, formal or non-formal.

Termination of employment: dismissal at the initiative of the employer.[6]

Universal precautions: a simple standard of infection control practice to be used to minimize the risk of blood-borne pathogens.[7]

Violence, verbal or physical: Any action, incident or behaviour that departs from reasonable conduct in which a person is assaulted, threatened, harmed, injured in the course of, or as a direct result of, his or her work.

4. APPLICATION AND SCOPE

This policy should be used as the basis for a national policy for the education sector and as the basis of policy for individual education and training institutions at all levels: early childhood, primary, secondary, tertiary, technical/vocational and adult education, except as otherwise stated in this policy.

5. PROCESS, AVAILABILITY AND REVIEW OF POLICY

5.1 Social dialogue

In accordance with the key principles set out in section 6 of this Policy, its provisions have been decided in consultation or negotiation, as appropriate, between the public education authorities as public employers, or private education employers, and worker representatives acting on behalf of employees. This Policy, resulting from such agreement, has been established in accordance with national law or practice and education service provisions for information sharing, consultation or negotiation between employers and employees and their representatives, as well as relevant HIV/AIDS policies.

In view of its importance within education institutions, agreement on this Policy, its application and its revision should involve representatives of students and parents or the community in the most appropriate manner.

The education institution should appoint an HIV/AIDS coordinator and where practicable establish an HIV/AIDS committee, as appropriate to its size and resources, in order to help apply and monitor this Policy. A committee should be composed of at least one representative each of the management, teachers, other employees, students, parents and a community-based HIV/AIDS association. The committee or coordinator should:

- be responsible for promoting the HIV/AIDS policy in the institution
- support the implementation of the education programme
- access and develop resources and partnerships for assistance and support
- work with parents and the wider community to disseminate information about HIV and AIDS and combat HIV- and AIDS-related stigma and discrimination
- adhere strictly to the confidentiality issues of this policy (see Article 11);
- help evaluate the objectives, processes and outcomes of the HIV/AIDS programme.

5.2 Availability of Policy

A copy of this Policy is to be kept on display in the institution and made available to all employees and students for reading and for reproduction. All forms of communication normally used in the institution – for example, posters, circulars to employees, staff meetings, notice boards, student body meetings, institution assemblies and electronic mail – should be used to make the Policy known and help ensure its application.

5.3 Review of Policy

This Policy should be reviewed regularly to take account of new developments in medical information or experience in the management and care of HIV and AIDS in educational institutions. The results of such reviews and changes in the Policy will be made known on the same basis as set out section 5.2 above.

The management should provide opportunities at staff meetings, Parent-Teacher Association meetings, institutional assemblies or other meetings as appropriate to discuss the policies and the effectiveness of their application.

6. KEY PRINCIPLES

The adoption of this policy implies commitment to the following key principles.

6.1 Recognition of HIV and AIDS as an issue affecting the education sector

HIV/AIDS is an issue for all education institutions, not only because the virus affects employees and students, but also because the education institution can play a vital role in limiting the spread and effects of the infection.

6.2 Non-discrimination and reduction of stigma

In the interests of decent work and respect for human rights, there should be no discrimination against an employee or student who has, is perceived to have, or who is affected by HIV/AIDS. Discrimination and stigmatization inhibit efforts for prevention, care, treatment and support.

6.3 Gender equality

HIV and AIDS impact on male and female employees and students differently, and women and girls are often more adversely affected by the epidemic, due to physiological, socio-cultural and economic reasons. Women and girls may also be more vulnerable due to unequal gender relations, in particular when faced with sexual harassment by the more influential males in the educational setting. Any discrimination and/or action that may put an employee or student of any sex at risk of HIV because of their sex strictly violates the basic principles of this policy. Education programmes should address the roles and responsibilities of men and boys in promoting gender equality as well as the rights of women and girls. Application of this policy is designed to take account of these unequal gender relations and enable all employees and students to successfully avoid risks, the spread of HIV infection and to cope with the impact of HIV and AIDS.

6.4 Supportive and caring environment

The employee or student who has contracted HIV needs compassion, care, treatment and support. There should be no discrimination against employees or their families in access to affordable health services and statutory or occupational benefits. There should be no discrimination against students with respect to the normal health benefits accessed and enjoyed by other students. Education institutions should set up programmes of care and support that guarantee access to treatment, and provide for reasonable accommodation, provision of or referral to counselling and healthy living information, notably HFLE.

6.5 Healthy work environment

The teaching/learning and work environment should be healthy and safe, so far as is practicable, for all concerned parties in order to reduce risk of HIV infection and transmission. While there is no risk of HIV transmission through normal casual contact, universal precautions should be applied to avoid transmission in the event of accidents, and risks reduced or eliminated.

6.6 Screening for purposes of exclusion from employment or studies

HIV screening should not be required of job applicants, students who wish to enrol, or current employees or students. Testing for HIV should not be carried out at the education institution except as specified in section 11 of this policy.

6.7 Continuation of employment relationship

HIV infection is not a cause for the termination, suspension, involuntary transfer or denial of career advancement of an employee or the expulsion or suspension of a student. Persons living with HIV-related illnesses should be able to work or study for as long as medically fit in appropriate work or studies.

6.8 Confidentiality

All personal medical information, whether oral, written, or in electronic format, obtained from an individual or third parties will be treated as confidential. No employee, student, or parent on behalf of the student, is compelled to disclose HIV status to authorities at the education institution.[8]

6.9 Prevention

HIV infection is preventable through information, education, and the creation of a climate that gives assistance and encouragement to all individuals in assessing and reducing their risk to HIV. Education institutions should set up programmes to provide information and behaviour change communication, promote voluntary (and confidential) testing with counselling (VCT), and provide practical means of prevention, including access to condoms, disposable syringes, etc.

6.10 Social dialogue

A successful HIV/AIDS policy and programme requires cooperation, trust and dialogue between government officials, the board of the education institution, administrators, employees, students, and parents.

7. RIGHTS AND RESPONSIBILITIES

7.1 Respect for rights

The rights of all members of education institutions must be respected. Education authorities, the board, administrators, teachers and other employees and their representatives, students and their representatives and parents of students in the institution are expected to respect the rights of all members of the education institution, regardless of their actual or perceived HIV status.

7.2 Public education authorities

The public education authorities should monitor and evaluate the implementation of this policy in all education institutions, and assist institutions with capacity building, training and implementation of the Policy.

The public education authorities should provide all institutions access to items necessary for implementation of universal precautions.

7.3 The institution board

The board of the education institution where applicable should ensure that the institution develops a policy on HIV/AIDS - based on the principles set out in section 6, that the process includes consultation between the representatives of managers, employees, students and parents, and that appropriate measures are taken for its implementation, including making it known to all staff and students. The board is expected to promote an educational climate that protects the rights of every student and employee living with or affected by HIV and AIDS.

7.4   Administrators

The administrators or management should:

- Advise the board of the implications of HIV and AIDS for the institution, and, in accordance with the social dialogue provisions of this Policy (Chapter 5), develop successful strategies to reduce stigmatization and eliminate discrimination against those infected and/or affected by HIV and AIDS, prevent the spread and mitigate the effects of HIV in the institution, and create a supportive and caring environment for employees and students;
- Take the necessary steps to develop, through social dialogue, a policy on HIV/AIDS, a plan for its implementation and a programme for prevention and care;
- Agree on the appointment of an HIV/AIDS focal point or committee (in larger institutions), in consultation with the representatives of the employees and the students, in accordance with section 5 of this Policy;
- Ensure a safe and healthy work and study environment, including the application of universal precautions as part of first aid provisions.

7.5 Teachers

Teachers are expected to adhere to the policy and support its implementation. They are responsible for the provision of accurate and up-to-date information on HIV and AIDS, the promotion of caring and supportive relationships between students - especially where some are living with HIV, and the provision of pastoral and professional care and support to orphans and other children in the institution affected by HIV/AIDS, in accordance with the agreed programme and subject to adequate training and working time provided for these responsibilities.

7.6 Employee and student representatives

Representatives of employees and (where they exist) representatives of student bodies have a responsibility to protect those they represent from any form of discrimination related to HIV status, and to help implement the institution's HIV/AIDS policy and programme by monitoring and promoting the information, education, health and safety and other practices and provisions set out in the Policy.

8. EMPLOYEE-STUDENT RELATIONSHIPS

All education institutions must develop and adhere to a code of conduct that contains clear guidelines for staff/student interactions and relationships, and is consistent with the provisions of 10.2 of this Policy.

The underlying principles must be:

- mutual respect and trust;
- cognisance of unequal positions of authority and the increased risk or vulnerability to HIV;
- adherence to the principles of the

International Convention on the Rights of Child.

9. PREVENTION: EDUCATION, INFORMATION AND TRAINING

A single presentation about HIV and AIDS is insufficient to ensure that employees and students develop the complex understanding and skills needed to cope with or avoid infection through the necessary risk-reducing behavioural changes. It is therefore essential that the education institution allocate sufficient time within the work hours and the curriculum to assist employees and students to gain the knowledge and skills needed to prevent HIV, and if infected, to live with HIV in a safe, secure and supportive working and learning environment. The HIV/AIDS education programme should be sensitive to cultural, developmental and socio-economic contexts, gender sensitive, involve people living with HIV if possible, form part of an integrated Health and Family Life Education (HFLE) programme and fit within an education sector conceptual framework for dealing with HIV/AIDS. It will require a coordinator and a cadre of peer educators/counsellors. Where possible, the HIV/AIDS education programmes should also be extended to parents of students.

9.1 Peer educators

The institution should identify, train and support at least two groups of HIV/AIDS peer educators: (i) for employees and (ii) for students. Peer educators should receive training in accordance with their roles and responsibilities in this Policy and reasonable release time from other duties so as to carry out their responsibilities.

The following are broad principles for HIV-related education/counselling:

- The peer educator is well acquainted with the following information: how the transmission of HIV occurs and may be prevented; the attitudes and behaviour choices that put people at risk for HIV; universal precautions; accurate information that dispels myths and combats AIDS-related stigma and discrimination; and services and benefits available within the institution or the community generally that enable employees and students to cope with HIV and AIDS, including V(C)CT and other forms of support, among which, means of risk reduction such as condoms. The educator should be knowledgeable and available to provide information, and counselling if trained to do so, for anyone concerned with or affected by HIV and AIDS;
- Counselling (where appropriate) is offered in a private and confidential setting, with sufficient time available and by a trained professional;
- The peer educators support but are not solely responsible for the implementation of the institution's HIV/AIDS education programme.

9.2 Employees

All employees will be given the opportunity to participate during working time in a planned HIV/AIDS education programme that addresses their concerns concerning coping strategies with regard to risk, as well as care, treatment and support, and:

- provides factual and current information on HIV transmission and prevention
- helps employees assess their own risk and understand means of prevention and universal precautions
- provides guidance on behaviour change

- assists staff to maintain productive, non-discriminatory and stigma-free staff, student, parent and community relations
- informs employees on rights and benefits of care, treatment and support provided in the institution or education service as well as in the local community environment
- includes means for monitoring, evaluation and annual review sessions
- is part of required, ongoing professional development at all levels
- is the subject of consultations or negotiation between employers and employees and their representatives, and appropriate government and other stakeholders, in accordance with the social dialogue provisions in section 5 of this Policy.

The content will include, but will not be necessarily limited to, the elements listed in Appendix 2.

9.3 Students

All students in education institutions should have access to HIV/AIDS education programmes. The goals of HIV/AIDS education are to promote healthy living, provide a supportive and caring environment to those affected by HIV and AIDS, and discourage behaviours that place students at risk for HIV infection. The education programme for students will:

- be appropriate to student's developmental levels
- be gender responsive and in accordance with universal human rights
- annually build upon knowledge and skills developed previously
- use instructional methods known to be effective, participatory and culturally appropriate
- promote an understanding of basic human

biology (including reproductive health and risks involved with drug use) and ARV treatment
- develop supportive attitudes towards those infected with and/or affected by HIV and work against stigma and discrimination
- stress the benefits of abstinence and safe sex, including the use of condoms, and faithfulness to one partner, and avoidance of drug and alcohol abuse
- address students' own concerns
- include means for monitoring and evaluation
- be an integral part of a coordinated education institution HFLE or comparable programme
- provide information on health care, counselling and support services within and outside the education institution, notably from other education stakeholders, including FBOs
- be taught by well-prepared instructors with adequate support
- be sensitive to the psycho-social environment in which the learner lives and the context of their home life
- involve parents and families as partners in education.

The programme for students will include culturally sensitive, gender responsive and developmentally appropriate information on (though not limited to) the elements listed in Appendix 2.

9.4 Parents

Parents will be given opportunities to preview HIV/AIDS programme prevention curricula and materials, and be provided with opportunities to discuss HIV infection issues with administrators, teachers, counsellors and peer educators.

10. PREVENTION: A SUPPORTIVE, SAFE AND HEALTHY WORK ENVIRONMENT

The environment at the education institution should be safe in order to prevent the transmission of HIV and be supportive to those living with or affected by HIV and AIDS. Every education institution should also foster and maintain a social climate wherein health, well-being, non-violence and safety are an important part of everyday work and learning.

10.1 Non-violence

Administrators and other employees (teaching and non-teaching staff) will make all reasonable attempts to maintain an environment free of violence and intimidation. No administrator, teaching or non-teaching staff employee or student should engage in or tolerate the physical or verbal abuse of persons living with HIV, a person associated with someone living with HIV, or a person perceived as living with HIV. Incidents of such behaviour should be subject to the rules governing behaviour at the education institution, contractual obligations of employees, and national law, and should be handled in accordance with sections 5 and 13 of this Policy with a view to improving respect for these provisions.

10.2 A Code of conduct

A Code of conduct consistent with the provisions of Chapter 8 of this Policy should be developed for employees and students by means of social dialogue mechanisms, which addresses ethical behaviour at the education institution, including the unacceptability of behaviour that discriminates against students on any basis, including HIV/AIDS.

10.3 First Aid

First Aid kits and necessary protective equipment (for example latex and heavy-duty gloves) should be available for emergency use and for routine protection against the risk of HIV transmission at the education institution at all times according to universal standards. All employees and students, especially physical education instructors and technical/vocational education teachers, must complete an approved first aid and injury prevention course that includes implementation of infection control guidelines (see Appendix 3 on universal precautions).

10.4 Exposure to blood

Administrators, other employees and students will follow universal precautions, as described in Appendix 3, in order to avoid accidental exposure to blood or body fluids. The institution must also have a post-exposure prophylaxis (PEP) procedure in place, including counselling and guidance for the employee or student and access to antiretroviral treatment (ART). A checklist for such a procedure applied in health services and of relevance to education sector workplaces is provided in Appendix 4.

10.5 Management of sharp instruments

Where sharp instruments must be used for work or educational purposes, use of these items should be carefully monitored and controlled. The administrators are responsible for ensuring that there is no unauthorized or unsupervised use of sharps, and that any found on institution property are removed and safely stored. Guidelines are provided in Appendix 4.

10.6   Employees and students with open wounds

Any wound that is bleeding or discharging should be kept covered. Any employee or students with wounds which cannot be covered will, as a precaution, be asked to stay away from the education institution until the wound has been healed or may be covered, unless the education institution receives a certificate from a physician that states that the employee or student does not pose a risk and may return to the institution.

10.7.   Hygiene

Education institutions should promote and implement rigorous procedures relating to hygiene and school health in accordance with national or international norms.[9]

10.8   Practical measures to support risk reduction

In addition to education, information and training on risk reduction in accordance with section 9 of this policy, latex condoms will be available at the education institutions free or at affordable prices to employees, or information provided on how to obtain them through local health providers. Risk reduction measures in relation to students will be determined in collaboration with parents, guardians and students of legal age in accordance with the social dialogue provisions of this Policy (Chapter 5).

11. TESTING, CONFIDENTIALITY AND DISCLOSURE

11.1   Testing and medical advice

The education institution will not engage in the mandatory testing for HIV of employees or students as a condition for employment or admission, for continued employment or enrolment, or for purposes of work assignments, benefits or educational activities. Routine fitness testing related to employment or educational activities will not include HIV testing.

Employees or students who wish to be tested as part of voluntary testing or 'Know your status' programmes should be provided with information on where to do so and on what the procedures entail. Such testing should normally be carried out by community health services and not in the education institution. If such programmes are organized by health services within the institution, testing should only be carried out at the request of and with the written consent of the employee or student (or parent or guardian on their behalf as appropriate), be performed by suitably qualified health personnel, adhere to strict confidentiality and disclosure requirements (as set out in this Policy), and be accompanied by gender-sensitive pre- and post-test counselling on the nature and purpose of the test, and on post-test options and services whether the result is positive or negative.

11.2   Ensuring confidentiality

All health records, notes, and other documents that make reference to an employee or student living with HIV, including those with AIDS, should be kept confidentially in a secure place accessible only in accordance with provisions of the International Labour Organisation code of practice on the protection of workers' personal data (Appendix 5). Only those persons who have received written permission from the employee, student, parent or emergency medical personnel may have access to those records. Information regarding HIV status will not be added to a student's permanent educational record.

Confidentiality should also be assured

by providing a private environment for personal interviews, and by working out arrangements for care and support with the person concerned.

Medical certificates do not have to specify an employee or student's HIV status.

11.3   Disclosure

Disclosure should always be voluntary; if information on the HIV status of an employee or student needs to be communicated by anyone other than the person concerned it should be only on the basis of their written consent. Procedures should be established to ensure confidentiality on HIV status in the institution based on the social dialogue processes set out in section 5 of the Policy, and in accordance with national laws and education service regulations. Breaches of confidentiality will be the subject of sanctions in accordance with Chapter 13.

12. EMPLOYMENT, CARE, TREATMENT AND SUPPORT

12.1   Recruitment and admission

HIV infection should not be taken into consideration as part of the employment or admission procedure or decision for any individual applying to the education institution for work or studies.

12.2   Employee rights, careers and right to study

a)   Employees

Employees living with HIV should not be discriminated against in decisions concerning their job security or tenure, renewal of fixed term contracts, opportunities for professional development or promotion. They may, however, be transferred from work positions that have been determined by their physician to be too strenuous for their condition [see

provisions for reasonable accommodation, Section 12.4] or where specific duties may carry a risk of infection to the employee or to others. Such transfers should occur in consultation with the employee living with HIV, in accordance with the principles of social dialogue of this policy, and may be subject to the grievance procedure provisions of the Policy (Chapter 13).

b)   Students

Administrators and teachers should follow established policies and procedures for students with chronic health problems. HIV or AIDS are not causes for denial of normal study opportunities or segregation in the education institution. Administrators and teachers, following consultations with the student and where not of legal age, parent as defined by this policy, must consult with and obtain the consent of the student's physician before the transfer or removal of a student from normal institutional activities. If a student becomes incapacitated and unable to follow normal education coursework, the education institution should apply the principles of reasonable accommodation to ease their workload as would be the case for any major illness, disability or incapacity, including - if possible and in cooperation with the education services and HIV/AIDS support networks in the community - making home study available to them.

12.3   Care and treatment

The education institution should facilitate access to medical services and healthy living programmes, including condom provision and ARVs, treatment to relieve HIV-related symptoms and common opportunistic infections, nutritional advice and supplements, and stress reduction measures. This may take the form of provision of such services, where possible, or referral to services in the community.

12.4 Statutory benefits and reasonable accommodation

Employees living with HIV and AIDS should enjoy the same social protection, including social security benefits under national law, education service regulations or education institution provisions, as employees with other chronic or serious illnesses. In accordance with national education service regulations, the education institution, or the human resource department of the education service if more appropriate, should also examine the sustainability of new benefits packages addressing the specific nature of HIV infection and AIDS as part of its human resource strategy.

Measures should be taken to reasonably accommodate employees with severe ARV side effects or AIDS-related illnesses to enable them to continue working as long as possible. Needs should be established by the administration of the education institution, or the human resource department of the education service if more appropriate, on a case-by-case basis, in consultation with the physician of the individual concerned. Reasonable accommodation may include: rearrangement of working hours; modified tasks or jobs; adapted work equipment; provision of rest periods; part-time or other flexible work arrangements; and leave provisions.

Employees living with HIV, including those with AIDS, may request sick leave without pay to have the appropriate medical care or recuperate from symptoms of their medical condition, in accordance with the relevant labour laws of the specific Caribbean country.

12.5 Employee, student and family assistance programmes

To reduce the impact of HIV and AIDS on work and study, education institutions should consult with representatives of employees and students to establish or extend employee, student and family services, in cooperation with education authorities at other levels and/ or community-based organizations. Services may include: compassionate leave; referrals to support groups or to tutorial programmes for students; financial counselling, including advice on social security and other forms of financial support; and legal information and assistance. [See also section 9 of the *ILO Code of practice on HIV/AIDS and the world of work*].

Special attention should be paid to the needs of employees and students who assume a relatively larger burden for care of HIV-positive relatives, to employees of both sexes who are single parents and affected by HIV and AIDS, and to students who are orphans and/or vulnerable in other ways.

13. DISCIPLINARY PROCEDURES AND GRIEVANCE RESOLUTION

The procedures for discipline and grievance-resolution for employees in relation to HIV/AIDS should be carried out in accordance with the relevant legislation (criminal, discrimination and labour acts), institutional policy and regulations, and negotiated/collective bargaining agreements of [*insert name of relevant country*]. Complainants may have recourse to normal appeal procedures related to unfair dismissal, denial or unjustified restriction of employment or work related rights and benefits, and may refer in this regard to the provisions and related jurisprudence of the ILO Discrimination (Employment and Occupation) Convention, 1958 (No. 111). Similarly, the disciplinary procedures for students should be in line with the regulations of the education service.

13.1 Refusal to work or study with an individual living with HIV

There is no justification for refusing to work, study or be present in the education institution with HIV-positive individuals, since HIV cannot be transmitted through casual contact in a classroom or other learning environment. Employees or students who are not prepared to work or engage in learning activities with an HIV-positive individual will be offered education and counselling by the institution or from the community – major/ key stakeholders in the school/education institutions, e.g., denominational boards, school boards, civic organizations, private sector – or education service.

If after counselling, the individual refuses to carry out contractual duties or to participate in the learning programmes of the education institution with HIV-positive employees or students, the education institution's disciplinary procedures concerning refusal to work or study should be followed.

Where discrimination occurs in the form of physical or verbal abuse, the employee or student who has experienced any form of discrimination will have recourse to existing mechanisms for redress, including regulations governing physical attacks and bullying. The appropriate representative of the Committee or Coordinator should be informed to ensure that proper measures are taken.

13.2 Violation of medical confidentiality

Employees or students who acquire personal information about the real or perceived HIV status of other employees or students must not disclose such information unless the person concerned has given her/his written consent. In accordance with section11 of this Policy, the violation of medical privacy may be the cause for disciplinary action to be taken against an administrator, teacher, other employee, or student.

APPENDIX 1:
EXAMPLES OF DISCRIMINATION AGAINST EMPLOYEES AND STUDENTS BASED ON ACTUAL OR PERCEIVED HIV STATUS

Discriminatory Action	Against Whom
Denial of employment	Employee (candidate)
Dismissal	Employee
Denial of promotion opportunities	Employee
Not given access to employee benefits	Employee
Not given access to professional development or work-related social activities	Employee
Compulsory transfer from a job function in which the person with HIV does not pose any form of medical threat to other employees "is not incapable of performing work to a reasonable standard, and is not afforded reasonable accommodation in an alternative work assignment"	Employee
Denial of admission to study	Student (candidate)
Expulsion, suspension, denial of student privileges	Student
Not given the opportunity to advance to the next grade/level	Student
Not given the opportunity to engage in social activities sponsored by the education institution	Employee and student
Breach of privacy or confidentiality	Employee and student
Not receiving protection from physical and verbal abuse	Employee and student

APPENDIX 2:
RECOMMENDED CONTENT FOR EMPLOYEE AND STUDENT EDUCATION PROGRAMMES

EMPLOYEES

- The HIV epidemic, how HIV is contracted and prevented, what is AIDS, risk assessment and reduction, including reference to other STIs, available ARV treatment medication
- Differences in risk between men and women, unequal power relations in education institutions - particularly affecting girls and young women, and rights and responsibilities of both men and women
- How to communicate with other employees and students about HIV and AIDS
- How to communicate with other employees and students living with HIV
- How to communicate with parents, guardians and other relatives of students living with HIV
- How to dispel myths relating to HIV and AIDS and avoid discriminatory practices and stigmatisation of those living with HIV
- Basic occupational health and safety and first aid procedures, the application of universal precautions, and strategies on creation of a safe, enabling environment
- How to cope with an HIV-positive diagnosis, healthy living (wellness) management programmes, rights, care, treatment and support benefits and responsibilities arising from HIV infection

or diagnosis, including continuing means of preventing transmission.

STUDENTS

• Accurate and up-to-date information about HIV and AIDS (transmission, prevention (including abstinence), care, treatment, support)
• The links between HIV, AIDS and other STIs
• The rights of persons living with HIV/AIDS
• How to support fellow students living with HIV and other illnesses
• How to live a healthy life through an HFLE or comparable programme
• Basic first aid procedures and the use of universal precautions
• How to cope, lead a healthy life, receive treatment and support if living with and/or affected by HIV.

APPENDIX 3:
UNIVERSAL PRECAUTIONS AND CHECKLIST OF PRECAUTIONS TO PREVENT HIV TRANSMISSION

UNIVERSAL PRECAUTIONS (EXTRACT FROM THE ILO CODE OF PRACTICE, APPENDIX II)

A. Universal blood and body fluid precautions

Universal blood and body-fluid precautions (known as "Universal Precautions" or "Standard Precautions") were originally devised by the United States Centers for Disease Control and Prevention (CDC) in 1985, largely due to the HIV/AIDS epidemic and an urgent need for new strategies to protect hospital personnel from blood-borne infections. The new approach placed emphasis for the first time on applying blood and body fluid precautions universally to all persons regardless of their presumed infectious status. Universal Precautions are a simple standard of infection control practice to be used in the care of all patients at all times to minimize the risk of blood-borne pathogens. Universal Precautions consist of:

– careful handling and disposal of sharps (needles or other sharp objects);
– hand-washing before and after a procedure;
– use of protective barriers – such as gloves, gowns, masks – for direct contact with blood and other body fluids;
– safe disposal of waste contaminated with body fluids and blood;
– proper disinfection of instruments and other contaminated equipment; and
– proper handling of soiled linen.

ADDITIONAL CHECKLIST OF PRECAUTIONS TO PREVENT HIV TRANSMISSION

1. First Aid Kits

- Store first aid kits in selected rooms in the education institution.
- Ensure that the first aid kits contain at least 4 disposable single-use latex-gloves, gauze, scissors, and materials to help heal the wound.
- Check the contents of first aid kits every week.
- Ensure that the responsible persons know where the first aid kits are stored.

2. Emergencies and Mouth-to-Mouth Resuscitation

- If you are trained to do so, perform mouth-to-mouth resuscitation in emergencies with persons living with

HIV/AIDS.

- Although saliva has not been implicated in HIV transmission, to minimize the need for contact with the mouth, you may use mouthpieces, or other ventilation devices.

3. How to Manage Injuries Involving Blood

- Put on your gloves.
- Cover any abrasions or cuts on your arms with a waterproof dressing.
- Clean the wound.
- Remove the gloves and place in a resealable bag.
- Do not touch your eyes before washing up.
- Wash hands immediately after touching blood, body fluids, and contaminated items, whether or not gloves had been worn.
- Wash hands with soap and water for at least 15-20 seconds.
- Change any bloodstained clothes as quickly as possible.
- Immediately discard contaminated sharps and materials in resealable bags.

4. Disinfecting

- Prior to disinfecting, ensure that adherent blood is scraped from surfaces and objects.
- HIV does not survive in the environment. None the less, potentially contaminated spills should be disinfected by using household bleach, 1 part bleach to 10 parts water. Pour the solution around the periphery of the spill.
- Ensure that mops, buckets and other cleaning equipment are disinfected with fresh bleach solution.

5. Cleaning Staff

- Inform all cleaning staff about the universal precautions for handling bodily fluids.

APPENDIX 4:
WHO FACT SHEET - MANAGEMENT OF OCCUPATIONAL EXPOSURE TO BLOOD-BORNE PATHOGENS

Provide immediate care to the exposure site:

- Wash wounds and skin with soap and water.
- Flush mucous membranes with water.

Determine risk associated with exposure by:

- Type of fluid (e.g. blood, visibly bloody fluid, other potentially infectious fluid or tissue and concentrated virus).
- Type of exposure (i.e. percutaneous injury, mucous membrane or non-intact skin exposure and bites resulting in blood exposure).

Evaluate exposure source:

- Assess the risk of infection using available information.
- Test known sources for HBsAg, anti-HCV and HIV antibody (consider using rapid testing).
- For unknown sources, assess risk of exposure to HBV, HCV or HIV infection.
- Do not test discarded needles or syringes for virus contamination.

Evaluate the exposed person:

- Assess immune status for HBV infection (i.e. by history of hepatitis B vaccination and vaccine response). Give PEP for exposures posing risk of infection transmission:

- HBV: PEP dependant on vaccination status:
  - unvaccinated: HBIG + HB vaccination;
  - previously vaccinated, known responder: no treatment;
  - previously vaccinated, known non-responder: HBIG + HB vaccination;
  - antibody response unknown: test and administer HBIG + HB vaccination if results are inadequate.
- HCV: PEP not recommended.
- HIV: Initiate PEP as soon as possible, preferably within hours of exposure. Offer pregnancy testing to all women of childbearing age not known to be pregnant:
  - seek expert consultation if viral resistance is suspected;
  - administer PEP for four weeks if tolerated.

Perform follow-up testing and provide counselling:

- Advise exposed persons to seek medical evaluation for any acute illness occurring during follow-up.
  HBV exposures:
- Perform follow-up anti-HBs testing in persons who receive hepatitis B vaccine: - test for anti-HBs one to two months after last dose of vaccine;
  - anti-HBs response to vaccine cannot be ascertained if HBIG was received in the previous three to four months.

HCV exposures:

- Perform baseline and follow-up testing for anti-HCV and alanine aminotransferase (ALT) four to six months after exposure.
- Perform HCV RNA at four to six weeks if earlier diagnosis of HCV infection desired.

- Confirm repeatedly reactive anti-HCV enzyme immunoassays (EIAs) with supplemental tests.

HIV exposures:

- Perform HIV-antibody testing for at least six months post-exposure (e.g. at baseline, six weeks, three months, and six months).
- Perform HIV antibody testing if illness compatible with an acute retroviral syndrome occurs.
- Advise exposed persons to use precautions to prevent secondary transmission during the follow-up period.
- Evaluate exposed persons taking PEP within 72 hours after exposure and monitor for drug toxicity for at least two weeks.

Source: Joint ILO/WHO guidelines on health services and HIV/AIDS, 2005, *Fact Sheet No. 10*

Safe handling of disposable sharps and injection equipment

Employers should develop procedures for the safe handling and disposal of sharps, including injection equipment, and ensure training, monitoring and evaluation. The procedures should cover:

(a) placement of clearly marked puncture-resistant containers for the disposal of sharps as close as practicable to the areas where sharps are being used or are found;

(b) regular replacement of sharps containers before they reach the manufacturer's fill line or when they are half full; containers should be sealed before they are removed;

(c) the disposal of non-reusable sharps in safely positioned containers that comply with relevant national regulations and technical guidelines;

(d) avoiding recapping and other hand manipulations of needles, and, if recapping is necessary, using a single-handed scoop technique;

(e) responsibility for proper disposal by the person using the sharp;

(f) responsibility for the proper disposal and for reporting the incident by any person finding a sharp.

Source: Joint ILO/WHO guidelines on health services and HIV/AIDS, 2005, paragraph 43

APPENDIX 5:
PROTECTION OF WORKERS' PERSONAL DATA

General principles from the *Protection of workers' personal data: An ILO code of practice (1997)*

5. General principles

5.1.   Personal data should be processed lawfully and fairly, and only for reasons directly relevant to the employment of the worker.

5.2.   Personal data should, in principle, be used only for the purposes for which they were originally collected.

5.3.   If personal data are to be processed for purposes other than those for which they were collected, the employer should ensure that they are not used in a manner incompatible with the original purpose, and should take the necessary measures to avoid any misinterpretations caused by a change of context.

5.4.   Personal data collected in connection with technical or organizational measures to ensure the security and proper operation of automated information systems should not be used to control the behaviour of workers.

5.5.   Decisions concerning a worker should not be based solely on the automated processing of that worker's personal data.

5.6.   Personal data collected by electronic monitoring should not be the only factors in evaluating worker performance.

5.7.   Employers should regularly assess their data processing practices:

(a)   to reduce as far as possible the kind and amount of personal data collected; and

(b)   to improve ways of protecting the privacy of workers.

5.8.   Workers and their representatives should be kept informed of any data collection process, the rules that govern that process, and their rights.

5.9.   Persons who process personal data should be regularly trained to ensure an understanding of the data collection process and their role in the application of the principles in this code.

5.10.   The processing of personal data should not have the effect of unlawfully discriminating in employment or occupation.

5.11.   Employers, workers and their representatives should cooperate in protecting personal data and in developing policies on workers' privacy consistent with the principles in this code.

5.12.   All persons, including employers, workers' representatives, employment agencies and workers, who have access to personal data, should be bound to a rule of confidentiality consistent with the performance of their duties and the principles in this code.

5.13.   Workers may not waive their privacy rights.

APPENDIX 6:
CHECKLIST FOR IMPLEMENTATION OF AN HIV/AIDS POLICY FOR EDUCATION SECTOR WORKPLACES[10]

AT NATIONAL LEVEL

1. Ministry of Education and Labour jointly establish a review committee composed of representatives of government, education sector unions and private school employers/managers, and other stakeholders as agreed among the tripartite partners, to consider application of the policy's provisions at institutional level in accordance with existing national laws and the education sector strategic framework, regulations, policies and collective bargaining agreements, as well as human resource (HR) policies.

2. Employers' organizations and education sector unions review the policy framework in order to reflect its principles and guidelines into collective agreements.

3. Review committee revises the policy as needed and organizes distribution of the agreed policy to all education sector workplaces: schools, TVET and tertiary institutions, adult and non-formal learning centres, etc.

4. Review committee establishes implementation support mechanisms to assist institutions to apply the policy.

AT EDUCATION INSTITUTION LEVEL

1. In consultation with other major stakeholders, the governing body or Principal [Director] of the institution appoints an HIV/AIDS coordinator/committee - depending on the size and resources of the institution - to coordinate the implementation of the policy and design a monitoring mechanism. Where

a workplace committee already exists, this should be used (e.g. occupational safety and health or health advisory committees etc.)

2. The HIV/AIDS coordinator/committee in consultation with the HR department of the institution and/or the education service, the governing body or Principal, students' and teachers and other education sector workers' representatives:
   a. identifies specific institutional needs by reviewing the policy framework adopted at national level and considering how to adapt it to the specific workplace setting;
   b. identifies the needs of students and educators, prior to planning the institutional programme.

3. The HIV/AIDS coordinator/committee assesses what health, social and support services, information services and other resources are already available in the education institution or in the surrounding community.

4. On the basis of the needs assessments and mapping of available services, the coordinator/committee drafts possible revisions of the policy framework and a work plan in consultation with students' and teachers' and other education sector workers' representatives. The work plan should include: time frame and lines of responsibility.

5. The draft policy and plan are circulated for comments to the governing body and the Principal.

6. When the workplace policy and work plan are finalised, the coordinator/committee draws up a list of resources – human, financial and technical - that are necessary for implementation, in consultation with the governing body and principal.

7. The implementation of the workplace

policy should happen through the established planning and budgeting cycles of the institution.

8. The Coordinator/committee organizes the dissemination of the policy and work plan through the governing body, teachers' assemblies and education sector union meetings, students' assemblies, induction courses and training sessions.

9. The Coordinator/committee, in consultation with representatives of teachers and other education sector workers and students, designs a monitoring mechanism to ensure the implementation of the work plan and review the impact of the policy as needed.

SELECTED REFERENCES

An ILO Code of Practice on HIV/AIDS and the world of work, International Labour Organization, 2001. http://www.ilo.org/public/english/protection/trav/aids/code/languages/hiv_a4_e.pdf

Barnett, Grant, Kitty; Ann Strode and Rose Smart (2002) *Managing HIV/AIDS in the Workplace: A Guide for Government Departments*. South Africa: The Department of Public Service and Action Project on HIV/AIDS

Draft National Policy on HIV/AIDS for the Education Sector. Prepared by the Ministry of Basic Education, Sport and Culture and the Ministry of Higher Education, Training and Employment Creation of the Government of Namibia http://www2.ncsu.edu/ncsu/aern/aidpol.html

Education International, World Health Organisation, Education Development Center, Inc. (2004), *Teachers' Exercise Book for HIV Prevention*, WHO Information Series on School Health www.who.int/school-youth-health

Focusing Resources on Effective School Health (FRESH). United Nations Educational, Scientific and Cultural Organization. www.unesco.org/education/fresh

Joint ILO/WHO guidelines on health services and HIV/AIDS, International Labour Organization and World Health Organization, Geneva, 2005

ILO/UNESCO Recommendation concerning the Status of Teachers, 1966 http://www.ilo.org/public/english/dialogue/sector/techmeet/ceart/teache.pdf

ILO, *Implementing the ILO Code of Practice on HIV/AIDS and the world of work: an education and training manual*, International Labour Organization, 2002 http://www.ilo.org/public/english/protection/trav/aids/publ/manualen.htm

ILO, *Protection of workers' personal data: An ILO code of practice*, International Labour Organization, 1997

ILO and UNESCO, Report of the Joint ILO/UNESCO Caribbean sub-regional workshop: Improving responses to HIV/AIDS in Education Sector Workplaces, September 28-30, 2005, Kingston, Jamaica, Geneva, 2005 http://www.ilo.org/public/english/dialogue/sector/papers/education/ed-hiv-carib-workshop.pdf

National Policy for HIV/AIDS Management in Schools, Ministry of Education, Youth and Culture, Jamaica, 2004

Position Statement: HIV/AIDS: The Professional Educational institution Counsellor and HIV/AIDS (2001) American Educational institution Counselor Association

UNESCO *Recommendation concerning the Status of Higher-Education Teaching Personnel*, 1997 http://portal.unesco.org/en/ev.php-URL_ID=13144&URL_DO=DO_TOPIC&URL_SECTION=201.html

World Health Organization's Universal Precautions, including injection safety. http://www.who.int/hiv/topics/precautions/universal/en/print.html

21

HIV AND AIDS EDUCATION THROUGH HFLE FOR
10-14 YEAR OLDS

THE CARICOM SECRETARIAT

A Framework for the development of Health and Family Life Education *(HFLE) curricula in Caribbean schools as developed by the Caribbean Community Secretariat (CARICOM) under the leadership of Dr Morella Joseph, with support from UNICEF and the Education Development Centre (EDC). The curriculum was finalised in 2005 and comprises standards and outcomes for each of the four themes: Sexuality and Sexual Health, Self and Interpersonal Relationships, Appropriate Eating and Fitness and Managing the Environment, guidelines for using the framework, and sample modules and lesson plans. The standards and outcomes for two of the four themes -* Sexuality and Sexual Health *and* Self and Interpersonal Relationships *and reprinted in this chapter, as these provide a framework for teaching about HIV and AIDS in upper primary and lower secondary classrooms.*

BACKGROUND

Society expects schools to assist in the education of children and youth in such ways as to prepare them to assume and practise responsible and positive roles in all aspects of personal, family, and community living. This is also a prerequisite for national and regional development. Because many of the problems affecting students impact negatively on learning, it is incumbent upon schools to go beyond their traditional boundaries to meet the challenge. The time has come for vigorous, coordinated and sustained effort to support the implementation and strengthening of HFLE in the Region.

In 1994, the Caribbean Community (CARICOM) Standing Committee of Ministers of Education passed a resolution supporting the development of a comprehensive approach to Health and Family Life Education (HFLE) by CARICOM and the University of the West Indies (UWI). In order to reduce the overlap of programmes already being implemented – and to reduce the risk of curriculum overload – support was also solicited from United Nations agencies working in the Region.

This commitment gave rise to the CARICOM Multi-Agency Health and Family Life Education (HFLE) Project. The objectives are:

- To develop policy, including advocacy and funding, for the overall strengthening of HFLE in and out of schools
- To strengthen the capacity of teachers to deliver HFLE programmes
- To develop comprehensive life-skills based teaching materials
- To improve coordination among all the agencies at the regional and national levels in the area of HFLE

In 1996, the CARICOM Standing Committee of Ministers of Health and Education endorsed the document, *A Strategy for Strengthening Health and Family Life Education (HFLE) in CARICOM Member States*. The Ministers also reaffirmed their commitment to HFLE as a priority for achieving national development goals, as well as to putting into place measures to ensure its sustainability. The Ministers agreed to make every effort to ensure the formulation and review of national policies on HFLE. More recently the Sixth Special Meeting of the Council for Human and Social Development (COSHOD), held in April 2003, further endorsed the need for urgent strengthening of the HFLE programme and for making it a core area of instruction at the primary, secondary, and tertiary levels. Additionally, COHSOD recommended that the focus of HFLE programmes should shift from an information-based model to a skills-development model, and that a Regional Curriculum Framework should be developed which could be adapted by Member States to meet their specific needs.

Partner agencies in the HFLE project include: the CARICOM Secretariat, Caribbean Child Development Centre (CCDC), UWI Schools of Education and the Advanced Training and Research in Fertility Management Unit (FMU), PAHO/WHO, UNESCO, UNDCP, UNFDA, UNDP, UNIFEM and UNICEF. The current operational mechanism for the project is a Regional Working Group. UNICEF has been carrying out overall coordination. Additionally, over the past two years, the Education Development Center, Inc. (EDC) has been involved in providing technical support to the project.

WHY HFLE?

There is the perception that traditional curricula do not ensure that children and youth achieve their full potential as citizens. In addition, increasing social pressures are impacting on young persons in ways that make teaching a challenge. Teachers are finding that young people are more disruptive, are more likely to question authority, and see little relevance of schooling that fails to adequately prepare them for their various life roles. The paradox is that schools are now seen as key agencies to redress some of these very issues. HFLE, then, is a curriculum initiative that not only reinforces the connection between health and education, but also uses a holistic approach within a planned and coordinated framework. It 'is perceived as the viable way to bridge existing gaps to enable young persons to attain the high levels of educational achievement and productivity required for the 21st century.' (UNICEF/CARICOM, 1999, p 15.)

THE HEALTH AND SOCIAL PROFILE OF CARIBBEAN CHILDREN AND YOUTH

The World Bank Country Study reveals that young persons, 10 to 24 years, make up about 30% of the population in the Caribbean (World Bank, 2003). The data for available countries indicate that the proportion of youth 10 to 24 years varies from as high as 34% in St. Lucia, to 24% in St. Kitts and Nevis.

This group has historically always been 'at risk.' In the past, it was infectious diseases that ravaged this group. Today, however, emotional and behavioural disabilities rank high among the health conditions that affect young persons in the Region. Increasingly, Caribbean youth are being adversely affected by a number of social, psychological, and physical problems.

Evidence of this is substantiated by the findings of Dicks (2001); Halcon, Beuhring &

Blum (2000); Heath (1997); PAHO (1998); UWI-Cave Hill (1998); and The World Bank (2003). The findings identify certain key social and environmental concerns: poverty, unemployment, high academic failure rates, family instability, fragmented communities, child abuse and neglect, violence, stress and alienation, negative influence of the media, questionable sub-cultures, and unavailability of physical education and recreational facilities. Health threats include such lifestyle-related conditions as diabetes, hypertension, obesity; HIV/AIDS/STDs, sexual abuse, substance abuse, suicide and teenage pregnancy.

WHAT IS HFLE?

HFLE is a comprehensive, life skills-based programme, which focuses on the development of the whole person in that it:

- Enhances the potential of young persons to become productive and contributing adults/citizens.
- Promotes an understanding of the principles that underlie personal and social well-being.
- Fosters the development of knowledge, skills and attitudes that make for healthy family life.
- Provides opportunities to demonstrate sound health-related knowledge, attitudes and practices.
- Increases the ability to practice responsible decision-making about social and sexual behaviour.
- Aims to increase the awareness of children and youth of the fact that the choices they make in everyday life profoundly influence their health and personal development into adulthood.

WHAT ARE LIFE SKILLS?

Life skills are abilities for adaptive and positive behaviour that enable individuals to deal effectively with the demands and challenges of everyday life (WHO 1997). This concept is premised on the assumption that there are certain life roles that are fundamental to life situations, for example, growing and developing as a healthy individual; living with and relating to others; managing resources, including the capacity to maximise one's potential; and receiving from, and contributing to, local, national, regional and global communities.

THEORETICAL FOUNDATIONS OF THE LIFE SKILLS APPROACH

Theories about the way human beings, and specially, children and adolescents grow, learn and behave provide the foundation for the life skills approach. These include child and adolescent development, social learning, problem behaviour, social influence, cognitive problem solving, multiple intelligences, and risk and resiliency theories (Mangrulkar, Whitman & Posner 2001).

There is a dearth of documented research evidence on the evaluation of health-related school intervention programmes in the Caribbean. However, results of programme evaluation studies in other countries reveal that competence in the use of life skills can:

- Delay the onset of drug abuse
- Prevent high-risk sexual behaviours
- Facilitate anger management and conflict resolution
- Improve academic performance, and
- Promote positive social adjustment.

Children and adolescents who fail to acquire the skills for interacting with others in a socially acceptable manner early in life can be rejected by their peers and often engage in unhealthy behaviours, such as violence or abuse of alcohol and drugs, to compensate for their rejection (Patterson1986). Research has also found that children with social deficits or aggressive behaviour are at a higher risk of poor academic performance (Parker and Ashe 1987).

Life skills may be classified in various ways. The following is one approach to classifying key skills:

- **Social and interpersonal skills** – for example, communication, refusal, assertiveness, and empathy skills.
- **Cognitive skills** - for example, decision-making, critical thinking, and self-evaluation skills.
- **Emotional coping skills** – for example, stress management skills, and skills for increasing internal locus of control.

Another approach is as follows:

- **Communication skills** – for example, empathy, verbal and non-verbal communication, assertiveness, refusal, negotiation and conflict management, advocacy, and relationship building skills.
- **Values analysis and clarification skills** – for example, skills for understanding different norms, beliefs, cultures and so on, and self assessment skills for identifying what are important influences on values and attitudes, and aligning values, attitudes and behaviours.
- **Decision-making skills** - for example, critical and creative thinking, and problem solving.
- **Coping and stress-management skills** – for example, self-awareness and self-control; coping with pressure, coping with emotions, conflict resolution, and goal setting.

In practice the skills are not separate or discrete, and more than one skill may be used simultaneously.

VALUES

Another justification for the life skills approach is that it is a natural vehicle for the acquisition of the educational, democratic and ethical values reflected in National and Regional policy documents. In the delivery of HFLE, the fostering of laudable attitudes and values is set alongside the knowledge and skill components. Some of the commonly held values are respect for self and others; empathy and tolerance; honesty; kindness; responsibility; integrity; and social justice. The teaching of values in HFLE is to encourage young people to strive towards accepted ideals of a democratic, pluralistic society such as self-reliance, capacity for hard work, cooperation, respect for legitimately constituted authority, and ecologically sustainable development. This is done in the context of existing family, spiritual, cultural and societal values, and through critical analysis and values clarification, in order to foster the intrinsic development of values and attitudes.

ETHICAL GUIDELINES FOR THE DELIVERY OF HFLE

RESPONSIBILITY TO STUDENTS

Teachers and other resource persons involved in the delivery of HFLE should:

- Have primary responsibility to the student, who is to be treated with respect, dignity, and with concern for confidentiality.
- Make appropriate referrals to service providers based on the needs of the student, and monitor progress.
- Maintain the confidentiality of student records and exchange personal

information only according to prescribed responsibility.

- Provide only accurate, objective, and observable information regarding student behaviours.
- Familiarise themselves with policies relevant to issues and concerns related to disclosure. Responses to such issues should be guided by national and school policies, codes of professional organisations/unions, and the existing laws.

RESPONSIBILITY TO FAMILIES

- Respect the inherent rights of parents/ guardians for their children and endeavour to establish co-operative relationships.
- Treat information received from families in a confidential and ethical manner.
- Share information about a student only with persons authorised to receive such information.
- Offer ongoing support and collaboration with families for support of the child.

RESPONSIBILITY TO COLLEAGUES

- Establish and maintain a cooperative relationship with other members of staff and the administration.
- Promote awareness and adherence to appropriate guidelines regarding confidentiality and the distinction between private and public information.
- Encourage awareness of and appropriate use of related professions and organisations to which the student may be referred.

RESPONSIBILITIES TO SELF

- Monitor one's own physical, mental and emotional health, as well as professional effectiveness.
- Refrain from any destructive activity leading to harm to self or to the student.

- Take personal initiative to maintain professional competence.
- Understand and act upon a commitment to HFLE.

THE ORGANISATION OF THE CURRICULUM FRAMEWORK

INTRODUCTION

The main thrust of HFLE is to improve human development and the quality life for all. If we are to prevent, reduce, and control the various health-related and social ills that pervade the Region, we must begin by addressing the common, underlying contributory factors, of which the manifested behaviours are but the symptoms. Promotion of Health and Wellness, therefore, underpins the entire HFLE curriculum. This approach is based on the premise that health is a product of the choices made at the levels of the individual, family, community and nation, and that health is not an end in itself, but a resource for living and development.

CONTENT

The content is organised around **four** themes. These themes have been adopted from the core curriculum guide developed for teachers' colleges as part of a PAHO initiative (see PAHO/Carnegie, 1994). Standards and core outcomes have been developed for each of these themes. This thematic approach marks a departure from the traditional topic centered organisation of curricula. For example, the use of alcohol and drugs, as well as premature sexual activity, represent maladaptive responses to coping with poor self-worth, boredom, failure, isolation, hopelessness, and fragmented relationships. The thematic approach, therefore, addresses the complexity and connectedness between the various concepts and ideas, goals, components and standards, which are associated with attitude and behaviour change.

THE THEMATIC AREAS

- Self and Interpersonal Relationships
- Sexuality and Sexual Health
- Eating and Fitness
- Managing the Environment

SELF AND INTERPERSONAL RELATIONSHIPS: KEY IDEAS

- Human beings are essentially social, and human nature finds its fullest expression in the quality of relationships established with others.
- Self-concept is learned, and is a critical factor in relationship building.
- Effective or healthy relationships are dependent on the acquisition and practice of identifiable social skills.
- Supportive social environments are critical to the development of social skills in order to reduce feelings of alienation, and many of the self-destructive and risk-taking tendencies, such as violence and drug-use among children and youth in the region.
- Teachers have a critical role to play in creating supportive school and classroom environments that preserve and enhance self-esteem, a critical factor in the teaching/learning process.

SEXUALITY AND SEXUAL HEALTH: KEY IDEAS

- Sexuality is an integral part of personality, and cannot be separated from other aspects of self.
- The expression of sexuality encompasses physical, emotional, and psychological components, including issues related to gender.
- Sexual role behaviours and values of teachers and children are conditioned by family values and practices, religious beliefs, and social and cultural norms, as well as personal experiences.
- Educational interventions must augment the socialisation role of the family and other social and religious institutions in order to assist in preventing/minimising those expressions of sexuality that are detrimental to emotional and physical health and well-being.

EATING AND FITNESS: KEY IDEAS

- Dietary and fitness practices are influenced by familial, sociocultural and economic factors, as well as personal preferences.
- Sound dietary practices and adequate levels of physical activity are important for physical survival.
- The quality of nutritional intake and level of physical activity are directly related to the ability to learn, and has implications for social and emotional development.
- The eating and fitness habits established in childhood are persistent, conditioning those preferences and practices, which will influence quality of health in later life.
- Teachers are well poised to assist students in critically assessing the dietary choices over which they have control, using the leverage provided by classroom instruction and the provision of nutritionally-sound meals in the school environment.

MANAGING THE ENVIRONMENT: KEY IDEAS

- All human activity has environmental consequences.
- Access to, and current use of technologies have had an unprecedented negative impact on the environment.
- Human beings are capable of making

the greatest range of responses to the environment, in terms of changing, adapting, preserving, enhancing, or destroying it.

- There is a dynamic balance between health, the quality of life, and the quality of environment.

TEACHING/LEARNING STRATEGIES

The objective of any teaching/learning approach in the HFLE classroom is the creation of an environment conducive to active, participatory or experiential learning. The learner is the active agent in creating knowledge in that he/she constructs and reconstructs his/her system of knowledge, skills, and values. In this way, 'meaning' is attached to his/her real life experiences.

A model of the *Active Learning Process* would include the following learning stages:

- Understanding the issue and the life skills required (e.g., risks of drugs).
- Relating to personal experiences.
- Practising the situation in a safe, supportive environment (e.g., role play).
- Applying knowledge and skills to real life situations.
- Reflecting on the experience gained.
- Strengthening life skills for further use.

This approach to learning:

- Utilises the experience, opinions, and knowledge of the students.
- Provides a creative context for the exploration and development of options.
- Provides a source of mutual comfort and security, which is important for the learning and decision-making process.
- Promotes the development of action competence for use in the real world.

METHOD OF DELIVERY

The approach adopted in the delivery of life skills-based HFLE should take into account context, needs, and availability of resources.

There are two major approaches to delivery:

- *Discipline-based* - HFLE is taught as a separate subject.
- *Integration* - HFLE is integrated with other subjects in the school curriculum. Models of integration include the following:
  - *Infusion* - An HFLE topic area and related skills are infused into another subject area. For example, strategies for developing healthy interpersonal relationships skills may be infused into a biology lesson that critiques the range of relationships found in living organisms. Decision-making and goal-setting skills related to promoting abstinence or delaying sexual activity may be infused into a mathematics lesson that explores statistical data related to the rates of incidence of HIV/AIDS among young persons of various age groups.
  - *Multidisciplinary* – Two or more subjects are organised around the same theme and skills. For example, subjects such as social studies, biology or science, language arts, physical education, and home economics, are subject areas that can be organised around the theme of 'Eating and Fitness.' The core skills are identified, and specific areas are allocated among the identified subject areas.
  - *Interdisciplinary* – Skills form the focus of the integration among two

or more subject areas. For example, if core skills such as critical thinking, communication, and problem-solving are selected as the focus, then content may be selected from two or more subject areas that are appropriate for the teaching of these skills. In this case, the content areas may or may not be directly related, since the focus is on skill acquisition.

- *Trans-disciplinary* – This is used in problem-based learning. For example, a problem may be loosely structured around an environmental issue in a community, which has implications for health and the quality of life of persons living in that community. The assumption is that different subject areas are embedded in the problem. Students then brainstorm to determine what they know, what they need to know, and how they are going to find out. Learning objectives, including the implicated life skills, are then determined. Students have to access the available resources and demonstrate the identified skills in coming up with strategies for solving the problem.

All of these approaches have advantages, as well as disadvantages, and have implications for teacher training. The obvious advantage of the discipline-based approach is wider coverage of HFLE. This approach requires a core of teachers specially trained to deliver life skills-based HFLE.

The integrated approaches are more economical, with respect to resource demands - human resources, material resources, and time resources. However, in addition to special training in life skills teaching and methods/strategies for integration, they require a high level of organisation, with respect to planning and collaboration across subject areas. For example, infusion, which is the simplest form of integration, requires that topics to be infused be developed and inventoried, that they be linked to the subjects in which they would be infused, that staff be rationally located to the tasks, and so on. In the case of trans-disciplinary integration, teachers would need additional training in problem-based learning methodologies. The major disadvantage with the integrated approaches is that key learning outcomes, from either HFLE, or the other subject/s area/s, or all, may be sacrificed.

Whether HFLE is integrated into existing curricula, taught as a separate subject or as a mix of both methods, will ultimately be a choice to be made by each country. Most countries have found a mixture of both to be effective.

INSTRUCTIONAL RESOURCES

Instructional resources should:

- Encourage active learning
- Provide all students with opportunities for participation, recognition, and successful achievement in order to foster confidence and self-acceptance
- Provide opportunities for all students to practise the life skills
- Allow for varied patterns of interaction among students, and between students and teacher
- Direct students to the use of available technology
- Recognise diversity among students
- Provide teachers with general and lesson-specific advice to support learning, based on current research on learning styles and effective instruction
- Bring the student's environment and daily experiences into the classroom
- Promote teacher sensitivity

ASSESSMENT/EVALUTION

Student Assessment

The primary aim of assessment is to foster learning for all students. In HFLE, meaningful assessment should focus on the four areas: attitudes, behaviours, knowledge and skills. The school should use assessment results in a formative way to determine how well they are meeting instructional goals, and how to alter curriculum and instruction so that goals can be better met.

All efforts should be made to ensure that there is a valid match between what is being assessed, how it is being assessed, what is taught, and how it is taught. A wide range of assessment strategies is available, and should be built into the curriculum design from the beginning. A critical factor is that it must be ongoing and varied.

A major challenge to teachers is to minimise the focus on the solely traditional and cognitive methods of assessment to which they have become accustomed. HFLE encompasses all the domains of learning, especially the affective domain. Profound challenges in our societies relate to our social unity, ethical standards and moral values, to our courage and compassion. Feeling is as real and as important a part of human nature, as is cognition or knowing. Alternative Assessment strategies are suggested, which test across the domains. Examples include performance-based assessment, portfolios, journal writing, and student-designed assessments, among others.

Teacher Assessment

Some of the areas to assess teacher performance might include:

- Knowledge of the subject area
- Knowledge/modelling of life skills

- The extent to which he/she permits expression of different viewpoints
- Teacher/student/student interaction
- Linkages made between what is taught and real life situations
- Establishment of home/school/community linkages
- Knowledge/application of alternative assessment
- Knowledge/application of interactive teaching methodologies
- Establishment of supportive classroom environments

Programme Evaluation

It is important that mechanisms be put in place to monitor and evaluate different components of the HFLE programme, and to use the feedback provided to improve programme quality and implementation, as well as support systems. These might include:

- Surveys to determine how much HFLE is actually taught across the school
- Evaluation of the effectiveness of new teaching techniques and materials
- Evaluation of the effectiveness of programme delivery
- Evaluation of the quality of reporting of results
- Evaluation of programme impact within the school environment
- Evaluation of the degree of fidelity in programme delivery.

HOME, SCHOOL, AND COMMUNITY LINKAGES

Schools today play important and varied roles in children's lives. In addition to fostering the development of academic skills, schools also equip students with the skills needed to lead safe and healthy lives. Yet, schools cannot and should not be the sole source of solutions to the varied social and health-related problems of students, nor can they work in isolation. Schools require the investment, support, and commitment of family and community to achieve their multifaceted goals.

The success of HFLE, therefore, depends on building strong home, school, and community collaboration. This collaboration will help to:

- Educate and empower parents so that they are better positioned to make informed decisions, with respect to the health and well-being of their families.
- Acknowledge and respect differences among communities.
- Make appropriate use of available community resources and expertise.
- Provide a vehicle for communication.
- Contribute to the development of local HFLE curricula.

THE HEALTH PROMOTING SCHOOL

The school, therefore, has a mandate that goes beyond the provision of providing life skills-based HFLE curricula. The school must adopt a holistic approach to promoting the health and well-being of all its members. One such approach is the Health Promoting School concept.

WHO defines the Health Promoting School (HPS) as one that is constantly strengthening its capacity as a healthy setting for living, learning, and working. An HPS fosters health and learning at all times through school policy; curriculum, teaching and learning; school organisation, ethos and environment (both physical and psychosocial); and partnerships and support services. HPS, therefore, provides a supportive learning environment, and links its efforts with families and communities.

STANDARDS FOR TWO THEMES

STANDARDS FOR THEME 1: SEXUALITY AND SEXUAL HEALTH

The standards are

1) Demonstrate an understanding of the concept of human sexuality as an integral part of the total person that finds expression throughout the life cycle.
2) Analyse the influence of sociocultural and economic factors, as well as personal beliefs on the expression of sexuality and sexual choices.
3) Build capacity to recognise the basic criteria and conditions for optimal reproductive health.
4) Develop action competence to reduce vulnerability to priority problems, including HIV/AIDS, cervical cancer, and STIs.
5) Develop knowledge and skills to access age-appropriate sources of health information, products, and services related to sexuality and sexual health.

REGIONAL STANDARD 1

Demonstrate an understanding of the concept of human sexuality as an integral part of the total person that finds expression throughout the life cycle.

Descriptor:

A differentiation needs to be made between the terms *sex* and *sexuality*. Sexuality is presented as including biological sex, gender, and gender identity. One's sexuality also encompasses the many social, emotional, and psychological factors that shape the expression of values, attitudes, social roles, and beliefs about self and others as being male or female. It is important to have students develop positive attitudes about self and their evolving sexuality.

Key Skills:

- Coping Skills (healthy self-management, self-awareness)
- Social Skills (communication, interpersonal relations, assertiveness, refusal)
- Cognitive Skills (critical and creative thinking, decision-making)

Core Outcomes Age Level 9–10	Core Outcomes Age Level 11–12	Core Outcomes Age Level 13–14
1. Explore personal experiences, attitudes, and feelings about the roles that boys and girls are expected to play. 2. Demonstrate awareness of the physical, emotional, and cognitive changes that occur during puberty.	1. Develop strategies for coping with the various changes associated with puberty. 2. Assess traditional role expectations of boys and girls in our changing society. 3. Assess ways in which behaviour can be interpreted as being "sexual."	1. Assess the capacity to enter into intimate sexual relationships. 2. Demonstrate use of strategies for recognising and managing sexual feelings and behaviours.

REGIONAL STANDARD 2

Analyse the influence of socio-cultural and economic factors, as well as personal beliefs on the expression of sexuality and sexual choices.

Descriptor:

Young people make daily decisions about their sexual behaviour, values, and attitudes. Family, religion, culture, technology—including media, and peers, influence these decisions. It is critical to provide students with knowledge and skills that will assist them in understanding their own sexuality and realising their potential as effective and caring human beings.

Key Skills:

- Coping Skills (healthy self-management, self-awareness)
- Social Skills (communication, interpersonal relations, assertiveness, refusal, negotiation)
- Cognitive Skills (critical thinking, creative thinking, problem-solving, decision-making, critical viewing)

Core Outcomes Age Level 9–10	Core Outcomes Age Level 11–12	Core Outcomes Age Level 13–14
1. Demonstrate an understanding of the ways in which sexuality is learned. 2. Demonstrate ways to respond appropriately to the key factors influencing sexual choices and experiences. 3. Demonstrate knowledge of the various types of sexual abuse and exploitation.	1. Critically analyse the key factors influencing sexual choices and experiences. 2. Demonstrate skills in communicating about sexual issues with parents, peers, and/or significant others.	1. Critically analyse the impact of personal beliefs, media, money, technology, and entertainment on early sexual involvement. 2. Demonstrate skills to counter the negative influences reaching youth through personal beliefs, media, money, marketing, and technology.

REGIONAL STANDARD 3

Build capacity to recognise the basic criteria and conditions for optimal reproductive health.

Descriptor:

Young people are facing a variety of risks that compromise their sexual and reproductive health. Acquisition of requisite skills to counteract these risks will increase the opportunity to maximise learning and provide a foundation for a healthy population.

Key Skills:

- Coping Skills (healthy self-management)
- Social Skills (communication, interpersonal relations, assertiveness, refusal, negotiation)
- Cognitive Skills (critical thinking, creative thinking, problem-solving, decision-making)

Core Outcomes Age Level 9–10	Core Outcomes Age Level 11–12	Core Outcomes Age Level 13–14
1. Demonstrate knowledge of factors that influence reproductive health. 2. Demonstrate knowledge of the basic health and social requirements of raising a child.	1. Demonstrate knowledge of the impact of raising a child. 2. Critically analyse the risks that impact on reproductive health.	1. Make appropriate choices to avoid risks to reproductive health. 2. Evaluate the social and biological factors that support healthy pregnancy and child rearing.

REGIONAL STANDARD 4

Develop action competence to reduce vulnerability to priority problems, including HIV/AIDS, cervical cancer, and STIs.

Descriptor:

Beyond knowledge of HIV/AIDS, cervical cancer, and STIs as a disease, efforts have to be intensified to render students less vulnerable to contracting and spreading HIV, cervical cancer, and STIs. Addressing issues related to the physical and emotional aspects of HIV/AIDS, stigma of living with HIV/AIDS, and discrimination against people living with HIV/AIDS is critical. Importantly, students are encouraged to examine a range of options for reducing vulnerability to these problems such as abstinence, a drug-free lifestyle and so on.

Key Skills:

- Coping Skills (healthy self-management, self-monitoring)
- Social Skills (communication, assertiveness, refusal, negotiation, empathy)
- Cognitive Skills (critical thinking, creative thinking, problem-solving, decision-making)

Core Outcomes Age Level 9–10	Core Outcomes Age Level 11–12	Core Outcomes Age Level 13–14
1. Identify the risk behaviours/ agents that are associated with contracting HIV, cervical cancer, and STIs. 2. Demonstrate skills to assist and respond compassionately to persons affected by HIV.	1. Make appropriate choices to reduce risk associated with contracting HIV, cervical cancer, and STIs. 2. Set personal goals to minimise the risk of contracting HIV, cervical cancer, and STIs. 3. Demonstrate ways of empathising and supporting persons and families affected by HIV/ AIDS.	1. Critically examine abstinence, fidelity, and condom use (if permitted) as preventive methods in transmission of HIV and STIs. 2. Make appropriate choices to reduce risk associated with contracting HIV, cervical cancer, and STIs. 3. Critically examine social norms and personal beliefs in light of current knowledge of the transmission and spread of HIV. 4. Advocate for reducing the stigma and discrimination associated with HIV, cervical cancer, and STIs.

REGIONAL STANDARD 5

Develop knowledge and skills to access age-appropriate sources of health information, products, and services related to sexuality and sexual health.

Descriptor:

Students should be capable of identifying a range of age-appropriate health services in their communities. Through an informed use of these services, they should acquire the necessary knowledge, skills, and attitudes needed for a lifelong commitment to the promotion of personal, family, and community health, including advocacy. Age-appropriate health services in the community may address the following: sexuality, child abuse, sexual assault/ harassment, and domestic violence.

Key Skills:

- Coping Skills (healthy self-management)
- Social Skills (communication)
- Cognitive Skills (critical thinking, creative thinking, problem-solving, decision-making)

Core Outcomes Age Level 9–10	Core Outcomes Age Level 11–12	Core Outcomes Age Level 13–14
1. Identify sources of accurate information. 2. Identify family, school, and community resources that deal with health, social, and emotional issues.	1. Demonstrate the ability to locate and utilise community resources that support the health, social, and emotional needs of families.	1. Evaluate the availability and appropriateness of the resources to address reproductive health and parenting issues. 2. Demonstrate an understanding of the basic tenets that address the sexual health of children and youth.

STANDARDS FOR THEME 2: SELF AND INTERPERSONAL RELATIONSHIPS

The standards are

1) Examine the nature of self, family, school, and community in order to build strong healthy relationships.
2) Acquire coping skills to deter behaviours and lifestyles associated with crime, drugs, violence, motor vehicle accidents, and other injuries.
3) Respect the rich differences that exist among Caribbean peoples as a valuable resource for sustainable development of the region within the framework of democratic and ethical values.

REGIONAL STANDARD 1

Examine the nature of self, family, school, and community in order to build strong, healthy relationships.

Descriptor:

Acceptance of self, the need to belong, and the need to be loved are some of the universal needs and rights that contribute to the shaping of our individual selves. Students need to develop a healthy self-concept in order to foster healthy relationships within the family, school, and community. They also need to be assisted in developing resiliency—the capacity to assess, cope, manage, and benefit from the various influences that impact on relationships.

Key Skills:

- Coping Skills (healthy self-management, self-awareness)
- Social Skills (communication, interpersonal relations)
- Cognitive Skills (critical thinking, creative thinking, problem-solving, decision-making)

Core Outcomes Age Level 9–10	Core Outcomes Age Level 11–12	Core Outcomes Age Level 13–14
1. Demonstrate an understanding of self. 2. Identify ways to promote healthy relationships with family and friends.	1. Analyse the influences that impact on personal development (media, peers, family, significant others, community, etc.). 2. Demonstrate an understanding of issues that impact on relationships within the family, school, and community.	1. Demonstrate ways to use adverse experiences for personal growth and development. 2. Recognise risks to mental and emotional well-being.

REGIONAL STANDARD 2

Acquisition of coping skills to deter behaviours and lifestyles associated with crime, drugs, violence, motor vehicle accidents, and other injuries.

Descriptor:

Students need to practise skills that reduce their involvement in risky behaviours. Crime, violence, bullying, alcohol and other drugs, and motor vehicle accidents and other injuries threaten the very fabric of Caribbean society and the lives of Caribbean youth. The acquisition of these skills will increase students' ability to assume a responsible role in all aspects of personal, family, and community living.

Key Skills:

- Coping Skills (healthy self-management, self-awareness)
- Social Skills (communication, interpersonal relations, assertiveness, conflict resolution, mediation, anger management)
- Cognitive Skills (critical thinking, creative thinking, problem-solving, decision-making)

Core Outcomes Age Level 9–10	Core Outcomes Age Level 11–12	Core Outcomes Age Level 13–14
1. Identify ways of coping with feelings and emotions in adverse situations. 2. Demonstrate skills to cope with violence at home, school, and in the community.	1. Develop resilience for coping with adverse situations (death, grief, rejection, and separation). 2. Analyse the impact of alcohol, and other illicit drugs on behaviour and lifestyle. 3. Demonstrate skills to cope with violence at home, school, and in the community.	1. Demonstrate skills to avoid high-risk situations and pressure to use alcohol and other illicit substances. 2. Demonstrate skills to cope with violence at home, school, and in the community.

REGIONAL STANDARD 3

Respect the rich diversity that exists among Caribbean peoples as a valuable resource for sustainable development of the region within the framework of democratic and ethical values.

Descriptor:

Survival in a global economy demands that we pool our individual and collective resources in order to be productive as a people. Students must be committed to valuing and respecting the rich diversity (cultural, ethnic, and religious) of the people of the Caribbean. Additionally, they must be encouraged to realise their fullest potential as contributors to sustainable development while embracing core values and democratic ideals.

Key Skills:

- Coping Skills (healthy self-management)
- Social Skills (communication, interpersonal relations, assertiveness, refusal, negotiation)
- Cognitive Skills (critical thinking, creative thinking, problem-solving, decision-making)

Core Outcomes Age Level: 9–10	Core Outcomes Age Level 11–12	Core Outcomes Age Level 13–14
1. Affirmation of persons who are different from oneself (ethnic and cultural). 2. Appreciate that resources among diverse people are essential to developing positive relationships.	1. Assess ways in which personal and group efforts can be enhanced by the interactions and contributions of persons of diverse cultural and ethnic groupings. 2. Recognise the value of personal commitment and hard work to the improvement of self, others, and the wider community.	1. Critically examine how relationships can be affected by personal prejudices and biases. 2. Advocate for acceptance and inclusion of persons from diverse groupings at all levels of society. 3. Recognise that the development of the region depends on individual and collective efforts at all levels of society.

22

SELF-ASSESSMENT CHECKLIST FOR UNIVERSITY RESPONSES TO HIV/AIDS

DAVID PLUMMER

Commonwealth/UNESCO Regional Chair in Education (HIV/AIDS), University of the West Indies

This 'self-assessment' checklist was developed in response to the global review of University HIV/AIDS strategies undertaken by UNESCO in 2005. It was first presented at the annual meeting of the Association of Caribbean Universities and Research Institutes (UNICA) in November 2005. It was apparent that (with some notable exceptions) many universities have not shown leadership in HIV/AIDS that would have been shown by universities on other important social issues. There are a variety of reasons why this is so, but it is likely that the foremost reason is because of the stigma and taboo associated with HIV/AIDS, which has lead to a qualitatively different response from many key institutions, not just universities. It is clear that universities would benefit from some additional guidance and models concerning how they should respond to HIV/AIDS.

The self-assessment checklist offers an implicit model for responding; a simple mechanism whereby universities can use to check their track record; and a basis for audit by umbrella bodies and quality assurance agencies if desired. The checklist is divided along the usual lines of responsibility accepted by universities: teaching, research and service:

Section 1: HIV and the education and training role of the University
Section 2: HIV and the research and inquiry role of the University
Section 3: HIV and service to the university and to society roles

SECTION 1:
EDUCATION AND TRAINING

What curriculum modifications have been made in response to HIV/AIDS?

What curriculum modifications are planned in response to HIV/AIDS?

To what extent has HIV/AIDS been mainstreamed into the general curriculum?

List courses; estimate % of teaching time with HIV-related content

What evidence is there for curriculum response in all faculties?

What specialised HIV/AIDS courses are currently available?

What specialised HIV/AIDS courses are planned?

SECTION 2: RESEARCH AND INQUIRY

What HIV/AIDS-related research outputs have there been?

List published research reports and papers in last 12 months

What other mechanisms are being used to feed results back to society? List.

List disciplines currently engaged in HIV-related research?

Is HIV/AIDS-related research balanced and found across disciplines?

SECTION 3A: SERVICE TO THE UNIVERSITY AND SOCIETY

Is there evidence of a coherent proactive university response to HIV/AIDS?

What is the evidence of senior staff and administrative support?

What leadership roles are taken by senior staff in HIV/AIDS?

What administrative support is provided for HIV-related activities?

Is the university largely pro-active or reactive?

List evidence of university initiatives

Is HIV mentioned in the staff recruitment policy? What?

Is HIV mentioned in the student intake policy? What?

Does the university have workplace policies for HIV? What?

Is there an infection control policy in clinical/laboratory settings? What?

Does the university have anti-discrimination provisions relevant to HIV; sexual harassment policy; gender equity? What?

Is there a policy on privacy and confidentiality for HIV? What?

SECTION 3B: SERVICE TO THE UNIVERSITY AND SOCIETY

Does the university have an HIV/AIDS response steering committee?

Is there a University HIV/AIDS steering Committee?

If so, how functional is it?

Frequency and duration of meetings

Meeting minutes available?

Breadth of membership:

Senior staff;

Student guild reps;

People from 'risk groups' and 'risk settings';

HIV+ membership;

External links (eg NGO reps)

Is there a HIV/AIDS committee work plan?

Does the committee receive any funding for activities?

Does the committee disburse any funds for activities?

Are there year-round health promotion activities? What?

Are posters, pamphlets on HIV/AIDS available around the University?

Are condoms freely available for students? Distribution rates?

Is sharps disposal freely available for students? Utilisation rates?

Are there year-round de-stigmatization activities? What?

What research for government, community and wider society is done?

What information has been put in public domain, reports, papers published?

SECTION 3C: SERVICE TO THE UNIVERSITY AND SOCIETY

Does the university have staff & student welfare provisions?

What evidence is there that the university accepts its duty of care for staff and students?

Is there monitoring of HIV-related absenteeism; student withdrawal & staff resignation (de-identified, aggregated & gender disaggregated)

What policy and facilities for welfare, support, care and treatment for staff and students affected by HIV/AIDS are there?

Policy on role of HIV testing in: recruitment of staff or students; worker's compensation; sick leave; superannuation; insurance (note this point is intended to prevent inappropriate testing and inappropriate use of results, not to promote testing in these settings)

SECTION 3D: SERVICE TO THE UNIVERSITY AND SOCIETY

What evidence is there of University contribution to and leadership on HIV related issues in wider society?

Does the university demonstrate leadership in HIV/AIDS? Evidence?

Does the university formally provide support and advice for government, community and wider society? What?

What university membership of external HIV/AIDS-related groups and committees is there?

23

Making bold moves in the Caribbean Education Sector: Establishment of the First Regional Network of Education Sector HIV and AIDS Coordinators

Sherlene Neal Tablada

Ministry of Education, Belize
First elected president, Caribbean Regional
Network of Education Sector HIV and AIDS
Coordinators

At a regional meeting in May 2006, supported by UNESCO and CARICOM, Ministry of Education HIV/AIDS and HFLE Coordinators formed their own association. The terms of reference and initial work plan are outlined here. Ministers of Education, in the Port of Spain Declaration (Chapter 19) endorsed 'the establishment and support development of the Caribbean Network of HIV Coordinators in the education sector as a CARICOM-led regional resource'.

BACKGROUND

When one examines the region's HIV situation closely it becomes evident that those most affected by HIV and AIDS are young people. Statistics indicate that upward of forty per cent of newly diagnosed HIV infections annually in the Caribbean are found among young persons aged between 15 and 24. (CAREC, 2004). The World Bank estimates that another 250,000 children in the region have been made vulnerable by HIV and AIDS.

As James Wolfensohn, former president of the World Bank Group said 'HIV/AIDS is reversing decades of development gains, increasing poverty and undermining the very foundations of progress and security. The epidemic demands a response that confronts the disease in every sector, but education has a particular role to play'.

Without question, the education sector is critical in the region's response to HIV and AIDS. The sector plays host to thousands of students whose lives are impacted daily, some in unimaginable ways, by HIV and AIDS. As a workplace, the sector employs thousands of teachers and support staff, many of whom are impacted either directly or indirectly by HIV and AIDS.

Based on the recognition that HIV and AIDS are critical issues for the education sector and that the sector has the potential to shape skills, attitudes and behaviours of students, staff and parents, the Caribbean education sector has been making many bold moves in its response to HIV and AIDS.

One such bold move is the establishment of the first Regional Network of Education Sector HIV and AIDS Coordinators. The call for such a network came from education sector coordinators who felt that there was a vital need to establish a platform to coordinate the HIV response of education sectors in the region by engaging in joint planning, sharing information and best practices, and continuous collaboration to ensure a truly comprehensive regional approach to HIV and AIDS.

This network was realised during a meeting of education sector coordinators, hosted by UNESCO, CARICOM, IDB and UWI and facilitated by the Education Development Centre (EDC), in Kingston, Jamaica from 25–28 April, 2006.

Delegates from 14 CARICOM countries, together with representation from the British and Dutch Overseas Countries and Territories, all affirmed that the network has significant potential to strengthen the contribution of the Caribbean's education sector to the overall HIV and AIDS response. The network is led by a seven-member executive comprising – chair (Belize), deputy chair (Trinidad and Tobago), secretary (St Vincent and the Grenadines), deputy secretary (the Bahamas), public relations officer (Jamaica) and two ex officio officers (Antigua and Barbuda, and the British and Dutch Overseas Countries and Territories). This network will work alongside regional organisations – the CARICOM Secretariat, the Caribbean Coalition of National AIDS Programme Coordinators (CCNAPC), the Caribbean Regional Network of Seropositives (CRN+), the University of the West Indies (UWI), and the Caribbean Union of Teachers to strengthen the regional response to HIV and AIDS.

TERMS OF REFERENCE OF THE NETWORK

Vision The network's vision is to transform the response of the region's education sector's to HIV and AIDS.

Mission To advocate for a comprehensive, coordinated and sustained regional response

to HIV and AIDS by Caribbean education sectors.

Goal To strengthen the Caribbean education sector's policy and programme response to HIV and AIDS.

OBJECTIVES

The network will:

- Seek to influence policymaking and programme implementation in the education sector that address HIV prevention, and the care, support and treatment of persons infected with HIV, and create environments that are free from discrimination,
- Provide a platform for communication and information sharing among network members and other stakeholders in the education sector,
- Provide mechanisms for identifying research needs, commissioning basic and applied research and ensuring evidence-based practice in education,
- Advocate for increased allocation of resources and support for the education sector response to HIV and AIDS,
- Identify and advocate for opportunities to increase capacity of network members in strategic areas, and
- Monitor the national and regional response of the education sector to HIV and AIDS.

GUIDING PRINCIPLES AND PHILOSOPHY

These include:

- Recognition of HIV and AIDS as critical issues affecting the education sector
- Recognition of the key role the education sector plays in the HIV and AIDS response

- Advancement of GIPA principles (Greater Involvement of Persons Living with HIV and AIDS)
- Promotion of a culture of non-discrimination and continued advocacy for the rights of PLWHA
- Promotion of a culture of mutual sharing of information and resources
- Commitment and passion for the mission and objectives of the network
- Sensitivity to the socio-economic and cultural context of member countries

MAKING BOLD MOVES

STRUCTURE AND MANAGEMENT OF THE NETWORK

The network will be led by an executive committee comprising a chair, deputy chair, secretary, deputy secretary, public relations officer and two advisors. The terms of office for the executive committee will not exceed two years.

The executive will hold monthly meetings via the Internet or teleconference and at least one face-to-face meeting per year. The secretary will be responsible for communicating the outcome of meetings to other members of the network no later than one week after the conclusion of the executive meeting. Quarterly meetings of the larger network will be conducted via teleconference. A face-to-face meeting of the network will be held at least once per year.

MEMBERSHIP

The network will comprise all education sector HIV/AIDS coordinators, representatives from supporting regional agencies such as CCNAPC, CRN+, CARICOM, UWI, OECS and CAREC. Representatives from UNESCO, PAHO, UNICEF, CUT and private sector organisations will be invited to special meetings and will be called upon by

the network to provide technical support.

INITIAL WORK PLAN

First six months. Although the network has been in existence for just over a month, much has already been achieved through the passion and commitment of its members.

- An executive was elected at the end of the first meeting and a draft Terms of Reference for the network was developed.
- With the technical support of EDC, an interactive website has been established to facilitate dialogue and information sharing among network members.
- Network members have also been engaged in advocacy activities at the national level to promote the network and gain support and commitment from Ministers and other policy- and decision-makers.

Other short-term activities include:

- Development and signing of pledges by members (by end-June)
- Intention for establishment of network and lobbying support and endorsement communicated at the highest level (COHSOD meeting in June)
- Presentation at COHSOD (June)
- Ministers communiqué endorsing network (June)
- Launch network regionally and nationally (by August)
- Three working meetings of the committee (two teleconferences and Internet meetings in May and June and one face-to-face meeting in July to finalise work)
- Commence drafting work plan based on groundwork done this week (to be completed by August)
- Development of website (by September)
- Submission of one example of best practice to be posted on website (by July)

Next three to five years. Key long-term activities include:

- Establishment of a fully staffed secretariat
- Establishment of subcommittees responsible for various areas of the regional response
- Advocacy for the establishment of full-time HIV and AIDS Coordinator in all Ministries of Education

CALL TO ACTION

Because of the direct involvement of network members in policy and programmatic responses to HIV and AIDS, the Caribbean Regional Network of Education Sector Coordinators is well-positioned to contribute significantly to the region's HIV and AIDS response. However, the success of the network is dependent on political support at the highest levels in the region. The network needs to be recognised and endorsed as an essential component of the region's education sector response by Ministers of Education, other policy- and decision-makers in the education sector, and regional and international organisations.

This endorsement needs to be accompanied by efforts at the regional and national level to strengthen the capacity of all education sectors to establish a comprehensive response to HIV and AIDS. This includes ensuring the provision of adequate technical, human and financial resources.

Many coordinators are responsible for a multiplicity of roles and functions within Ministries of Education, which minimises the time they can dedicate to the HIV response. HIV units in many Ministries of Education also remain understaffed and underfunded. In addition, many education sectors lack clear policies on HIV and AIDS, which limits their capacity to mount a comprehensive response to HIV and AIDS. It is essential for local, regional and international agencies to increase support to the education sector to ensure that they are viable entities in the region's response to HIV and AIDS.

With the dedication and commitment of the network and the political support of regional education leaders and regional and international partners, the Caribbean education sector can lead the way in demonstrating how an effective education sector response can change the course of HIV and AIDS and save millions of lives.

24

GIPA and the Education Response to HIV and AIDS in the Caribbean

Suzette M. Moses-Burton	Christoforos Mallouris
Chair, Executive Board, Caribbean Regional Network of People Living with HIV/AIDS (CRN+)	UNESCO and member of United Nations System HIV-Positive Staff Group (UN+)

In the Caribbean, there have been advances in realisation of GIPA, greater involvement of people living with HIV/AIDS, in the education sector response. In this chapter, progress is charted, challenges explained, and proposals are made for the way forward .

GIPA: THE BACKGROUND

The movement to involve people living with HIV in the response to HIV and AIDS was first articulated by HIV-positive people during the earliest stages of the epidemic in Denver, Colorado. The 1983 *Denver Principles* was drafted by members of the HIV-positive community who had been advocating for increased participation in decision-making and development initiatives aimed at responding to the epidemic. With a strong emphasis on the fundamentality of people's human rights, the principles denounce stigma and discrimination against people living with HIV and AIDS (PLWHA) and call for the support and inclusion of PLWHA in decision making.

Networks of people living with and/or affected by HIV/AIDS since that time have continued their advocacy for their continued involvement and inclusion in all aspects of the response to the epidemic.

However, it was not until December 1994 that a formal statement was made promoting the idea of PLWHA providing leadership in the areas of policy development as well as in the implementation of projects and programmes. The 42 governments that adopted the *Paris AIDS Declaration* outlined the need for the greater involvement of people living with HIV/AIDS (GIPA). The declaration called to 'Support a greater involvement of people living with HIV/AIDS through an initiative to strengthen the capacity and coordination of networks of people living with HIV/AIDS and community-based organisations. By ensuring their full involvement in our common response to the pandemic at all – national, regional and global – levels, this initiative will, in particular, stimulate the creation of supportive political, legal and social environments.'[1]

In June 2001 at the United Nations General Assembly Special Session (UNGASS) on HIV/AIDS, UN Member States signed the 'United Nations Declaration of Commitment on HIV/AIDS', which makes reference to the principle of GIPA and the recognition of its impact when applied: 'Acknowledging the particular role and significant contribution of people living with HIV/AIDS, young people and civil society actors in addressing the problem of HIV/AIDS in all its aspects, and recognising that their full involvement and participation in the design, planning, implementation and evaluation of programmes is crucial to the development of effective responses to the HIV/AIDS epidemic.'

The concept of GIPA therefore is based on two primary tenets: capacity building for PLWHA and effectiveness of responses to HIV and AIDS – emphasising the mutually beneficial partnerships between the communities of people living with HIV and the institutions involved in the response to HIV and AIDS. The GIPA principle advocates for the recognition of the important role people living with HIV can play in the response to the epidemic; but its application requires countries, societies and communities to create the space for the full and active participation of people living with HIV at every level of the design and implementation of HIV- and AIDS-related programmes and policies.

While GIPA generally refers to the involvement of persons *infected* with HIV, there are those who feel and continue to advocate for the inclusion of people *affected* by HIV and AIDS, such as family and partners. This is based on the premise that while they may not encounter the same type of discrimination as persons with HIV, they do share in the associated stigma through their experiences by virtue of association.

According to a four-country study (Burkina Faso, Ecuador, India and Zambia,) on the involvement of PLWHA in responses to HIV and AIDS, outlining the challenges and benefits of applying GIPA, the involvement

of those living with HIV can take one of four levels of participation:[2]

1. **Access to services** – PLWHA take part in activities as beneficiaries or users of services, such as health care, counselling or training. This is the most common type of PLWHA involvement.

2. **Inclusion** – PLWHA serve as staff and volunteers in non-HIV- and AIDS-related activities, or as occasional volunteers in HIV- and AIDS-related service delivery, such as providing informal peer support and community outreach. Formal training at this stage is limited.

3. **Participation** – PLWHA deliver services on a formal, regular basis. Their expertise is officially recognised by the organisation offering the services as volunteers or staff members and could receive remuneration.

4. **Greater Involvement** – considered to be the highest level of involvement of PLWHA and can be in management, policymaking and strategic planning as directors, trustees or programme managers. As PLWHA may represent their organisation externally, this level of involvement may expose them to risk of stigma and discrimination due to the higher visibility.

GIPA IN THE CARIBBEAN

No Caribbean country (with the exception of the Bahamas) is signatory to the *1994 Paris AIDS Declaration*. However, the Caribbean was represented at the 2001 UNGASS meeting and Caribbean countries are signatories to the *UN Declaration of Commitment on HIV/AIDS*. Following this, Caribbean Community (CARICOM) Heads of State during a meeting in Nassau, Bahamas in July 2001 signed the *Nassau Declaration on Health 2001*, which recognises 'the critical role of health in the economic development of Caribbean people and overawed by the prospect that our current health problems, especially HIV/AIDS, may impede such development',[3] proclaiming 'The Health of the Region is the Wealth of the Region'.

Despite the recognition in the *Nassau Declaration* that the sustainability of regional efforts will require the involvement of civil society and other specialised stakeholders, there was no clear or formal commitment to the involvement of people living with HIV or, more specifically, the GIPA principle in the response to the epidemic in the region – a region where there exists a high level of stigma and discrimination towards HIV and AIDS and, more importantly, against those living with HIV and key populations most vulnerable to HIV.

The Pan Caribbean Partnership Against HIV/AIDS (PANCAP), established at the February 2001 meeting of the CARICOM Heads of State and endorsed by the Nassau Declaration, has been identified by UNAIDS as a 'best practice' and this model of regional cooperation and collaboration in the response to HIV and AIDS is currently used to inform the responses of other regions of the world. According to PANCAP,[4] the Partnership aims to scale up the response to HIV/AIDS in the region. Its specific mandate is:

- To advocate for HIV/AIDS issues at government and highest levels.
- To coordinate the regional response and mobilise resources both regional and international.
- To increase country-level resources, both human and financial, to address the epidemic.

GIPA AND EDUCATION IN THE CARIBBEAN

In his keynote address to the CARICOM meeting on *Stigma & Discrimination* in 2004, Sir George Alleyne, UN Secretary-General's Special Envoy for HIV/AIDS to the Caribbean, noted that an important aspect of accelerating the education sector's response to the epidemic is the 'embracing of persons living with HIV/AIDS. The Caribbean Network of [PLWHA] is strong and growing but it would be ideal if it was recognised more publicly, embraced and supported by leaders in our society'.[5]

The application of GIPA in the education sector's response, which could take place at all stages of the development, dissemination and implementation of policies could, make the following contributions:

- *Contributing to the reduction of stigma and discrimination* – Developing policies for the education sector with the input of the infected community ensures that policies are developed in accordance with basic human rights, taking into account the right to education and a safe learning environment for HIV-positive children, as well as ensuring a safe workplace environment for teachers, learners and staff infected with and/or affected by HIV/AIDS with zero tolerance for discrimination against both students and staff. Persons living with HIV can serve as role models which also help to de-stigmatise the disease. The rights-based and meaningful involvement of PLWHA could also contribute, not only to the reduction of stigma and discrimination against those living with and/or affected by HIV, but also to the reduction of stigma and discrimination against vulnerable key populations at most risk to HIV, particularly important for concentrated epidemics such as those seen in the CARICOM countries.

- *Delivering more effective prevention programmes* – Behaviour Change Communication programmes developed in collaboration with, and/or implemented by, persons living with HIV as resource persons will be more effective as people living with HIV act as peer educators and put a human face to the epidemic. Children also generally learn more effectively by example. First-hand accounts of living with HIV also provide a broader understanding for students and faculty of the challenges of living with HIV, breaking down myths about HIV transmission and prevention, and dissociation of personal risks and vulnerabilities based on perception of membership to particular key populations.

- *Creating a supportive environment* – Persons living with HIV working within the education sector can also assist with the provision of formal or informal counselling services to students and staff, which helps to create a supportive environment within the school setting for those most affected by HIV to become more involved. The involvement of HIV-positive teachers, learners and staff in the design, dissemination and implementation of education sector workplace policies on HIV and AIDS will promote and support safer learning environments and workplace settings, not only for those PLWHA directly involved during the process, but more importantly those infected with and/or affected by HIV who are not in a position to be meaningfully involved due to fear of stigma and discrimination based on real and/or perceived HIV status.

A quick review of several member networks of the Caribbean Regional Network of CRN+ vis-à-vis their collaboration with the education sector in national responses to HIV and AIDS revealed that, for the most part, national networks have neither formal nor informal partnerships with the education sector. There are a few exceptions, with some networks that work directly with a small number of schools in their countries during HIV- and AIDS-related sensitisation activities with students, giving a face to the epidemic and allowing the students the opportunity to interact with someone living with HIV, to learn first hand about prevention, stigma, discrimination and the challenges of living with HIV. Much of this work, however, is not structured and is very ad hoc; there is often no follow-up or regular frequency for conducting such sessions. In addition, because there are no formal agreements or clear guidelines for involving people living with HIV in the education response, there is a lack of capacity-building that can help to ensure the effective implementation of the GIPA principle. Furthermore, persons taking part in this type of educational outreach often do so voluntarily and are not compensated.

CRN+

HISTORY

The Caribbean Regional Network of People Living with HIV/AIDS (CRN+) was established on September 28, 1996. It is part of the Global Network of People Living with HIV/AIDS (GNP+), whose overall aim is to improve the quality of life of people living with HIV.

CRN+ is dedicated to raising awareness of PLWHA primarily, but not exclusively, within the Caribbean Basin through advocacy, lobbying and sensitisation strategies. Indeed, its main thrust is to improve access to information exchange, advocacy, and to build capacity among PLWHA and their networks in the region.

In order to effectively achieve its mission, the establishment of national networks in its member territories has been undertaken. CRN+ has initiated a strategy that emphasises skills training and capacity building (both human and institutional) in all the above-mentioned focus areas. Its long-term goal envisages empowered regional/national networks of PLWHA who will:

1. Create/influence policy and legislative decisions;
2. Establish links and maintain these through spirited cooperation and coordination with key national and international stakeholders in both the public and private sphere;
3. Improve their access to treatment, care and support;
4. Reduce and eliminate stigma and discrimination, and
5. Encourage research and development with respect to HIV and AIDS.

VISION STATEMENT

"CRN+ is the authentic voice of Caribbean people living with HIV/AIDS. As a full and equal partner in the collaborative fight against HIV/AIDS, CRN+ is driven by [PLWHA] making a meaningful difference to their lives"

MISSION STATEMENT

"The Caribbean Regional Network of people living with HIV/AIDS (CRN+) is committed to empowering and supporting persons affected and infected with HIV/AIDS through advocacy, research, partnership, capacity building and resource mobilization".

JAMAICA NETWORK OF SEROPOSITIVES (JN+) AND EDUCATION SECTOR

JN+

HISTORY

The Jamaican Network of Seropositives (JN+) was formed in 1997 following the establishment of CRN+ the previous year. JN+ now has offices in all six (6) regions of Jamaica and is part of CRN+. Currently JN+ receives the support from the National AIDS Programme (currently managed by the Ministry of Health), GTZ, UNV GIPA Project, PAHO, UNAIDS, JRC, NAPWA and NHCP. Funding for JN+ is primarily through Jamaica's grant from the Global Fund to fight AIDS, Tuberculosis and Malaria, currently managed by the Ministry of Health.

JN+ MAIN ACTIVITIES (IN ADDITION TO THE SUPPORT TO ITS MEMBERS AND OTHER PLHIV)

- Member of the National AIDS Committee and collaboration with the Committee's member institutions.
- Member of the UN Theme Group on HIV/AIDS.
- Collaboration with UNAIDS Jamaica office; UNAIDS is represented on the technical advisory board of JN+
- Recent collaborative work with ILO and the National AIDS Committee acting as resource in a "behavioural change" campaign for the private sector (in the workplace)
- Participation in the World AIDS Day-related events with the Ministry of Education and UNICEF on a series of activities, which included a "Lesson For Life"
- JN+ members contribute regularly to the Ministry of Education trainings of school administrators (mainly through testimonials of PLHIV)

VISION STATEMENT

"Persons living with HIV/AIDS accepted and recognized as full members of society"

MISSION STATEMENT

"To advocate for the rights and concerns of people living with HIV/AIDS, through empowerment, partnership and resource mobilization."

SUCCESSES AND CHALLENGES OF JN+

The recent collaborative work of JN+ with the National AIDS Committee and, more importantly, through its active participation in Country Coordinating Mechanisms, is changing the 'tokenism' engagement of PLWHA in Jamaica to a stronger application of GIPA in policy areas.

JN+ has also built collaborative relationships with UNAIDS Cosponsors (mainly UNICEF, ILO and UNESCO), UNAIDS Secretariat and the Jamaica Red Cross. In 2006, JN+ took part in a capacity building retreat for JN+ board members and members of the Jamaica AIDS Support.

The main challenges faced by JN+ are the high level of stigma attached to HIV and the capacity of JN+ and its members. One of the results of stigma is the limitation of outreach work to treatment centres. Expanding outreach work to public spaces requires addressing stigma and discrimination faced by PLWHA in the country.

The capacity needs of JN+ are directly related to the Network's level of involvement and contribution to national policies. Addressing the capacity needs of JN+ is considered by the Network as a more urgent need than resource mobilisation. Capacity-building opportunities for JN+ are mostly available in Kingston, which poses additional difficulties to those JN+ members from other regions.

In addition to capacity needs, the current membership of JN+ does not represent the full sociocultural and socio-economic spectrum of society – with the most economically vulnerable currently forming the JN+ membership.

Achieving a critical mass of members, especially when it comes to representativity, is not only a challenge to Jamaica, however, but to any low HIV prevalence country.

JN+ COOPERATION WITH MINISTRY OF EDUCATION, YOUTH AND CULTURE (MOEYC)

The collaboration of JN+ with the Ministry of Education, Youth and Culture lies mostly within the framework of the Ministry's Education Department. In particular, in the Education's sensitisation and awareness-raising activities with school administrators, as well as the scaling-up of dissemination and implementation efforts of the Jamaica HIV/AIDS workplace policy in education institutions.

Following formal requests by the Ministry of Education, JN+ members give testimonial presentations for school principals, administrative staff, parents and teachers in all regions of the country. As a result, JN+ participation has enhanced the quality and effectiveness of activities, but also contributed to JN+ capacity building.

JN+ has also collaborated with the Ministry of Education in individual cases of discrimination against HIV-positive children in schools, including refusal of admission. Following the action of JN+ outreach officers and the Ministry of Education, through collaborative efforts, the Ministry of Education was able to achieve the re-admission of the HIV-positive children to school. These cases of discrimination, however, remain undocumented.[6]

JN+ AND NON-FORMAL EDUCATION

JN+ and its members have also participated in many non-formal education activities, such as the recent anti-stigma campaign launched by the Ministry of Health, and outreach work at treatment centres and support groups. It is worth noting that HIV and AIDS education outside the classroom in primary through secondary education is managed by the Ministry of Health.

CHALLENGES OF GIPA APPLICATION IN THE JAMAICAN EDUCATION SECTOR

The placement of the National AIDS Committee within and the management of Jamaica's grant from GFATM by the Ministry of Health reinforces the impression that HIV and AIDS in Jamaica is a health sector issue. Similarly, the UWI's HIV and AIDS Response Programme (HARP) is located within the Medical Faculty. The above, have consequences on the ability of the Ministry of Education and the tertiary education institutions' ability to advocate for HIV- and AIDS-related policies and programmes and the national response to HIV and AIDS of the Jamaican education sector. Despite this, the Ministry of Education has managed to scale-up HIV- and AIDS-related policy and programme development in schools. Activities include development of curricula, early childhood development and HIV/AIDS, adaptation of HFLE to include HIV and AIDS content, development of HIV/AIDS workplace policies, and promotion of its HIV and AIDS policy for schools.

Further scale-up efforts and the application of GIPA in the Education Sector will require a continuous and increased commitment from high-level decision makers at both Ministerial level as well as school level.

In regard to JN+, the main challenges as mentioned above are capacity of JN+ members, representativity of JN+ membership, and the stigma and discrimination faced by those living with HIV.

FUTURE POSSIBLE ENTRY POINTS FOR COOPERATION BETWEEN MOEYC AND JN+

- Incorporate JN+ into the working group for implementation of the national education sector HIV/AIDS workplace policy
- The involvement of HIV-positive teachers in the implementation of workplace policies.
- The use of local cultural context to define the structure and content of responses to HIV and AIDS that include the participation of PLWHA. This includes the use of non-formal learning environment.
- A formalised partnership between MoE and JN+ to reflect a long-term relationship, with clear expectations, targets, deliverables and terms of reference for each party.
- The recent restructuring of CRN+ and the recent formal structuring of JN+ can serve as opportunities to enhance the capacity of JN+.
- The fact that UCC Jamaica serves on the board of JN+, as well as the fact that UNICEF, UNESCO, ILO and World Bank are key partners of the MoE in HIV and AIDS Education, can provide additional entry points to support JN+ empowerment and its contribution to Education Sector responses.
- Addressing the needs of HIV-positive children – treatment, care and support, as well as cases of discrimination.
- HIV-positive teachers, parents and/ or community members can serve as participants to Health Advisory Committees at school level.

In addition, there is a need to develop guidelines for MoE to bring GIPA in action:

advocacy, technical guidelines, multi-sectoral response opportunities, best practice and good policy assessment and guidelines on adaptation to local context of other country experiences.

To develop such guidelines, an assessment needs to be undertaken of what are possible entry points within and obstacles to be overcome for governmental bodies, ministries and other national institutions. Past, current and future work that can inform such assessment include:

- the work commissioned by UNESCO on the UWI institutional response to HIV and AIDS,
- the current work by the UNESCO Chair, Prof. Plummer, on assessing GIPA for education,
- as well as documenting cases of stigma.

The actual procedures followed by PLWHA networks such as JN+ when they receive a request for contribution by one of their members can also help to inform those guidelines. For example, upon reception of a request from Ministry of Education to JN+, JN+ takes the following steps:

- Formal form requested by JN+ on background information on the meeting
- JN+ determines its member able to contribute to the meeting given the location, date and more importantly the expected contribution from JN+
- Ministry of Education signs an agreement on its obligation vis-à-vis JN+ such as travel and participation costs
- Ministry of Education signs an agreement on its responsibilities vis-à-vis the JN+ representative's rights
- When member returns from session, he/she provides feedback to the Network on

session content as well as issues arising.

The above steps ensure respect for JN+ member's rights, and will inform future collaboration and how to improve the relationship between the two organisations,

Lastly, JN+ like many other PLWHA networks, has shown success in advocacy and entering National AIDS teams. Their experience and lessons learned can serve to inform Ministries of Education to determine entry points to national HIV- and AIDS-related bodes.

CHALLENGES TO ACHIEVING GIPA IN EDUCATION IN THE CARIBBEAN

Even though the Governments of CARICOM have not taken an official stand on the issue of the greater involvement of people living with HIV/AIDS in the Caribbean response to the epidemic, national AIDS responses have sought to increase the level of participation of PLWHA through continued advocacy by national networks as well as CRN+. The PLWHA community is involved at all levels of HIV/AIDS programmes from decision-making and policy development to implementation of programmes and projects.

Despite the success stories, there continue to be challenges in applying the GIPA principle and, in some cases where there is involvement it remains tokenistic, prompting the HIV-positive global community to speak out for the *more meaningful* involvement of people living with HIV/AIDS (MIPA).

While there are many reasons that contribute to the challenges in applying GIPA in the Caribbean – such as the high stigma and discrimination attached to HIV and AIDS – some of the challenges identified by PLWHA national networks particular to the education response to HIV and AIDS are:

1. *Level of involvement of the education sector* – Despite the critical role education plays in both the prevention of HIV as well as the reduction of stigma and discrimination, the education sector has been slow in designing and implementing a sectoral response to HIV and AIDS and/or scaling-up of efforts. In some cases it is still not involved in any formal way in the national HIV/AIDS programme.

2. *Absence of policies* – The absence of HIV- and AIDS-specific policies within the education sector is another challenge. Few countries in the region have HIV/AIDS workplace policies for the education sector which set out clear guidelines for a safe environment (workplace and learning) for persons living with and/or affected by HIV that includes the right to education and a safe learning environment for HIV-positive children. In the cases where HIV/AIDS workplaces exist, the principle of GIPA is generally not reflected in policies, and there is a lack of mechanisms that encourage sharing of experiences and skills of persons living with HIV.[7]

3. *Absence of HIV- and AIDS-related curricula* – HIV and AIDS education is often not included in the school formal curriculum. Curricula on HIV and AIDS could provide entry points for the application of GIPA in the education sector.

4. *Lack of leadership for the education sector* – Although many persons in health ministries have shown clear leadership on the issues related to HIV throughout the region, the education sector faces challenges not only in clearly defining its role but also in taking up the mantle of leadership in the response to the epidemic. In National Strategic Plans, responses to HIV and AIDS remain largely the responsibility of the health sector.

5. *Poor communication* – National networks of PLWHA continue to face difficulties working with Ministries, in particular, Ministries of Education. There is poor communication between the two bodies as well as a lack of understanding of the GIPA principle and determining entry points for its application.

6. *Inability to provide supportive health care management within the school setting* – Educational institutions lack the capacity to provide the necessary management, care and treatment for HIV-positive children. This is of particular concern to members of the staff for whom providing education and not care and support is seen as their primary responsibility to students. Fostering an understanding of the medical and social support needs of HIV-positive children in the school setting may help to address this issue and bring about a better understanding of the needs of these children. Proper student and teacher health is essential for high academic performance.

7. *Limited capacity of persons living with HIV* – Many people living with HIV are enthusiastic and motivated to share their experiences in order to promote better understanding of the disease or to assist in programme implementation. However, motivation and enthusiasm cannot sustain programmes, and many people living with HIV have a need to develop their individual capacity in order to strengthen their contributions and also enable them to overcome their fears to disclose their status.

The above challenges, although brought up by PLWHA networks in the Caribbean, apply to other regions in the world.

RECOMMENDATIONS FOR THE WAY FORWARD

1. Draft a Caribbean GIPA Declaration as an addendum to the Nassau Declaration that clearly formalises and endorses the commitment to the principle of GIPA.

2. Develop policies and introduce supportive legislation that will seek to enforce the rights of students as well as educators (zero tolerance for discriminatory behaviour and stigmatisation of students, teachers and staff). Involve people living with HIV in this policy development as well as in programme implementation and research.

3. Develop a model for the education sector for working with people living with HIV, clearly defining recruitment and training strategies, normative guidelines for the process of involvement of PLWHA, remuneration, incentives, monitoring and evaluation and supportive mechanisms. Use educational institutions to deliver training programmes. (See Annex 2 – Suggestions for a draft model)

4. Encourage partnerships and formalise agreements between Ministries of Education and National PLWHA networks, clearly defining joint planning strategies, procedures, and shared roles and responsibilities in programme implementation.

5. Develop a more comprehensive approach to a healthy educational environment including psycho-social support for teachers and children

infected and/or affected by HIV/AIDS, the educational needs of orphans and vulnerable children (OVC) and how to address stigma and discrimination through education.

CONCLUSION

Since 1983, when the idea of involving people living with HIV in all aspects of the response to HIV and AIDS was first articulated by the community of HIV-positive people themselves, GIPA, even though it has been formalised in principle by governments in the Paris Declaration, has struggled to move meaningfully from principle to practice.

The leading role in the realisation of the GIPA principle continues to lie largely among communities infected with and/or affected by HIV/AIDS. This persists despite the numerous studies showing that the involvement of people living with HIV in a meaningful way is an essential element of effective responses.

Strengthening and sustaining the role of PLWHA in the Caribbean's education response will require a multisectoral and comprehensive national and regional response. With the greater availability of anti-retroviral therapies (ART) and the low HIV prevalence (concentrated mainly in distinct key populations), the National Strategic Plans of the Caribbean countries may require revision to support the education sectors to develop and cultivate entry points for PLWHA involvement and to address the following:

1. HIV and AIDS is not only a health issue but a socio-economic and cultural issue. Thus, the role of other sectors in addition to the health sector, such as

education, can greatly contribute to HIV and AIDS responses;

2. the particular needs of vulnerable populations, and more importantly, the social exclusion and marginalisation of these key populations, leads to dissociation with real vulnerabilities to HIV by the general population. Therefore, addressing stigma and discrimination towards PLWHA and key populations and ensuring a rights-based approach is crucial to the effectiveness of HIV-prevention programmes;

3. the particular needs of women and girls in regard to HIV and AIDS, which include traditional gender roles and gender-based vulnerabilities;

4. the particular needs of HIV-positive children, which include documenting and addressing cases of stigma and discrimination, availability of and capacity to provide antiretroviral treatment for children, and treatment-related education for the teachers and parents;

5. effective responses to HIV and AIDS need to be inclusive and provide necessary linkages between prevention, treatment, care and support;

6. increasing access to voluntary and confidential counselling and testing facilities;

7. providing access to and availability of antiretroviral treatment to all those who need it so they can remain active in their chosen fields of work;

8. creating the practical and political space for people living with HIV to expand their role and contribution by addressing HIV-related stigma and discrimination; promoting appropriate legal and policy environments; building

the capacity and skills of PLWHA involved in responses to HIV and AIDS, and supporting participation with resources, including organisational development;

9. the role tertiary education institutions can play in the response to HIV and AIDS, which include teacher training programmes and training of healthcare workers;

10. Linking schools with communities and community institutions, including faith-based organisations, parents–teachers associations, youth centres and other institutions involved in non-formal education. Developing strategies to form linkages as well as developing programmes to deliver HIV- and AIDS-related sensitisation and awareness are equally important.

HIV/AIDS organisations already exist in many forms, from support and service-delivery bodies to advocacy and representational organisations. In the face of a long-standing but constantly changing epidemic, the range of these organisations needs to be extended even further. HIV/AIDS organisations are reaching out beyond PLWHA networks, to non-health-care settings – to workplaces, faith-based settings, schools and other institutions.

Networks of people living with HIV are demonstrating their commitment to forging new partnerships. However, for the commitment to translate into the application of GIPA, there is a need for support in order to enhance their organisational capacities and meet the challenges.

No single approach to implementing GIPA can be successful given the various challenges. Nevertheless, there is sufficient evidence from around the world to inform on how GIPA can be effectively translated into action.

The experience of JN+, and CRN+ in general, can serve to inform how to improve the level of GIPA application and the effectiveness of responses to HIV and AIDS, not only for the Caribbean region, but for other regions and countries with high levels of stigma and discrimination.

SELECTED REFERENCES

CRN+. 2006. Operation Manual.

UNESCO. 2005. *The "GIPA" Principle and Accelerating the Response of the Education Sector in the Caribbean to HIV/AIDS.* Kingston: UNESCO Office for the Caribbean.

UNESCO. 2004. *Education and HIV/AIDS.* Quarterly report to United Nations HIV/AIDS Theme Groups in the Caribbean, Issue 8, December. Kingston: UNESCO Office for the Caribbean.

UNAIDS. 1999. *From principle to practice: Greater Involvement of People Living with or Affected by HIV/AIDS (GIPA).* UNAIDS Best Practice Collection.

UNAIDS. 2002. *The faces, voices and skills behind the GIPA workplace wodel in South Africa.* UNAIDS Case Study. UNAIDS Best Practice Collection

International HIV/AIDS Alliance, Horizons-Population Council, and USAID. 2003. *The involvement of people living with HIV/AIDS in community-based prevention, care and support programs in developing countries – A multi-country diagnostic study.*

ANNEX 1
Declaration of the Paris AIDS Summit
1 December 1994
(Note: statements directly related to GIPA are in italics)

We the Heads of Government or Representatives of the 42 States assembled in Paris on 1 December, 1994:

I.   MINDFUL that the AIDS pandemic, by virtue of its magnitude, constitutes a threat to humanity, that its spread is affecting all societies that it is hindering the social and economic development, in particular of the worst affected countries, and increasing disparities within and between countries, that poverty and discrimination are contributing factors in the spread of the pandemic, that HIV/AIDS inflicts irreparable damage on families and communities, that the pandemic concerns all people without distinction but that women, children and youth are becoming infected at an increasing rate, that it not only causes physical and emotional suffering, but is often used as a justification for grave violations of human rights,

MINDFUL ALSO that obstacles of all kinds – cultural, legal, economic and political – are hampering information, prevention, care and support efforts, that HIV/AIDS prevention and care support strategies are inseparable, and hence must be an integral component of an effective and comprehensive approach to combating the pandemic, that new local, national and international forms of solidarity are emerging, involving in particular people living with HIV/AIDS and community based organisations,

II. SOLEMNLY DECLARE our obligation as political leaders to make the fight against HIV/AIDS a priority, our obligation to act with compassion for and in solidarity with those with HIV or at risk of becoming infected, both within our societies and internationally, *our determination to ensure that all persons living with HIV/ AIDS are able to realise the full and equal enjoyment of their fundamental rights and freedoms without distinction and under all circumstances, our determination to fight against poverty, stigmatisation, and discrimination, our determination to mobilise all of society – the public and private sectors, community-based organisations and people living with HIV/AIDS –* in a spirit of true partnership, our appreciation and support for the activities and work carried out by multilateral, intergovernmental, nongovernmental and community-based organisations, and our recognition of their important role in combating the pandemic, our conviction that only more vigorous and better coordinated action worldwide, sustained over the long term – such as that to be undertaken by the joint and co-sponsored United Nations programme on HIV/AIDS – can halt the pandemic,

III. UNDERTAKE IN OUR NATIONAL POLICIES TO *protect and promote the rights of individuals, in particular those living with or most vulnerable to HIV/AIDS, through the legal and social environment, fully involve non-governmental and community-based organisations as well as people living with HIV/AIDS in the formulation and implementation of public policies, ensure equal protection under the law for persons living with HIV/AIDS with regard to access to health care, employment, travel, housing and social welfare*, intensify the following range of essential approaches for the prevention of HIV/AIDS:

- promotion of and access to various culturally acceptable prevention strategies and products, including condoms and treatment of sexually transmitted diseases,

- promotion of appropriate prevention education, including sex and gender education, for youth in school and out of school,

- improvement of women's status, education and living conditions,

- *specific risk-reduction activities for and in collaboration with the most vulnerable populations, such as groups at high risk of sexual transmission and migrant populations,*

- the safety of blood and blood products,

- strengthen primary health care systems as a basis for prevention and care, and integrate HIV/AIDS activities into these systems, so as to ensure equitable access to comprehensive care,

- make available necessary resources to better combat the pandemic, including adequate support for people infected with HIV/AIDS, nongovernmental organisations and community-based organisations working with vulnerable populations.

IV. ARE RESOLVED TO STEP UP THE INTERNATIONAL COOPERATION THROUGH THE FOLLOWING MEASURES AND INITIATIVES. We shall do so by providing our commitment and support to the development of the joint and co-sponsored United Nations programme on HIV/AIDS, as the appropriate framework to reinforce partnerships between all involved and give guidance and worldwide leadership in the fight against HIV/AIDS. The scope of each initiative should be further defined and developed in the context of the joint and co-sponsored programme and other appropriate fora:

1. *Support a greater involvement of people living with HIV/AIDS through an initiative to strengthen the capacity and coordination of networks of people living with HIV/AIDS and community-based organisations. By ensuring their full involvement in our common response to the pandemic at all – national, regional and global – levels, this initiative will, in particular, stimulate the creation of supportive political, legal and social environments.*

2. Promote global collaboration for HIV/AIDS research by supporting national and international partnerships between the public and private sectors, in order to accelerate the development of prevention and treatment technologies, including vaccines and microbicides, and to provide for the measures needed to help ensure their accessibility in developing countries. This collaborative effort should include related social and behavioural research.

3. Strengthen international collaboration for blood safety with a view to coordinating technical information, proposing standards for good manufacturing practice for all blood products, and fostering the establishment and implementation of cooperative partnerships to ensure blood safety in all countries.

4. Encourage a global care initiative so as to reinforce the national capability of countries, especially those in greatest need, to ensure access to comprehensive care and social support services, essential drugs and existing preventive methods.

5. Mobilise local, national and international organisations assisting as part of their regular activities, children and youth, including orphans, at risk of infection or affected by HIV/AIDS, in order to encourage a global partnership to reduce the impact of the HIV/AIDS pandemic upon the world's children and youth.

6. Support initiatives to reduce the vulnerability of women to HIV/AIDS by encouraging national and international efforts aimed at the empowerment of women: by raising their status and eliminating adverse social, economic and cultural factors; by ensuring their participation in all the decision-making and implementation processes which concern them; and by establishing linkages and strengthening the networks that promote women's rights.

7. *Strengthen national and international mechanisms that are concerned with HIV/AIDS related human rights and ethics, including the use of an advisory council and national and regional*

networks to provide leadership, advocacy and guidance in order to ensure that non-discrimination, human rights and ethical principles form an integral part of the response to the pandemic.

We urge all countries and the international community to provide the resources necessary for the measures and initiatives mentioned above.

We call upon all countries, the future joint and co-sponsored United Nations programme on HIV/AIDS and its six member organisations and programmes to take all steps possible to implement this Declaration in accordance with other multilateral and bilateral aid programmes and intergovernmental and non-governmental organisations.

Countries which were represented at the Paris Summit and signed the Declaration:

Argentina, Australia, Bahamas, Belgium, Brazil, Burundi, Cambodia, Cameroon, Canada, China, Côte d'Ivoire, Denmark, Djibouti, Finland, France, Germany, India, Indonesia, Italy, Japan, Mexico, Morocco, Mozambique, Netherlands, Norway, Philippines, Portugal, Romania, Russian Federation, Senegal, Spain, Sweden, Switzerland, United Republic of Tanzania, Thailand, Tunisia, Uganda, United Kingdom, United States of America, Viet Nam, Zambia, Zimbabwe.

ANNEX 2

Suggestions for draft model for working with PLWHA in the education sector

- **Select candidates according to their skills, which correspond to the needs of the organisations and/or programmes.**

This will improve the effectiveness of programmes and policy implementation.

- **Select candidates from within a partner organisation, or from support groups in the area,** to avoid the stresses of relocation, maximise local knowledge and build sustainability. This will also ensure building ownership of programmes and policies by local communities and stakeholders.

- **Select from all backgrounds,** because it is skills and competence profiles that define ability to take on a meaningful role in a workplace. This will also ensure the representation of PLWHA vis-à-vis their communities.

- **Building capacity and skills of PLWHA and their networks** so that GIPA fieldworkers can operate in a formal workplace and help implement formal workplace programmes. This will also allow the involvement of PLWHA to move from access to services, inclusion and/or participation to a greater involvement of PLWHA.

- **Demand management collaboration and commitment from decision- and policy-makers,** from divisions such as human resource management, unions, health care and employee benefits.

- **Build in performance appraisal and skill/performance-based remuneration** to attract the best-quality candidates and ensure appropriate job descriptions.

- **Clarify job descriptions** to direct GIPA fieldworkers to areas where they can make maximum impact and ensure that partner organisations provide the financial and management skills needed to define other elements crucial to workplace policies and programmes.

- **Provide health care and emotional support** as selection and employment involve constant public exposure and media attention, in addition to the demands of counselling. This is particularly important in areas of high stigma.

- **Set up a positive environment and methods of redress** so that national and corporate policy supports people with HIV on issues such as access to medical care and education.
- **Ensure confidentiality** because the involvement of a person living with HIV does not imply public disclosure of one's HIV status.
- **Set up mechanisms of addressing stigma and discrimination.**

participation of Ministries of Health, teachers' unions and other key stakeholders in the creation and adoption of a Caribbean HIV/AIDS workplace policy.

NOTES

1. Paris Declaration. December 1994. http://www.ecpp.co.uk/parisdeclaration.htm, accessed 4 June 2006.
2. International HIV/AIDS Alliance, Horizons-Population Council, and USAID, 2003.
3. Nassau Declaration on Health 2001, July 2001. http://www.caricom.org/jsp/communications/meeting_minutes/nassau_declaration_on_health.jsp?menu=communications, accessed 4 June 2006
4. PANCAP, http://www.pancap.org, accessed 7 June 2006.
5. UNESCO Office for the Caribbean. 2004.
6. There is anecdotal evidence of discrimination of HIV-positive children (e.g. refusal to admission, isolation of HIV-positive children by other children, etc.) but very few or no documented cases. In Jamaica, for example, the Ministry of Education, when such cases come to its attention, has worked with the schools and parents of HIV-positive children to allow admission to and create a more supportive learning environment for those children.
7. UNESCO and ILO began collaboration in 2005 on the elaboration and implementation of HIV/AIDS education sector workplace policies. Within the framework of this collaboration, a workshop was held in the Caribbean region, with the active

25

THE MASTERS IN EDUCATION (HEALTH PROMOTION)

DAVID PLUMMER

COMMONWEALTH-UNESCO REGIONAL CHAIR IN
EDUCATION (HIV/AIDS/HEALTH PROMOTION),
THE UNIVERSITY OF THE WEST INDIES, SCHOOL
OF EDUCATION, FACULTY OF HUMANITIES AND
EDUCATION, ST AUGUSTINE, TRINIDAD AND
TOBAGO

*The University of the West Indies established the first Chair in the world in Education & HIV/
AIDS in 2005, with the support of UNESCO and the Commonwealth Secretariat, to promote
teaching, research and public service in this emerging field. The first chair holder, Professor David
Plummer, designed a professional degree following extensive regional and international consultation.
The graduate programme in Health and Human Relationships,* Masters in Education (Health
Promotion), *outlined in this chapter, was approved by the university in June 2006, and the first
cohort of 30 enrolled in December 2006.*

BACKGROUND

The importance of health for Caribbean
people has long been acknowledged by
Caribbean governments and multilateral
agencies such as PAHO and CARICOM.
Disease prevention, health promotion and
health education have been widely recognised
as key strategies in strengthening the health
of the region. More recently, the inexorable
spread of HIV and the realisation that the
Caribbean people are second only to sub-
Saharan Africa in terms of HIV prevalence,
has introduced a new sense of urgency into
the health education and health promotion
fields.

In responding to HIV, Caribbean
governments initially looked to their
respective health authorities for guidance.
More recently, Caribbean education
ministries have started to recognise a greater
role for the education sector in responding to
HIV/AIDS. In part this has been prompted
by the realisation that schoolchildren have
among the lowest rates of infection in the
population, and that if they can be kept
uninfected into adulthood, then HIV can be
radically reduced within a generation. This
realisation is made even more compelling
given that infection rates rise rapidly in late
adolescence and early adulthood – the period
of low infection during the early school
years is immediately followed by a period
of extreme risk during the teens and early
adulthood.

Over the years, there have been various
programmes to promote better health among
schoolchildren and the wider community.
The current Caribbean framework for health
education in schools is known as Health
and Family Life Education (HFLE). This
programme has been in existence since the

1970s in one form or another. However, while HFLE has long been recognised as having great potential for assisting Caribbean societies to adjust to the changing social pressures of a modern world, it is fair to say that HFLE implementation is yet to live up to those expectations, particularly with respect to HIV. There are many reasons why this shortfall might have occurred, including social taboos, political pressures, sensitivity of the subject matter, competing educational priorities, lack of accredited subject status, lack of professional career paths, lack of formal qualifications, and so on.

In response to these issues, The University of the West Indies (UWI) has established a professional and academic stream in Health Education and Health Promotion at the School of Education, St Augustine, Trinidad. This programme has the following objectives:

1. to establish a credible and *internationally respected professional and academic stream* in Health and Human Relationships in Education with special emphasis on HIV/AIDS and HFLE;
2. to establish and promote *professional qualifications, skills, and standards* in Health and Human Relationships in the education sector, with special emphasis on HIV/AIDS and HFLE;
3. to *develop and promote research* into Health and Human Relationships in Education, with special emphasis on HIV/AIDS and HFLE; and
4. to *engage with policy makers in order to develop effective responses* to Health and Human Relationships in Education, with special emphasis on HIV/AIDS and HFLE.

OVERVIEW OF THE MASTERS IN EDUCATION (HEALTH PROMOTION)

The centrepiece of the UWI response to the need to strengthen Caribbean health education training is the M.Ed. (Health Promotion). This degree is intended to be the premiere professional qualification to work in health and human relationships education and health promotion in the region. The M.Ed. (Health Promotion) is designed to be cross disciplinary (reaching the health, welfare and education sectors); to include formal 'in-school' education and informal extra-mural, community and workplace education; and is based on the assumption that education is life-long.

The M.Ed. (Health Promotion) programme will:

- meet the demands of the HIV epidemic by producing highly skilled personnel with specialised advanced training, so that the Caribbean education sector can mount a vigorous response to HIV/AIDS and other priority health issues;
- advance scholarship in the area of HFLE so that the capacity and response of the Caribbean education sector to social development and change can be strengthened;
- be the flagship qualification for developing a professional career path in health and human relationships education in the education sector;
- be a flagship qualification for health promotion training in the Caribbean for the health, welfare, labour, and education sectors; and
- provide a strong foundation for progressing to research-only higher degrees in the field of health promotion, especially doctoral

research in health promotion and health and human relationships.

OBJECTIVES OF THE MASTERS IN EDUCATION (HEALTH PROMOTION)

- To develop a sound knowledge base and a strong sense of intellectual inquiry for working with people of all ages on issues relating to health promotion, and health and human relationships in the Caribbean
- To develop strong practical skills to address issues relating to health and human relationships in a variety of settings (individual, group, family, classroom, and population-level policy and programme development)
- To develop monitoring, evaluation, and research competencies that can be confidently applied in professional and academic settings and in the field
- To work within an ethical framework that emphasises human rights, social justice, and equity to promote good citizenship and social responsibility, and which values diversity in the Caribbean

TARGET AUDIENCE OF THE MASTERS IN EDUCATION (HEALTH PROMOTION)

The principal target audience will consist of people working in health promotion and health education; with adults and/or children; in the formal and informal education sectors; from health and educational sectors; and from the three main UWI countries as well as the 'UWI 12'. Participants will include:

- Professionals in the formal school sector
- Health and family life educators
- Tertiary sector staff, particularly in a train-the-trainer relationship, for example, with staff of teachers' colleges

- Workers in the non-formal education sector whose role includes health promotion
- Counselling, guidance, and social workers
- Nurse educators
- Creative arts and communication workers
- Youth workers and officers from the Ministry of Youth
- Workplace health and safety programmes
- Designated health promotion workers
- Health and education sector administrators, policy makers, planners, and implementers

STRUCTURE OF THE MASTERS IN EDUCATION (HEALTH PROMOTION)

Admission requirements: A bachelor's degree in health, education, or social sciences from an approved university with at least lower second-class standing.

Credits and attendance: 35 credit points and a 75% attendance are required to successfully complete the Masters programme.

Duration: The programme will run on a 2-year part-time basis.

Summary of programme structure: The programme is designed to maximise access to the programme by professionals working in health promotion/health education field; and to maximise access to the programme by professionals who are based elsewhere in the Caribbean, particularly in the 'UWI 12' countries. In order to achieve these outcomes, the programme will:

(a) be run part-time over two years to allow health and education professionals to continue their duties at their home base while undertaking advanced training;

(b) be delivered using a combination of intensive face-to-face teaching and distance modalities;

(c)   the face-to-face components will be delivered in residential school blocks in Trinidad during the Summer school and pre-Christmas periods;

(d)   the distance components will be possible from the person's home base, and include activities such as professional development, fieldwork and literature reviews.

Summary of programme content: The programme is divided into 6 components.

The main objective of year 1 is to establish a solid knowledge base in the relationships between health, behaviour and social life. This will be achieved primarily through components A and B of the curriculum. These components are primarily designed to equip candidates with the foundation knowledge and skills necessary to inform the design of meaningful health promotion interventions. The programme will be delivered in such a way as to foster the simultaneous development of suitable attitudes for working with sensitive issues.

There is a strong emphasis on sexual health in this initial year because: (1) there is an urgent need to strengthen the Caribbean response to the AIDS epidemic; (2) sexual health has been the most difficult element of HFLE to implement in the Caribbean to date; and (3) of the complexities of this area, mastery of sexual health promotion will result in solid skills for working in other areas of health promotion too. Year 1 will also include the first part of the component designed to develop academic skills in reviewing the literature, writing, and research and evaluation design (component D); professional development fieldwork (component E); and developing the student's research proposal (component F).

Component C is a year-long component that primarily aims to develop the necessary skills for designing and delivering health promoting interventions. These interventions and the skills developed will range from individual (counselling) skills through to group, community, and 'macro skills' for institutional responses such as public policy, programme, and campaign development. Component C and the remainder of components D, E, & F will be undertaken in Year 2.

OUTLINE OF NEW COURSES IN THE MASTERS IN EDUCATION (HEALTH PROMOTION)

THE HEALTH AND HUMAN RELATIONSHIPS KNOWLEDGE BASE

Rationale
Part 1: Nature and nurture – the social construction of health

Just as the literature review is the indispensable basis for sound research, a sound evidence-base is an essential foundation for any discipline. In the case of programmes to work with controversial and highly stigmatised conditions (such as HIV and STI) and for working with marginalised populations, starting with a sound knowledge base is obligatory. This unit, like the entire masters degree programme, is based on the premise that all knowledge is socially constructed and that it is never possible to separate nurture from nature without creating a false binary. This course will therefore cover both. Recognising that knowledge is socially constructed lays the groundwork for reflexive evaluation of the students' own values and attitudes, which will be encouraged throughout the course.

Part 2: Sexual and reproductive health

Within this unit there will be a special focus on sexual and reproductive health. This sub-theme builds on the earlier material in the unit and develops it to a much greater level of detail. The basis for this theme is to explore sensitive and taboo issues of sexuality, gender, and health more deeply. There are several reasons for highlighting sexual health in this course: (1) there is an urgent need to strengthen the Caribbean response to the AIDS epidemic; (2) sexual health has been the most difficult element of HFLE to implement in the Caribbean to date; and (3) because of the complexities of this area, strong skills in sexual health promotion will be extremely useful in other areas of health promotion too.

OBJECTIVES

At the end of the course, participants will:

- Demonstrate an understanding of the colonial and post-colonial basis for health and sexual health
- Be able to discuss the social contexts / social construction of health in the Caribbean
- Critique the theoretical and research bases of gender in development, particularly in relation to health
- Demonstrate a reflexive awareness of the nature and impacts of stigma, marginalisation, and discrimination
- Apply basic biomedical knowledge to inform the development of health promotion interventions
- Demonstrate an understanding of the milestones of human development from embryology through to ageing

- Have a detailed knowledge-base concerning the biomedical aspects of sexual health
- Have a detailed knowledge-base concerning the social construction of sexuality and health, particularly for the Caribbean
- Be able to talk comfortably and competently about sexual health in public settings
- Be skilled at being able to frame biomedical explanations to suit particular social and cultural contexts

CONTENT

- Human dignity
- What is health?
- Determinants of physical, social, and mental health
- Caribbean historical and social contexts
- Social construction of health in the Caribbean
- Gender and society
- Stigma theory, marginalisation, prejudice, discrimination
- Biomedical knowledge base
- Critique of purely biomedical approaches
- Human development & 'the 7 ages': embryology, childhood, puberty, early adulthood, ageing
- Infectious diseases
- Introduction to public health
- Introduction to sexual health:
  - Sexuality and health in Caribbean society
  - STI / HIV/AIDS
  - People with HIV
  - Infertility and contraception
  - Fertility, pregnancy, and parenthood
  - Sexual function and dysfunction
  - Sexuality in health and disease

MAJOR COMPETENCIES TO BE DEVELOPED

- Gain new perspectives on the relationship between nature and nurture
- A spirit of enquiry into the relationship between social contexts and health
- Reflexive and critical thinking in relation to social justice and health
- A biomedical knowledge-base to underpin future health promotion work, including sexual health promotion.
- Communication skills for discussing sexual health in a meaningful and accurate way
- A practical and grounded understanding of the relationships between stigma, marginalisation, and health and how these might affect health promotion

Assessment:

Group class presentations	50%
Examination	50%

REQUIRED READING

Chevannes,B. (2001). *Learning to be a man: Culture, socialistion and gender identity in five Caribbean communities.* Mona: UWI Press. (ISBN: 976 640 092 X)

Goffman, E. (1963). *Stigma: Notes on the management of spoiled identity.* Simone & Schuster. (ISBN: 06710622447)

Kelly, M. J., & Bain, B. (2005). *Education and HIV/AIDS in the Caribbean.* Kingston: Ian Randle Publishers.

Mac an Ghaill Mairtin (1994). *The making of men: Masculinities, sexualities and schooling.* Buckingham: Open University Press. (ISBN: 0-355-15781-5)

Reddock, R.ed. (2004). *Interrogating Caribbean Masculinities: Theoretical and empirical analyses.* Kingston: University of the West Indies Press. (ISBN: 062117110523)

Weeks, J. (1985). *Sexuality and its discontents.* London: Routledge. (ISBN: 0-415-04503-7)

RECOMMENDED READING

Bailey, W., Branche, C., McGarrity, G., Stuart, S. (1998). *Family and the quality of gender relations in the Caribbean.* Mona: Institute for Social and Economic Research. (ISBN: 9764000568)

Chevannes, B. (1999). *What we sow and what we reap: problems in the cultivation of male identity in Jamaica.* Kingston: Grace Kennedy Foundation. (ISBN: 9768041129).

Cooper, S. W., Kellogg, N. D., Giardino, A. P. (2006). *Child sexual exploitation quick reference: for health care, social service, and law enforcement professionals.* G. W. Medical Publishing. (ISBN: 187806021X)

Feldman, S. S., Rosenthal, D. A. eds. (2002). *Talking sexuality: parent-adolescent communication. New directions for child and adolescent development.* San Francisco: Jossey-Bass. (ISBN: 0787963259)

Halstead, J., Halstead M., & Reiss, M. J. (2002). *Sex education: Principles, policy and practice.* London: Routledge-Falmer. (ISBN: 0415232562)

Holmes, K. K., Sparling, P. F., Mardh P.-A., Lemon, S. M, Stamm W. E., Piot P., Wasserheit J. N. eds. (2006) *Sexually transmitted diseases.* McGraw-Hill (ISBN: 007029688X)

Leo-Rhynie, E., Bailey, B., Barrow, C. eds. (1997). *Gender: A Caribbean Multi-disciplinary Perspective.* Kingston: Ian Randle Publishers.

Libby, R. (2006) *The naked truth about sex: A guide to intelligent sexual choices for teenagers and twentysomethings.* California: Freedom Press. (ISBN: 1893910385)

McAnulty, R. D., Burnette, M. M. (2003). *Exploring human sexuality: Making healthy decisions* (2nd ed.). Boston: Allyn & Bacon. (ISBN: 020538059X)

Measor, L. (2000). Young people's views on sex education: Education, attitudes and behaviour. London: Routledge-Falmer. (ISBN: 0750708948)

Mohammed, P., Shepherd, C. (2002). *Gender in Caribbean development.* Mona, Jamaica: University of the West Indies Press. (ISBN: 9768125551)

Newburn, T., Stanko, E. A. eds. (1994). *Just boys doing business? Men, masculinities & crime.* London: Routledge. (ISBN: 0415903201)

Spong, J. S. (1990). *Living in sin? A bishop rethinks human sexuality*. San Francisco: Harper & Row. (ISBN: 0 06 067505 5)

Thorne, B. (1993). *Gender play: Girls and boys in school*. Buckingham: Open University Press. (ISBN: 0 355 19123 1)

WEBSITES

1. www.who.org
2. www.unaids.org
3. www.caricom.org
4. www.unesco.org
5. www.unfpa.org
6. www.unicef.org
7. www.undp.org
8. www.nlm.gov
9. www.cdc.gov

JOURNALS

1. Social Science and Medicine
2. The Lancet
3. The New England Journal of Medicine
4. Morbidity and Mortality Weekly Report

RISK IN THE CONTEXT OF MODERN SOCIAL LIVES

Rationale

Human behaviours are embedded in social relations and cultural forms. In early health promotion programmes, too little attention was paid to the role this 'embeddedness' plays in entrenching risk and generating resistance to protective change. The present course is built on assumptions that knowledge is socially constructed and that behaviours (safe and otherwise) are socially embedded. In order to deepen the candidate's understanding of the influence of embeddedness, this unit will focus on the role of relationships, relationship dynamics and networks in health promotion. The focus will also be on analysing, and understanding risk as it relates to these relationships and networks, and on the impact of these risks on health and well-being.

OBJECTIVES

At the end of the course, participants will:

- Demonstrate a clear understanding of social and cultural influences on behaviour and resistance to change
- Demonstrate understanding and insight into how cultural and social embeddedness can assist in transforming behaviour on a sustainable basis
- Demonstrate an understanding of the relationship between social systems and the promotion and entrenchment of dangerous and unhealthy patterns and practices
- Analyse and critique the social networks that health promotion workers will need to mobilise and work closely with
- Use knowledge of social diversity to work with, and advocate for, people from diverse backgrounds
- Be able to critically analyse health issues in their social context using the concept of 'risk' as an analytical tool
- Be able to critically analyse health issues in a framework of human rights and social justice, and to design health promotion strategies accordingly

CONTENT

- Adolescence, school-ground cultures, peer groups, and gangs
- Relationships in diverse cultures
- Strengthening families and family life
- Gender and power in relationships
- Gender and violence
- Sexual and gender diversity
- Ageing
- Disability
- Mass media and communication
- What is risk?
- Stigmatised conditions, marginalised populations, and unpopular issues

- Networks and socially embedded risks
- Protective networks, the potential of parents, teachers, & peers
- Bullying, violence, harassment, and hate crimes
- Domestic violence and sexual assault
- High-risk settings and special populations – understanding drug use, gay men and women, sex workers, and so on
- Drugs, alcohol, tobacco
- Mental health and suicide
- Poverty and power

MAJOR COMPETENCIES TO BE DEVELOPED

- Critical thinking about social relationships and networks
- Practical skills for working with social networks
- Sensitisation to human rights, social justice, and advocacy for marginalised populations
- Reflexive and critical insights into the candidate's own vantage point and how it might be biased (albeit inadvertently)
- Ability to analyse impacts on people's health and well-being using the lenses of risk, marginalisation, power dynamics and gender
- A capacity to use a risk assessment to plan interventions for improving community health
- Capacity to analyse the causes and social and health impacts of bullying, harassment, violence, sexual assault, and hate crimes
- Insights and skills to work effectively with marginalised and diverse populations, and to advocate for and with them
- Insights and skills to work effectively with key health issues that are traditionally marginalised (such as mental health and sexual health), and to advocate for

improved services and social justice in relation to them
- Understand the health implications of other key practices that impact on public health (such as smoking, drugs, alcohol)

ASSESSMENT

Assignments   100%

REQUIRED READING

Farmer, P. (2001) *Infections and Inequalities: The Modern Plagues* (Updated Edition). University of California Press. (ISBN: 0520229134)

Irvine, J. M. (1994). *Sexual cultures and the construction of adolescent identities* (Health, Society, and Policy Series). Temple University Press. (ISBN: 1566391369)

Klein, A., Day, M., Harriott, A. (2004). *Caribbean Drugs From Criminalisation to Harm Reduction.* Kingston: Ian Randle Publishers. (ISBN: 976 637 194 6)

Lupton, D. (1999). *Risk.* Routledge. (ISBN: 0415183340)

Rew, L. (2004). *Adolescent health: A multidisciplinary approach to theory, research, and intervention.* Sage. (ISBN: 0761929118)

RECOMMENDED READING

Berkman, L. F., Kawachi, I. (2000). *Social epidemiology.* Oxford: Oxford University Press. (ISBN: 0195083318)

Rundle, A., Carvalho, M., Robinson, M. (2002). *Cultural competence in health care: a practical guide.* Jossy-Bass. (ISBN: 078796221X)

Turner, B. (2004). *The New Medical Sociology: Social Forms of Health and Illness.* WW Norton. (ISBN: 0393975053)

STRATEGIES, SKILLS, AND INTERVENTIONS FOR PROMOTING HEALTH

Rationale
Part 1: Approaches to effective prevention and health promotion

This part introduces the major theme of the second year of coursework for the M.Ed.

(Health Promotion). The theme is: *developing interventions.* In order to develop effective and sustainable interventions, students must have a grasp of core theory and techniques of health promotion, health communication, behavioural development and change, social development and change, risk and risk reduction.

Part 2: Policy, strategy, and campaign development

Included in the target audience for the Masters programme are candidates drawn from government and non-government agencies whose role is to develop, administer, and deliver health education and health promotion programmes. The programme therefore needs to equip graduates with skills for developing strategies and for planning, delivering, and evaluating programmes. Moreover, there is a considerable need for professional and institutional strengthening in health promotion in the Caribbean. This part responds to those needs.

Part 3: Health promoting institutions

Extensive work on health promoting institutions (including schools) has been done elsewhere in the world. These activities appear to have had limited impact on the Caribbean education sector. This course will examine the experiences elsewhere to inform local and regional initiatives. This unit is the third of a set of four, which collectively examine the implementation of health promotion at various levels from macro to micro, with the current unit examining institutional units such as hospitals, schools, and workplaces. This unit also encourages students to look beyond health promotion, HFLE, and the formal education sector in order to find innovation and for problem-solving purposes.

Part 4: People skills and life skills

The practice of health promotion requires an holistic approach to analysing health issues and implementing meaningful interventions. The entire UWI M.Ed. (Health Promotion) course is based on the premise that health is socially constructed, that risks are socially embedded, and that health outcomes will also be likely to be sustainable if they are also embedded in the social and cultural fabric. The implication of this rationale is that effective health promoters and educators will need to have highly developed people skills: one-to-one, group, and macro institutional and public advocacy skills; and be able to model the key life skills: critical and creative thinking, problem solving and decision-making, and healthy self-management. It is not tenable for educators to implement public education without having core group work and individual skills. HFLE raises difficult social issues, and educators teaching HFLE will need basic counselling competencies in order to: recognise problems, provide support and where appropriate to organise follow-up and referral for participants who need additional assistance.

OBJECTIVES

At the end of the course, participants will:

- Be able to discuss the basic principles and theories that underpin health promotion, health communication, behavioural development and change, social development and change, risk and risk reduction
- Be able to knowledgably discuss the difference between prohibition-based approaches and harm-minimisation in relation to health and social problems
- Be able to knowledgably discuss the concept of health promotion and the key

differences between disease treatment, illness prevention, and health promotion

- Be able to identify and discuss the strengths and weaknesses of mainstreamed/ infused strategies and specialised stand-alone strategies, and appropriate combinations of both
- Demonstrate an understanding of the steps involved in developing macro-level responses including policy, strategy, and large scale campaigns
- Be able to plan, organise, coordinate, resource, and evaluate a major health promotion intervention
- Demonstrate an understanding of the importance of, and methods for, forming networks, partnerships, alliances to inform, resource, and support the programme
- Be able to utilise methods for advocacy, lobbying, community consultation, creating supportive public opinion to ensure programme viability and sustainability
- Apply health promotion principles at an institutional level
- Critically analyse health promotion at an institutional level for quality improvement purposes
- Extend the analysis of health promotion beyond institutional boundaries in a search for more effective approaches and innovation
- Communicate confidently and competently on sensitive issues
- Plan for and provide supplementary advice, support, and advocacy at an individual and group level using basic counselling, group work, and life skills
- Work confidently from a social justice and human rights framework with issues that attract stigma, prejudice, and discrimination

- Work with other professionals to develop health promotion training initiatives

CONTENT

- Education, communication, and health promotion theory
- Behavioural development and change theory and strategies
- Social development and change theory and strategies
- Risk and risk reduction; protective factors
- Behaviour change psychology; Models for behavioural intervention
- Safety, abstinence, prohibition, harm reduction, and harm minimisation
- Mainstreamed and specialised programmes
- Innovative pedagogical approaches to health promotion
- Understanding adult and childhood education
- Educating and supporting parents
- Developing strategies, campaigns, and social marketing
- Institutional partnerships and external assistance
- Communication for social and behavioural development and change
- Political strategies
- Creating a receptive social context
- Working with the mass media
- Graphics and communication/graphic design
- Piloting and refining messages
- Creativity and message design
- Developing the capacity of parents
- Costing interventions and fundraising
- Group, classroom, and schoolyard skills
- Students with special needs
- Key life skills and health management skills
- Counselling, guidance, and care
- Working with sexual and gender diversity

- Working with parents and communities
- Train the trainer and workforce development
- Stigma, prejudice, discrimination
- Talking about sensitive issues
- Health promoting schools
- Curriculum development and health promotion
- HFLE and beyond HFLE
- Out-of-school strategies
- Health promoting workplaces
- Health promoting health services
- Working with faith based organisations

MAJOR COMPETENCIES TO BE DEVELOPED

- A sound theoretical base in health promotion, health communication, prevention, and behaviour change
- Enhanced skills in application of key principles and issues for health promotion including: mainstreaming versus specialised programmes; prohibition versus harm minimisation approaches; behavioural development and change.
- A repertoire of pedagogical approaches to health promotion development
- Enhanced skills to develop health promotion policies, strategies, and interventions at community, institutional, and governmental levels
- Critical and creative thinking (e.g. in 'social marketing' strategies)
- Ability to identify, consult, and involve key stakeholders in planning and implementation, including members of marginalised populations such as people with HIV
- Practical skills for forming synergistic partnerships to strengthen health promotion strategies

- Skills for developing strategies for creating a pragmatic community understanding, and a receptive social context in which effective health promotion can be undertaken
- Enhanced skills for managing social prejudices and taboos, so that they don't impede important health promotion activities
- Insights into the political and ideological dimensions of health and be able to formulate advocacy and lobbying strategies
- Enhanced capacity to understand and manage human behaviours and social interactions
- Action competence in the use of basic counselling and life skills
- Enhanced confidence, comfort, and competency to deal with sexual and gender diversity
- Enhanced skills to infuse health promotion within a humanistic, human rights, and social justice principles
- The ability to evaluate health promotion at an institutional level
- The ability to think beyond institutional boundaries to seek innovation and improved outcomes
- The ability to plan and implement health promotion strategies at a local institutional level

Assessment

Examination	25%
Public presentation	25%
Simulated counselling exercises	25%
Class presentations	25%

Required reading

DiClemente, R. J., Crosby, R. A., Kegler, M. C. (2002) *Emerging theories in health promotion practice and research: strategies for improving public health*. Jossey-Bass. (ISBN: 0787955663).

Freire, P. (2000). *Pedagogy of the oppressed*. New York: Continuum International Publishing. (ISBN: 0826412769)

Glanz, K., Rimer, B. K., Lewis, F. M. Eds. (2002). *Health behaviour and health education: theory, research, and practice* (3rd edition). Jossey-Bass. (ISBN: 0787957151)

Maibach, E., Parrott, R. L. (1995). *Designing health messages: approaches from communication theory and public health practice*. Sage. (ISBN: 0803953984)

McKenzie, J. F., Neiger, B. Smeltzer, J. L. (2004). *Planning, implementing, and evaluating health promotion programs: a primer* (4th Ed.). Benjamin Cummings. (ISBN: 0805360107).

Naidoo, J. (2000). *Health Promotion: Foundations for practice* (2nd Ed.). New York: Baillière Tindall. (ISBN: 0 621 171105 2 3)

Nutbeam, D., Harris, E. (2004). *Theory in a nutshell: A practical guide to health promotion theories* (2nd Ed.). McGraw-Hill. (ISBN: 0074713329).

RECOMMENDED READING

Books

Barker, T. E., Roger, E. M., & Sopory, P. (1992). *Designing health communication campaigns: What works?* CA: Sage. (ISBN: 0803943326)

Downie, R. S., Tannahill, C., & Tannahill, A. (1996). *Health promotion: models and values*. (2nd Ed.) NY: Oxford University Press. (ISBN: 0192625918)

Freund, P. E. S., McGuire, M. B., & Podhurst, L. S. (2003). *Health, illness, and the social body: A critical sociology* (4th Ed.). NJ: Prentice Hall. (ISBN: 013098230X)

Glanz, K., Rimer, B. K., & Lewis, F. M. (Eds.). (2002). *Health behaviour and health education: Theory, research, and practice* (3rd Ed.). San Francisco: Jossey-Bass. (ISBN: 0787957151)

Morgan, O. (Ed.). (2005). *Health issues in the Caribbean*. Jamaica: Ian Randle. (ISBN: 9766372136)

Weare, K. (2000). *Promoting mental, emotional & social health: A whole school approach*. London: Routledge. (ISBN: 0415168759)

World Bank. (2003). *Caribbean youth development: Issues and policy directions*. Washington, DC: World Bank. (ISBN: NA)

World Health Organization (1997). *Promoting health through schools*. WHO Technical Report Series, 870. Geneva: WHO. (ISBN: 9241208708)

World Health Organization (2001). *Evaluation in health promotion: Principles and perspectives*. WHO Regional Publications European Series, no. 92. Denmark: WHO. (ISBN: 9289013591)

Journals

1. Journal of Adolescent Health
2. American Journal of Public Health
3. Journal of School Health

Databases

Sociological abstracts (sociofile) (NISC)
AIDSearch (MEDLINE AIDS/HIV Subset, AIDSTRIALS & AIDSDRUGS) FREE (NISC)
Child Abuse, Child Welfare & Adoption (NISC)
Gender Studies Database (NISC)

Websites

1. www.who.org

2. www.unaids.org
3. www.who.int/healthpromotion/conferences/previous/ottawa/en/index.html
4. www.who.int/healthpromotion/conferences/6gchp/bangkok_charter/en/index.html
5. www.who.int/healthpromotion/en/
6. www.caricom.org
7. www.unesco.org
8. www.unfpa.org
9. www.unicef.org
10. www.undp.org
11. www.nlm.gov
12. www.cdc.gov
13. www.social-research.org

ACADEMIC AND RESEARCH SKILLS

Rationale

Strengthening academic and research skills is a fundamental aspect of professional capacity building. This unit therefore constitutes a major component of the M.Ed. (Health Promotion) degree. The unit will lead students through the core elements of academic inquiry: working with the literature, research planning and implementation, writing and analysis, publishing and grants. A basic premise of the unit is that the course be useful in both professional, public administration and academic settings. Research coverage will include qualitative and quantitative paradigms, and monitoring and evaluation as key applied research activities.

Objectives

At the end of the course, participants will:
- Be able to conduct a literature search and write a detailed literature analysis
- Apply theoretical understanding and practical skills in monitoring and evaluation
- Design and implement a research project
- Use knowledge of research paradigms to select an appropriate methodology for a research question
- Be competent in academic writing and presentation skills
- Be able to prepare articles for publication and grant applications

Content

- Informatics
- Using databases
- Reading and reviewing the literature
- The monitoring, evaluation, research continuum
- Research methods & design
- Qualitative project design, including action research
- Quantitative project design
- Introductory statistics
- Writing skills, reports, theses & publishing
- Research proposal writing and presentation
- Grant applications
- Publishing: looking good in print
- Publishing: copy and content editing
- Progressing to doctoral studies

Major competencies to be developed
- Analytical and critical skills for reviewing the literature
- Research conceptualization, design, implementation, and analysis
- Academic writing skills

Assessment

Develop and publicly defend a research plan	25%
Literature review assignments	75%

Required reading

Crotty, M. (1998). *Foundations of social research*. Sydney: Allen & Unwin. (ISBN: 186448604X)

De Vauss, D. (2002). *Surveys in social research* (5th Ed.). London: Routledge. (ISBN: 0415268583)

Kvale, S. (1996). *InterViews: an introduction to qualitative research interviewing*. Thousand Oaks: Sage. (ISBN: 080395820X)

Parker, R. (2005). *Looking good in print* (6th Ed.). Paraglyph Press (ISBN: 193309706X)

Posavac, E. J., Carey, R. G. (2003). *Program Evaluation: methods and case studies* (6th Ed.). New Jersey: Prentice Hall. (ISBN: 0130409669)

Strunk, W. Jr., White, E.B., Angell, R. (2000). The Elements of style (4th Ed.). Longman. (ISBN: 020530902X)

Recommended reading

Any recent edition of Roget's Thesaurus.
Clarke, A. (1999). *Evaluation research: An introduction to principles, methods and practice*. Sage. (ISBN: 0761950958)

Fitzpatrick, J. L., Sanders, J. R., Worthen, B. R. (2003). *Program evaluation: Alternative approaches and practical guidelines* (3rd Ed.). Allyn & Bacon. (ISBN: 0321077067)

Hoffman, G., Hoffman, G. (2003). *Adios, Strunk and White: A handbook for the new academic essay*, (3rd Ed.). (ISBN: 0937363200)

Layder, D. (1993). *New strategies in social research*. Cambridge: Polity. (ISBN: 0745608817).

McLeod, J. (2002). *Qualitative research in counselling & psychotherapy*. London: Sage. (ISBN: 0761955062)

Owen, J. M, Rogers, P. (1999). *Program evaluation: Forms and approaches*. Sage. (ISBN: 076196178X)

Rossi, P. H., Lipsey, M. W., Freeman, H. E. (2003). *Evaluation : A systematic approach* (7th Ed.). Sage (ISBN: 0761908943).
Strauss, A., Corbin, J. (1990). *Basics of qualitative research: Grounded theory procedures and techniques*. Newbury Park, CA: Sage. (ISBN: 0803932502)

Trumble, W., & Brown, L. (Eds.). (2002). *Shorter Oxford English dictionary* (5th Ed.). Oxford: Oxford University Press. (ISBN: 0198604572).

Witkin, B. R., & Altschuld, J. W. (1995). *Planning and conducting needs assessments: A practical guide*. Thousand Oaks, CA: Sage. (ISBN: 0803958102)

Websites

1. www.wordnet.princeton.edu
2. www.en.wikipedia.org

PROFESSIONAL DEVELOPMENT ELECTIVES AND FIELD WORK

Rationale

Academic skills benefit from exposure to real world practices. Moreover, professional disciplines benefit from exposure to the practice of other professions. This unit aims to expose candidates to the problems of health promotion in applied settings. It also aims to encourage cross-fertilization of ideas by exposing students to the everyday activities of disciplines other than their own. This course will take place outside of formal teaching blocks and most activities can be undertaken at the student's home base, although a wider perspective will be encouraged.

Objectives

At the end of this course participants will:

- Understand the importance of widened professional experience, and exposure to alternative approaches
- Be able to examine the activities of other disciplines whose work is relevant to health promotion
- Be able to transfer and adapt the practices of other disciplines to improve your own practice where appropriate
- Be able to undertake critical reflection on personal practice and professional growth

Content

Students will be able to choose elective professional development assignments from the following fields:

- Sexual health
- Family planning
- Health promotion
- HFLE
- Nutrition, diet, obesity, anorexia, bulimia
- Exercise
- Environment
- Occupational Health and Safety
- Motor vehicles
- Weapons
- Smoking
- Drugs and alcohol

Alternative fieldwork proposals will be considered by the unit coordinator. All fieldwork must have prior approval of the unit coordinator.

Major competencies to be developed

- Skills in the observation and evaluation of professional practice
- Capacity for critical evaluation of personal knowledge and practice
- Positive attitudes to seeking alternative models and paradigms of practice
- Capacity to seek innovation and improvement, and to adapt and apply it to personal practice

Assessment

Submission and presentation of a fieldwork report consisting of field notes, analysis of the observations, analysis of the professional development benefits for the student	100%

Recommended reading

Bolton, G. (2005). *Reflective practice: Writing and professional development* (2nd edition) London: Sage. (ISBN: 1412908124)

Guskey, T. R. (2000). *Evaluating professional development*. Thousand Oaks: Sage, Corwin Press. (ISBN: 0761975616)

MASTERS LEVEL RESEARCH PROJECT

Rationale

The field of health and human relationships in education in the Caribbean has many aspects that are largely unexplored. The importance of deepening research in this field has become increasingly apparent in view of the relentless expansion of the HIV epidemic. For students gaining academic and research competencies, the research component of the M.Ed. (Health Promotion) degree will add substantially to the Caribbean evidence-base.

Objectives

At the end of this unit the candidate will be able to:

* Conceptualize, plan, execute, analyze, and write up a research project which makes a significant original contribution to the literature

Content

* Literature review topic
* Literature review methods & design
* Presentation of proposal
* Project design submission
* Data collection
* Data analysis
* Write-up
* Presentation of findings

Major competencies to be developed

* Research design, planning, execution, analysis, and write-up

ASSESSMENT

Thesis	100%

Required reading

While there is no compulsory reading, it should be noted that all academic theses require at least two literature reviews. The first consists of a comprehensive coverage of the subject area. The second explores the methodology. Careful attention should be given to the UWI's Rules and Regulations. Candidates should be careful to conform to these documents. This research project should also draw closely on the companion unit: Academic and research skills (Component D).

STAFFING, BUDGET, AND SUSTAINABILITY OF THE MASTERS IN EDUCATION (HEALTH PROMOTION)

STAFFING AND FACILITIES

* Coordination. A course coordinator will be required
* Staff from the School of Education. Particularly in the fields of educational theory and practice, internal staffing will be drawn upon
* Staff from other faculties in Trinidad. Staffing from key partners in the Health Economics Unit, St Augustine; UWI HARP; the Medical Faculty; the Centre for Gender and Development.
* Contributions will be actively sought from the Ministry of Education; the Ministry of Health; the National AIDS Coordinating Committee
* Contributions from campuses, Ministries, and organizations from other Caribbean countries are desirable, but will depend on budgetary considerations
* The possibility of involvement of personnel from outside the Caribbean will be pursued
* Residential facilities and costings for block teaching
* Availability of scholarships and bursaries

BUDGET - OUTGOINGS

* Funding will be required for a full-time course coordinator, office, and administrative support
* Funding for module development
* Funding will be required for external presenters
* Books will need to be purchased for the library
* Marketing and promotion

BUDGET - INCOMINGS

- Course fees are yet to be determined
- It is assumed that candidates from Trinidad and Tobago will be fully funded
- This programme is designed to support the CARICOM, UNESCO, and UNICEF initiatives in HIV/AIDS and HFLE, and donor funding will need to be explored

SUSTAINABILITY AND RISKS

- There is a clear need for leadership, training, professional development, qualifications, academic skills, and research into health and human relationships in the Caribbean

- There is a demand for advanced training and professional qualifications in health education and health promotion from both the health and education sectors. The target audiences for this programme are listed at the beginning of this document.
- There is limited capacity in the School of Education, St Augustine to sustain this programme, which will need to be addressed.
- This programme will benefit enormously from inputs from other faculties and key external bodies. It is envisaged that these contributions will form the 'backbone' of the programme.

TABLES

Table 25.1: The six components of the M.Ed. (Health Promotion)
Component A: The health and human relationships knowledge base • Nurture and nature • Sexual and reproductive health **Component B: Risk in the context of modern social lives** • People and their relationships in modern society • People and their risks in modern society **Component C: Strategies, skills, and interventions for promoting health** • Approaches to effective prevention and health promotion • Policy, strategy and campaign development • People and life skills • Health promoting institutions **Component D: Academic and research skills** • Monitoring & evaluation • Research methods & design • Reading & reviewing the literature • Report writing • Research proposal writing and presentation • Grant applications • Doctoral studies **Component E: Professional development electives and fieldwork** **Component F: Masters level research project**

Table 25.2: Course structure for the M.Ed. (Health Promotion)			
Year 1	**Component A: The health and human relationships knowledge base** • Nurture and nature • Sexual and reproductive health **Component B: Risk in the context of modern social lives** • People and their relationships in modern society • People and their risks in modern society	**Component D: Academic and research skills** • Monitoring & evaluation • Research methods & design • Reading & reviewing the literature • Report writing • Research proposal writing and presentation • Grant applications • Doctoral studies	**Component E: Professional development electives and fieldwork**	**Component F: Research project**
Year 2	**Component C: Strategies, skills and interventions for promoting health** • Approaches to effective prevention and health promotion • Policy, strategy and campaign development • People and life skills • Health promoting institutions			

Table 25.3: Credit points for the M.Ed. (Health Promotion)		Credits	Hours
Course 1 (Component A)	**The health and human relationships knowledge base**	4	48
Course 2 (Component B)	**Risk in the context of modern social lives**	4	48
Course 3 (Component C)	**Strategies, skills, and interventions for promoting health**	8	96
Course 4 (Component D)	**Academic and research skills**	5	60
(Component E)	**Professional development electives & fieldwork**	4	48
(Component F)	**Masters level research project**	10	NA
	Total	**35**	**300**

Table 25.4: Schedule for the M.Ed. (Health Promotion)		Hours	Total hours (working days)
1st Residential Block Year 1	• Part component A • Part component B • Part component D • Introduction to component E • Meet with supervisors about project	33 33 20 5 -	91 hours (15 working days)
Interim Activities	• Assignment for component A • Assignment for component B • Identify site, negotiate attachment, & prepare proposal for component E • Commence literature review for project	- - - -	-
2nd Residential Block Year 1	• Remainder component A • Remainder component B • Part component D • Submit proposal for component E • Meet with supervisors about project	15 15 10 - -	40 hours (5 working days)
Interim Activities	• Assignment for component A • Assignment for component B • Undertake professional development attachment • Finalize literature review for project	- - 30 -	30 hours (3 hours per week for 10 weeks)
1st Residential Block Year 2	• Part component C • Part component D • Report back component E • Meet with supervisors about project	72 20 7 -	99 hours (15 working days)
Interim Activities	• Assignment for component C • Data collection for project	- -	-
Final Residential Block Year 2	• Part component C • Part component D • Report back component E • Meet with supervisors about project	24 10 6 -	40 hours (5 working days)
Remaining time	• Complete write-up of masters level research project	-	-
		TOTAL	300

Table 25.5: Course content for the M.Ed. (Health Promotion)	
Nurture and nature	• Historical backgrounds • Caribbean social contexts • Ideological, political, legal, ethical, policy, economic, religious contexts • Social construction of health in the Caribbean • Gender and society • Sexuality, sexual identity, & sexual stigma • Stigma theory, marginalization, prejudice, discrimination • Biomedical knowledge base • Critique of biomedical approaches • Human development & 'the 7 ages': embryology, childhood, puberty, early adulthood, ageing • Infectious diseases
Sexual and reproductive health	• Sexuality and health in Caribbean society • STI / HIV/AIDS • People with HIV • Infertility and contraception • Fertility, pregnancy, and parenthood • Sexual function and dysfunction • Sexuality in health and disease
People and their relationships in modern society	• Adolescence, school-ground cultures, peer groups and gangs • Relationships in diverse cultures • Strengthening family life • Masculinities and violence • Diversity • Sexual and gender diversity • Ageing • Disability • Mass media and communication
People and their risks in modern society	• What is risk? • Stigmatized conditions, marginalized populations and unpopular issues • Networks and socially embedded risks • Protective networks, the potential of parents, teachers, & peers • Bullying, violence, harassment, and hate crimes • Domestic violence and sexual assault • High-risk settings and special populations • Drugs, alcohol, tobacco • Mental health and suicide • Poverty and power

Approaches to effective prevention and health promotion	• Education, communication, and health promotion theory • Understanding adult and childhood education • Innovative pedagogical approaches to health promotion • Educating and supporting parents • Curriculum development and health promotion • Behavioural development and change • Social development and change • Risk and risk reduction • Safety, abstinence, prohibition, harm reduction, and harm minimization • Mainstreamed and specialized programmes
Policy, strategy, and campaign development	• Developing strategies, campaigns, and social marketing • Institutional partnerships and external assistance • Communication for social and behavioural development and change • Working with parents and communities • Political strategies • Creating a receptive social context • Working with the mass media • Graphics and communication/ graphic design • Piloting and refining messages • Creativity and message design • Developing the capacity of parents • Costing interventions and fundraising
People and life skills	• Group, classroom, and schoolyard skills • Teaching on sensitive topics • Key life skills and health management skills • Counselling, guidance, and care • Working with sexual and gender diversity • Partnerships with parents • Working with communities • Train the trainer and workforce development • Stigma, prejudice, discrimination • Talking about sensitive issues
Health promoting institutions	• Health promoting schools • Curriculum development • HFLE • Beyond HFLE • Out of school • Health promoting homes • Health promoting workplaces • Health promoting health services • Working with faith-based organizations

Academic and research skills	• Reading and reviewing the literature • The monitoring, evaluation, research continuum • Research methods & design • Qualitative project design • Quantitative project design • Writing skills, reports, theses, & publishing • Research proposal writing and presentation • Grant applications • Publishing: looking good in print • Publishing: copy and content editing • Progression to doctoral studies
Professional development electives and field work	• Sexual health • Family planning • Health promotion • HFLE • Nutrition • Exercise • Environment • Occupational Health and Safety • Motor vehicles • Weapons • Smoking • Drugs and alcohol • Research priorities: prevention, stigma, gender, impact • Co-factors in HIV transmission: poverty, mobility, substance use
Masters level research project	• Literature review topic • Literature review methods & design • Presentation of proposal • Project design submission • Data collection • Data analysis • Write-up • Presentation of findings

Table 25.6: Due dates for assessments for the M.Ed. (Health Promotion)		Due date
Course 1 (Component A)	**The health and human relationships knowledge base**	End of academic Yr 1
Course 2 (Component B)	**Risk in the context of modern social lives**	
Course 3 (Component C)	**Strategies, skills, and interventions for promoting health**	End of academic Yr 2
Course 4 (Component D)	**Academic and research skills**	
(Component E)	**Professional development electives & fieldwork**	
(Component F)	**Masters level Research Project**	

Table 25.7: Organizational Chart for 2006-2007 Academic Year M.Ed. (Health Promotion)

Course Coordinator DP+					
Secretariat and Administrative Support SR					
Component Coordinators					
Component A	**Component B**	**Component C**	**Component D**	**Component E**	**Component F**
VJ	JM	JR	DP	SL	DP
Component Coordinator Support					
Head of School (CK)	Head of School (CK)	Course Coordinator (DP)	Post Graduate / Research Coordinator (JG)	Course Coordinator (DP)	Post Graduate / Research Coordinator (JG)
Responsibilities of Component Coordinator					
* Curriculum development * Updating reading materials * Timetabling * Identification and scheduling of presenters * Assessments	* Curriculum development * Updating reading materials * Timetabling * Identification and scheduling of presenters * Assessments	* Curriculum development * Updating reading materials * Timetabling * Identification and scheduling of presenters * Assessments	* Curriculum development * Updating reading materials * Timetabling * Identification and scheduling of presenters * Assessments	* Curriculum development * Updating reading materials * Timetabling * Identification of presenters * Approval of attachments * Assessments	* Assignment of supervision * Development of research proposal * Support for student * Oversight of project * Coordination of thesis examination

INDEX